Non-canonical Kinases and Substrates in Cancer Progression

Non-canonical Kinases and Substrates in Cancer Progression

Editor

Francisco M. Vega

MDPI • Basel • Beijing • Wuhan • Barcelona • Belgrade • Manchester • Tokyo • Cluj • Tianjin

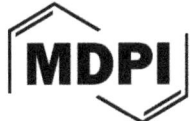

Editor
Francisco M. Vega
Cell Biology
Universidad de Sevilla
Seville
Spain

Editorial Office
MDPI
St. Alban-Anlage 66
4052 Basel, Switzerland

This is a reprint of articles from the Special Issue published online in the open access journal *Cancers* (ISSN 2072-6694) (available at: www.mdpi.com/journal/cancers/special_issues/KinSubCanPro).

For citation purposes, cite each article independently as indicated on the article page online and as indicated below:

LastName, A.A.; LastName, B.B.; LastName, C.C. Article Title. *Journal Name* **Year**, *Volume Number*, Page Range.

ISBN 978-3-0365-3055-0 (Hbk)
ISBN 978-3-0365-3054-3 (PDF)

© 2022 by the authors. Articles in this book are Open Access and distributed under the Creative Commons Attribution (CC BY) license, which allows users to download, copy and build upon published articles, as long as the author and publisher are properly credited, which ensures maximum dissemination and a wider impact of our publications.

The book as a whole is distributed by MDPI under the terms and conditions of the Creative Commons license CC BY-NC-ND.

Contents

About the Editor vii

Preface to "Non-canonical Kinases and Substrates in Cancer Progression" ix

Francisco M. Vega
Non-Canonical Kinases and Substrates in Cancer Progression
Reprinted from: *Cancers* **2021**, *13*, 1628, doi:10.3390/cancers13071628 1

Charles Pottier, Margaux Fresnais, Marie Gilon, Guy Jérusalem, Rémi Longuespée and Nor Eddine Sounni
Tyrosine Kinase Inhibitors in Cancer: Breakthrough and Challenges of Targeted Therapy
Reprinted from: *Cancers* **2020**, *12*, 731, doi:10.3390/cancers12030731 3

Jacopo Boni, Carlota Rubio-Perez, Nuria López-Bigas, Cristina Fillat and Susana de la Luna
The DYRK Family of Kinases in Cancer: Molecular Functions and Therapeutic Opportunities
Reprinted from: *Cancers* **2020**, *12*, 2106, doi:10.3390/cancers12082106 21

Víctor Mayoral-Varo, María Pilar Sánchez-Bailón, Annarica Calcabrini, Marta García-Hernández, Valerio Frezza and María Elena Martín et al.
The Relevance of the SH2 Domain for c-Src Functionality in Triple-Negative Breast Cancer Cells
Reprinted from: *Cancers* **2021**, *13*, 462, doi:10.3390/cancers13030462 47

Ana Colmenero-Repiso, María A. Gómez-Muñoz, Ismael Rodríguez-Prieto, Aida Amador-Álvarez, Kai-Oliver Henrich and Diego Pascual-Vaca et al.
Identification of VRK1 as a New Neuroblastoma Tumor Progression Marker Regulating Cell Proliferation
Reprinted from: *Cancers* **2020**, *12*, 3465, doi:10.3390/cancers12113465 71

Catalina Alamón, Belén Dávila, María Fernanda García, Carina Sánchez, Mariángeles Kovacs and Emiliano Trias et al.
Sunitinib-Containing Carborane Pharmacophore with the Ability to Inhibit Tyrosine Kinases Receptors FLT3, KIT and PDGFR-, Exhibits Powerful In Vivo Anti-Glioblastoma Activity
Reprinted from: *Cancers* **2020**, *12*, 3423, doi:10.3390/cancers12113423 87

Raúl García-González, Patricia Morejón-García, Ignacio Campillo-Marcos, Marcella Salzano and Pedro A. Lazo
VRK1 Phosphorylates Tip60/KAT5 and Is Required for H4K16 Acetylation in Response to DNA Damage
Reprinted from: *Cancers* **2020**, *12*, 2986, doi:10.3390/cancers12102986 109

Clara Reglero, Vanesa Lafarga, Verónica Rivas, Ángela Albitre, Paula Ramos and Susana R. Berciano et al.
GRK2-Dependent HuR Phosphorylation Regulates HIF1 Activation under Hypoxia or Adrenergic Stress
Reprinted from: *Cancers* **2020**, *12*, 1216, doi:10.3390/cancers12051216 133

María Belén Ortega-García, Alberto Mesa, Elisa L.J. Moya, Beatriz Rueda, Gabriel Lopez-Ordoño and Javier Ángel García et al.
Uncovering Tumour Heterogeneity through PKR and nc886 Analysis in Metastatic Colon Cancer Patients Treated with 5-FU-Based Chemotherapy
Reprinted from: *Cancers* **2020**, *12*, 379, doi:10.3390/cancers12020379 155

About the Editor

Francisco M. Vega

Dr Francisco M. Vega is an Associate professor in the department of Cell Biology at the University of Seville. Dr Vega is also co-leading researcher at the Instituto de Biomedicina de Sevilla. He leads the Cancer cell biology laboratory at the University, interested in exploring the contribution of cancer stem cells to cancer metastasis in solid tumors. Dr Vega developed his career as a research scientist in the fields of cellular signaling and cancer biology, working in the Center for Cancer Research in Salamanca, Spain, the Ludwig Institute for Cancer Research and King's College London in United Kingdom and the Moores Cancer Center at UCSD in USA. He has produced relevant works on the mechanisms of cell proliferation, cell adhesion, motility and invasion controlled by the Rho family of GTPases, ROCK and other kinases, with the goal of gaining new insights into the cancer metastasis process in solid tumors. He is currently interested in the cellular signalling that connects cell migration and stemness in aggressive neuroblastoma and other solid tumors.

Preface to "Non-canonical Kinases and Substrates in Cancer Progression"

Protein Ser/Thr or Tyr kinases mediate most signal transduction pathways in eukaryotic cells, being the favourite post translational modification for situations where a rapid response to extracellular or intracellular signalling is required. Many of the known oncogenic proteins are kinases and many tumour suppressor proteins are among their substrates. More than 15 years after the publication by Manning et al. of their landmark paper describing the human kinome, only a small proportion of the kinases potentially involved in cancer progression have received most of the attention. Moreover, only a few of the potential targets have been investigated in their cellular context. With an ever-pressing need for new druggable targets, the understanding of the biological function and contribution to cancer progression of the lesser known cancer-related kinases represents an unavoidable asset.

This Special Issue of *Cancers* pretends to bring together the latest views and original research on non-canonical protein kinases, substrates, and scaffolds. Topics include protein structure and regulation, scaffolding and complex formation, cellular signalling, non-canonical substrates, inhibition and targeting, and biological function.

Francisco M. Vega
Editor

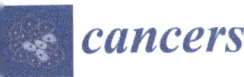

Editorial

Non-Canonical Kinases and Substrates in Cancer Progression

Francisco M. Vega [1,2]

1 Departamento de Biología Celular, Facultad de Biología, Universidad de Sevilla, 41012 Seville, Spain; fmvega@us.es
2 Instituto de Biomedicina de Sevilla (IBiS), Hospital Universitario Virgen del Rocío, CSIC, Universidad de Sevilla, 41013 Seville, Spain

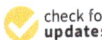

Citation: Vega, F.M. Non-Canonical Kinases and Substrates in Cancer Progression. *Cancers* **2021**, *13*, 1628. https://doi.org/10.3390/cancers13071628

Received: 23 March 2021
Accepted: 25 March 2021
Published: 1 April 2021

Publisher's Note: MDPI stays neutral with regard to jurisdictional claims in published maps and institutional affiliations.

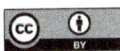

Copyright: © 2021 by the author. Licensee MDPI, Basel, Switzerland. This article is an open access article distributed under the terms and conditions of the Creative Commons Attribution (CC BY) license (https://creativecommons.org/licenses/by/4.0/).

Cellular protein kinases remain the target of choice when the intention is to intervene in a particular signaling pathway leading to cancer progression. Their reversible mode of action, tight regulation, and molecular structure allows for the design of specific inhibitors. However, from the more than 500 protein kinases identified, many potentially involved in important cancer-related signaling cascades, only a few have received most of the attention over the years. This is either due to their central role on essential processes, the facility of intervention, or their early discovery. This Special Issue tried to offer new insights into some of the lesser-known human protein kinases, their substrates, regulation, and involvement in cancer progression. The published articles offer good examples of the important cellular functions that the so-called non-canonical kinases develop and their contribution to cancer. They also discuss some of the therapeutical opportunities and challenges.

The vaccinia-related kinase (VRK) proteins are structurally related to the casein kinase family and the viral protein B1R. This family of protein kinases has revealed itself as an important mediator of tumor progression and cell proliferation. Although a role for VRK1 in normal cell division is granted, the high expression and activity of this protein in some cancers, including now pediatric neuroblastoma, is essential for malignization [1]. VRK1 synergizes with other oncogenes to drive cancer progression, notably with NMYC in neuroblastoma. Increasingly, data point to their possible use as a prognostic marker and therapeutical target. However, the complexity of its regulation and substrates makes detailed molecular studies about this chromatin remodeling enzyme necessary. Here, García-González et al. also report a role for VRK1 in chromatin acetylation leading to DNA damage response, indicating that VRK1 could also be involved in increased genome instability [2]. It is now clear that the expression of some of these non-canonical kinases could be incorporated as new prognostic markers or biomarkers of therapy response in various cancers. Another example is offered by the study of the protein kinase R (PKR) and its regulator, the non-coding pre-mir-nc886, in colorectal cancer responses after chemotherapy [3].

Another family of pleiotropic protein kinases associated with cancer is dual-specificity tyrosine-regulated kinases (DYRK). Their molecular functions leading to tumor progression are discussed in another contribution to this Special Issue [4]. Interestingly, small DYRK inhibitors have been developed, offering new therapeutic avenues. Recent evidence has established the importance of the tumor microenvironment for cancer progression and there is a need to understand the signaling pathways mediating the response and adaptation of cancer cells to external stimuli. In their contribution to the Special Issue, Reglero et al. describe how a GRK2-dependent phosphorylation can modulate Hypoxia Inducible Factor (HIF)-dependent responses to hypoxia in cancer cells [5].

Specific tyrosine kinase inhibitors are being used with success in the treatment of some types of cancer. In addition to major signaling players, tyrosine kinase inhibitors also offer specificity against other tyrosine kinases. A revision of their use and targets could offer new opportunities for the treatment of tumors with poor prognosis and few therapeutic tools available [6]. For example, the inhibitor sunitinib is used as an antiangiogenic inhibitor, principally for its action against the VEGF receptors, VEGFR1 and VEGFR2, and the PDGF receptor. Sunitinib also inhibits other protein kinases such as Fms Related Receptor Tyrosine Kinase 3 (FLT3) or KIT. These kinases seem to be the main targets in glioblastoma and, when combined with a cytotoxic therapy such as boron neutron capture, offer a good response in these difficult-to-treat tumors [7]. This is an example in which well-known inhibitors use could be expanded for their action over non-canonical kinases. In most cases, the attention, even in widely studied protein kinases, has been focused on kinase activity, ignoring other protein domains with potentially important molecular functions. The Src tyrosine kinase was one of the first oncogenic kinases discovered. However, much less attention has been paid to the adapter domains SH2 and SH3 in the molecule. The results presented in this Special Issue by Mayoral-Varo et al. explore the functionality of these domains in breast cancer cells, suggesting a synergistic effect between their inhibition and the inhibition of the kinase activity [8].

In summary, this Special Issue of *Cancers* shows good examples of the functionality and therapeutic values that the study of non-canonical kinases or domains, their substrates, and inhibition can offer. With research on these lesser-known proteins, we will expand not only our knowledge about cancer progression, but our possibilities to halt it.

Funding: This research received no external funding.

Conflicts of Interest: The authors declare no conflict of interest.

References

1. Colmenero-Repiso, A.; Gómez-Muñoz, M.; Rodríguez-Prieto, I.; Amador-Álvarez, A.; Henrich, K.; Pascual-Vaca, D.; Okonechnikov, K.; Rivas, E.; Westermann, F.; Pardal, R.; et al. Identification of VRK1 as a New Neuroblastoma Tumor Progression Marker Regulating Cell Proliferation. *Cancers* **2020**, *12*, 3465. [CrossRef] [PubMed]
2. García-González, R.; Morejón-García, P.; Campillo-Marcos, I.; Salzano, M.; Lazo, P. VRK1 Phosphorylates Tip60/KAT5 and Is Required for H4K16 Acetylation in Response to DNA Damage. *Cancers* **2020**, *12*, 2986. [CrossRef] [PubMed]
3. Ortega-García, M.; Mesa, A.; Moya, E.; Rueda, B.; Lopez-Ordoño, G.; García, J.; Conde, V.; Redondo-Cerezo, E.; Lopez-Hidalgo, J.; Jiménez, G.; et al. Uncovering Tumour Heterogeneity through PKR and nc886 Analysis in Metastatic Colon Cancer Patients Treated with 5-FU-Based Chemotherapy. *Cancers* **2020**, *12*, 379. [CrossRef] [PubMed]
4. Boni, J.; Rubio-Perez, C.; López-Bigas, N.; Fillat, C.; de la Luna, S. The DYRK Family of Kinases in Cancer: Molecular Functions and Therapeutic Opportunities. *Cancers* **2020**, *12*, 2106. [CrossRef] [PubMed]
5. Reglero, C.; Lafarga, V.; Rivas, V.; Albitre, Á.; Ramos, P.; Berciano, S.; Tapia, O.; Martínez-Chantar, M.; Mayor, F., Jr.; Penela, P. GRK2-Dependent HuR Phosphorylation Regulates HIF1α Activation under Hypoxia or Adrenergic Stress. *Cancers* **2020**, *12*, 1216. [CrossRef] [PubMed]
6. Pottier, C.; Fresnais, M.; Gilon, M.; Jérusalem, G.; Longuespée, R.; Sounni, N. Tyrosine Kinase Inhibitors in Cancer: Breakthrough and Challenges of Targeted Therapy. *Cancers* **2020**, *12*, 731. [CrossRef] [PubMed]
7. Alamón, C.; Dávila, B.; García, M.; Sánchez, C.; Kovacs, M.; Trias, E.; Barbeito, L.; Gabay, M.; Zeineh, N.; Gavish, M.; et al. Sunitinib-Containing Carborane Pharmacophore with the Ability to Inhibit Tyrosine Kinases Receptors FLT3, KIT and PDGFR-β, Exhibits Powerful In Vivo Anti-Glioblastoma Activity. *Cancers* **2020**, *12*, 3423. [CrossRef] [PubMed]
8. Mayoral-Varo, V.; Sánchez-Bailón, M.; Calcabrini, A.; García-Hernández, M.; Frezza, V.; Martín, M.; González, V.; Martín-Pérez, J. The Relevance of the SH2 Domain for c-Src Functionality in Triple-Negative Breast Cancer Cells. *Cancers* **2021**, *13*, 462. [CrossRef]

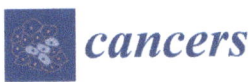

Review

Tyrosine Kinase Inhibitors in Cancer: Breakthrough and Challenges of Targeted Therapy

Charles Pottier [1,2,*], Margaux Fresnais [3,4], Marie Gilon [1], Guy Jérusalem [2], Rémi Longuespée [3,†] and Nor Eddine Sounni [1,†]

1. Laboratory of Tumor and Development Biology, GIGA-Cancer and GIGA-I3, GIGA-Research, University Hospital of Liège, 4000 Liège, Belgium; marie.gilon@student.uliege.be (M.G.); nesounni@uliege.be (N.E.S.)
2. Department of Medical Oncology, University Hospital of Liège, 4000 Liège, Belgium; G.Jerusalem@chu.ulg.ac.be
3. Department of Clinical Pharmacology and Pharmacoepidemiology, University Hospital of Heidelberg, 69120 Heidelberg, Germany; Margaux.Fresnais@med.uni-heidelberg.de (M.F.); remi.longuespee@med.uni-heidelberg.com (R.L.)
4. German Cancer Consortium (DKTK)-German Cancer Research Center (DKFZ), 69120 Heidelberg, Germany
* Correspondence: charles.pottier@student.uliege.be
† Equivalent contribution.

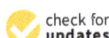

Received: 17 January 2020; Accepted: 16 March 2020; Published: 20 March 2020

Abstract: Receptor tyrosine kinases (RTKs) are key regulatory signaling proteins governing cancer cell growth and metastasis. During the last two decades, several molecules targeting RTKs were used in oncology as a first or second line therapy in different types of cancer. However, their effectiveness is limited by the appearance of resistance or adverse effects. In this review, we summarize the main features of RTKs and their inhibitors (RTKIs), their current use in oncology, and mechanisms of resistance. We also describe the technological advances of artificial intelligence, chemoproteomics, and microfluidics in elaborating powerful strategies that could be used in providing more efficient and selective small molecules inhibitors of RTKs. Finally, we discuss the interest of therapeutic combination of different RTKIs or with other molecules for personalized treatments, and the challenge for effective combination with less toxic and off-target effects.

Keywords: cancer; oncology; pharmacology; tyrosine kinase inhibitors

---

1. Introduction

1.1. Description of Receptor Tyrosine Kinases and Downstream Signaling Pathways

Receptor tyrosine kinases (RTKs) are key regulators of cellular processes and their role in the pathophysiology of many diseases is well recognized. The known human RTKs are classified into twenty subfamilies and have a similar molecular architecture (Figure 1), with an extracellular ligand-binding region and a single transmembrane helix. The cytoplasmic region contains the protein tyrosine kinase (TK) domain with additional carboxy-(C-)terminal and juxtamembrane regulatory regions.

Activation of RTK (Figure 1) involves ligand binding to stabilize connections between monomeric or oligomeric receptors and form active dimers or oligomers, which in turn activate the intracellular kinase. RTK activities are mainly dependent on signaling molecule phosphorylation and activation of transcription factors that mediate target gene expression in response to ligands [1]. These activities can also be regulated by receptor internalization and recycling during physiological and pathological processes.

The signaling pathways of the RTKs are complexes and involve an increasing number of biochemical reactions and molecular mediators in complex signaling networks. For instance, epidermal growth factor receptor (EGFR) signaling network involves 211-biochemical-reactions and 322 signaling molecules [2]. In fact, attempts of modeling of this network seem to be very complex due to the requirement of more sophisticated spatial and stochastic aspects. An example of RTK network modeling was proposed by Kitano's "bow tie" or "hourglass" (Figure 2) [1]. In this model, the set of RTKs (input layer) influences a small number of intermediaries, such as mitogen-activated protein kinases (MAPK), phosphoinositide 3-kinase (Pi3K), and Ca^{2+} signaling (core processes). RTKs mainly activate the Pi3K/protein kinase B (AKT)/mechanistic target of rapamycin (mTOR), rat sarcoma (RAS)/MAPK, Janus kinase (JAK)/signal transducer and activator of transcription protein family (STAT), and phospholipase C (PLC)/Ca^{2+}/calmodulin-dependent protein kinase-protein kinase C (CaMK-PKC) pathways, and downstream effectors of multicellular processes during cancer progression [3]. Pi3K/AKT/mTOR pathway controls cell growth, metabolism, and survival, and is essential for maintaining pluripotency. The RAS/MAPK pathway is a central regulator of metabolism, cell cycle, cell proliferation, differentiation, and migration. STAT is known to control the signaling activated by lymphokines, the platelet-derived growth factor (PDGF), the epidermal growth factor (EGF), or the fibroblast growth factor (FGF), and is therefore involved in many cellular changes Finally, PKC is also involved in the regulation of survival, proliferation and cell motility [3–5]. It is important to note the complex crosstalks between these pathways. For example, the Pi3K/AKT and RAS/MAPK pathways interfere in various nodes including extracellular signal-regulated kinases (ERK), and regulate themselves through a positive and negative feedback, depending on the cellular context. These two pathways can also be activated by molecules of the STAT pathway, and finally, PKC has been shown able to activate MAPK. Many neoplastic characteristics (proliferation, metabolic anomaly, migration, etc.) are therefore regulated at least in part by the intracellular signaling triggered by RTKs, and some key kinases of these pathways (Pi3K, RAS, JAK, STAT, etc.) are frequently mutated in cancers [6–8]. Since molecular deregulation of cell signaling is essential for the acquisition of cancer hallmarks, classifying tumors according to these anomalies is complementary to histological classification. This molecular classification is becoming more and more important. Thus, in certain clinical trials known as "agnostics", the therapeutic strategy no longer depends on the histology, but only on the molecular anomalies. These clinical trials are currently investigating inhibitors of BRAF, human epidermal growth factor receptor-2 (HER2), and Pi3K/AKT/mTOR or rapidly accelerated fibrosarcoma (RAF)/mitogen-activated protein kinase kinase (MEK) pathways on mutated tumors [9].

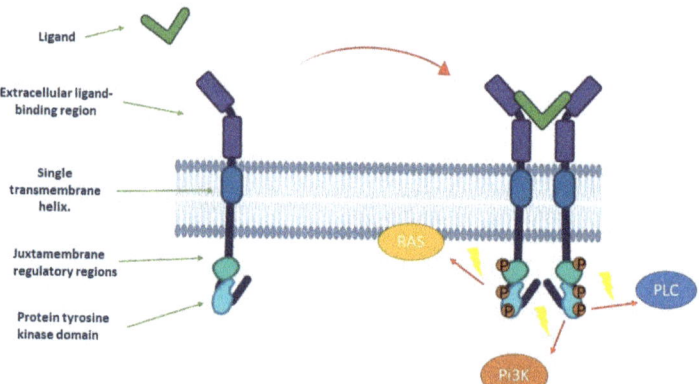

Figure 1. Activation of tyrosine kinase receptor. Ligand binding stabilizes connections between monomeric receptors to form an active dimer, which in turn activates the intracellular kinase. Three main effectors can be activated later: phosphoinositide 3-kinase (Pi3K), rat sarcoma (RAS), and phospholipase C (PLC).

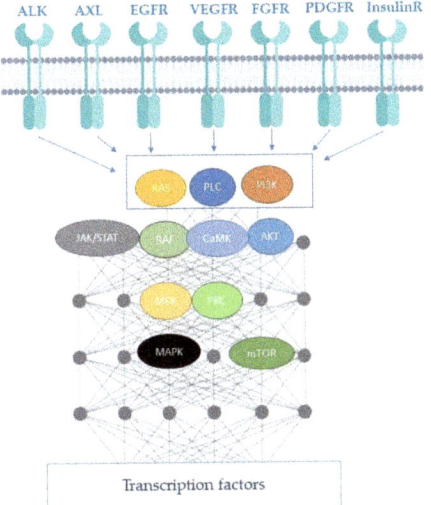

Figure 2. Receptor tyrosine kinase (RTK) network modeling proposed by the Kitano's "bow tie". The set of RTKs (input layer) influences a small number of intermediaries, such as mitogen-activated protein kinases (MAPK), phosphoinositide 3-kinase (Pi3K), and Ca^{2+} signaling (core processes), which leads to the activation of a complex signaling network implicating Pi3K/protein kinase B (AKT)/mechanistic target of rapamycin (mTOR), rat sarcoma (RAS)/MAPK, Janus kinase (JAK)/STAT, and phospholipase C (PLC)/Ca^{2+}/calmodulin-dependent protein kinase-protein kinase C (CaMK-PKC) pathways with their numerous crosstalks. The result of the signaling cascade leads to a transcriptional control.

1.2. Classification of Receptor Tyrosine Kinase Inhibitors

Cancer cell proliferation has been proposed to follow the Darwinian selection in order to continue proliferation in harsh conditions and changes imposed by tumor microenvironment (TME) [10]. Drug targeting intracellular signaling have been developed to target the hubs of these molecular pathways. Among these drugs, receptor tyrosine kinase inhibitors (RTKIs) are a large family within these targeted drugs and have been used clinically with numerous successes since 2001. They generally target the active site of the kinase and thereby prevent the phosphorylation of intracellular targets, which are often involved in cell proliferation or angiogenesis [11,12]. As of August 2019, 43 RTK inhibitors were approved by the Food and Drug Administration (FDA) for oncological indications (Table 1) [13]. Reversible inhibitors are usually distinguished from irreversible ones, which bind covalently with or near an adenosine triphosphate (ATP) binding site. Among the non-covalent inhibitors, the majority are ATP-competitive inhibitors that link to active conformations (type-I inhibitors). ATP binding sites are generally conserved, therefore selectivity can be achieved by targeting poorly preserved residues, particularly residues flanking the hinge. Type-II inhibitors bind to a site adjacent to the ATP site of inactive kinases and maintain their inactive conformation. This type of inhibitor is usually nonselective. Allosteric inhibitors (type III) inhibit kinases by binding to an allosteric site, remote from the ATP site and the hinge, and are highly selective [14]. New substrate-directed inhibitors or type-IV RTKIs, which target substrate-binding site in a reversible manner, are under development. Finally, covalent kinase inhibitors bound irreversibly with the kinase active site, also called type-V inhibitors, and have the advantage to be potent and have reduced off-target side effects [15].

This review discusses the current challenges of the use of RTKIs in clinic and the potential use of new emerging technological advances for the design of efficient RTKIs therapies.

Table 1. List of FDA-approved small molecule protein kinase inhibitors (updated by 18 August 2019). These inhibitors are sorted by their main targeted pathways and from signal initiation at cytoplasmic membrane of the cell to its propagation to the nucleus [13,15–19].

Name	Known Target	Inhibitor Class	Indications
Anaplastic lymphoma kinase (ALK)			
Alectinib	ALK and RET	II	ALK+ NSCLC
Brigatinib	ALK, ROS1, IGF-1R, Flt3, EGFR	I	ALK+ NSCLC after crizotinib
Ceritinib	ALK, IGF-1R, InsR, ROS1	II	ALK+ NSCLC as first-line treatment or after crizotinib resistance
Crizotinib	ALK, c-Met (HGFR), ROS1, MST1R	II	ALK+, ROS1+ NSCLC
Entrectinib	TRKA/B/C, ROS1, ALK	I	ROS1+ NSCLC; solid tumors with NTRK fusion proteins
Lorlatinib	ALK	I	ALK+ NSCLC
Fusion of breakpoint cluster region and Abelson (BCR-ABL)			
Bosutinib	BCR-ABL, Src, Lyn, Hck		CML
Dasatinib	BCR-ABL, EGFR, Src, Lck, Yes, Fyn, Kit, EphA2, PDGFRβ	I	Ph+ chronic ML and ALL
Imatinib	BCR-ABL, Kit, PDGFR	II	Ph+ CML or ALL, CEL, DFSP, HES, GIST, MDS/MDP
Nilotinib	BCR-ABL, PDGFR, DDR1	II	Ph+ CLL
Ponatinib	BCR-ABL, BCR-ABL T315I, VEGFR, PDGFR, FGFR, EphR, Src family kinases, Kit, RET, Tie2, Flt3	II	Ph+ CML or ALL
Epidermal growth factor receptor (EGFR)			
Afatinib	EGFR, ErbB2, ErbB4	Covalent (V)	NSCLC
Dacomitinib	EGFR/ErbB2/ErbB4	I	EGFR- mutated NSCLC
Erlotinib	EGFR	I	SCLC and PaC
Gefitinib	EGFR	I	NCLC
Lapatinib	EGFR, ErbB2	II	BC
Neratinib	ErbB2/HER2	Covalent (V)	HER2+ breast cancer
Osimertinib	EGFR T970M	Covalent (V)	NSCLC
Vandetanib	EGFRs, VEGFRs, RET, Brk, Tie2, EphRs, Src family kinases	I	MTC
FMS-like tyrosine kinase 3 (FLT3)			
Gilteritinib	FLT3	I	AML with FLT3 mutation5
Midostaurin	FLT3	I	ALL Flt3 mutation+
Fibroblast growth factor receptors (FGFR)			
Erdafitinib	FGFR1/2/3/4	I	Urothelial carcinoma
Janus kinase (JAK)			
Ruxolitinib	JAK1 and 2	I	MF and PV
Neurotrophic Tyrosine Receptor Kinase (NTRK)			
Larotrectinib	NTRK	I	Solid tumors with NTRK gene fusion proteins
Vascular endothelial growth factor (VEGFR)			
Axitinib	VEGFR1/2/3, PDGFRβ	II	RCC
Carbozantinib	RET, Met, VEGFR1/2/3, Kit, TrkB, Flt3, Axl, Tie2, ROS1	I	Metastatic MTC, advanced RCC and HCC
Lenvatinib	VEGFRs, FGFRs, PDGFR, Kit, RET	II	DTC
Pazopanib	VEGFR1/2/3, PDGFRα/β, FGFR1/3, Kit, Lck, Fms, Itk	I	RCC, STS
Regorafenib	VEGFR1/2/3, BCR-ABL, BRAF, BRAF(V600E), Kit, PDGFRα/β, RET, FGFR1/2, Tie2, Eph2A	II	CRC, GIST
Sorafenib	B/C-Raf, BRAF (V600E), Kit, Flt3, RET, VEGFR1/2/3, PDGFRβ	II	RCC, DTC and HCC
Sunitinib	PDGFRα/β, VEGFR1/2/3, Kit, Flt3, CSF-1R, RET	II	RCC, GIST, PNET

Table 1. Cont.

Name	Known Target	Inhibitor Class	Indications
BRAF			
Dabrafenib	BRAF	I	Melanoma and NSCLC with BRAF mutations
Encorafenib	BRAFV600E/K	I	BRAFV600E/K mutant melanoma with binimetinib
Vemurafenib	A/B/C-Raf, BRAF (V600E), SRMS, ACK1, MAP4K5, FGR	I	Melanoma with BRAFV600E mutation and ECD
Bruton tyrosine kinase			
Acalabrutinib	Bruton tyrosine kinase	Covalent (V)	MCL
Ibrutinib	Bruton tyrosine kinase	Covalent (V)	MCL, CLL, WM, graph vs host disease.
Mitogen-activated protein kinase kinase (MEK)			
Binimetinib	MEK1/2	III	BRAF V600E/K melanoma with encorafenib
Cobimetinib	MEK1/2	III	Melanoma with BRAF V600E/K mutations with vemurafenib
Trametinib	MEK1/2	III	Melanoma (2013) and NSCLC (2017) with BRAF mutations
Cyclin-dependent-kinase 4/6			
Abemaciclib	CDK4/6	I	HR+, HER− BC
Palbociclib	CDK4/6	I	ER+ and HER2− BC
Ribociclib	CDK4/6	I	HR+−EGFR− metastatic BC

Type-I inhibitors are ATP-competitive inhibitors that bind to active conformations, Type-II inhibitors bind to a site adjacent to the ATP site of inactive kinases and maintain their inactive conformation; Type-III inhibitors are allosteric inhibitors, they are highly selective and inhibit kinases by binding to an allosteric site, distant from the ATP site and the hinge; Type-IV inhibitors target substrate-binding site in a reversible manner (under development); Type-V inhibitors bind to their targets with covalent bonds. ALL: acute lymphoid leukemia; ALK: Anaplastic lymphoma kinase; BCR-ABL: breakpoint cluster region- Abelson; CDK: cyclin-dependent kinase; CML: chronic myeloïd leukemia; CLL: chronic lymphoid leukemia; CRC: colorectal carcinoma; CSFR: colony stimulating factor 1 receptor; DTC: differentiated thyroid carcinoma; ECD: Erdheim-Chester disease; EGFR: Epidermal growth factor receptor; EphR: Ephrin receptor; FGFR: fibroblast growth factor receptor; FKBP: FK506-binding protein; GIST: gastro intestinal stromal tumor; HCC: hepatocellular carcinoma; HER or ErbB: human epidermal growth factor receptor; HGFR or c-Met: hepatocyte growth factor receptor; InsR: Insulin receptor precursor; IGF insulin-like growth factor; Itk: interleukine 2 inducible T cell kinase; JAK: Janus kinase; MAPK: mitogen-activated protein kinases; MCL: mantle cell lymphoma; MEK: MAPK/extracellular signal-regulated kinase; MF: Myelofibrosis; ML: myeloid leukemia; MTC: medullary thyroid cancer; mTOR: mechanistic target of rapamycin; NSCLC: non-small-cell lung cancer; NTRK: neurotrophic tyrosine receptor kinase; PDGFR: Platelet-derived growth factor receptors; PNET: primitive neuroectodermal tumor; RCC: renal cell carcinoma; SGCAs: subependymal giant cell astrocytoma; SCLC: small cells lung carcinoma; SRMS: src-related kinase lacking C-terminal regulatory tyrosine and N-terminal myristylation sites; STS: soft tissue sarcoma; Tie2: tyrosine kinase with immunoglobulin and EGF homology domains; TRK: tropomyosin receptor kinase; TSGCTs: tenosynovial giant cell tumors VEGFR; WM: Waldenstrom's macroglobulinemia.

2. Current Place of Receptor Tyrosine Kinase Inhibitors in Oncological Treatments

RTKIs occupy an important place in precision oncology, even if their effectiveness is limited by the acquisition of resistance mechanisms. This section describes the advent of RTKIs in non-small cell lung cancer (NSCLC) and other types of cancer, and the mechanisms of resistance.

2.1. Evolution of Receptor Tyrosine Kinase Inhibitor Use in Non-Small Cell Lung Cancer

The use of RTKIs in NSCLC was reported in clinical trials with the first generation, EGFR reversible inhibitors of ATP-binding sites (gefitinib and erlotinib in cancer patients). Compared with chemotherapy, these treatments improved patient survival by 50% (overall survival (OS) of 30.5 months versus 23.6 months) [20]. The second generation of RTKIs is composed of irreversible inhibitors (afatinib and dacomitinib) with greater affinity for the EGFR kinase domain, which also inhibits other members of the HER family to which the EGFR belongs. Afatinib doubles survival compared to chemotherapy (median progression-free survival (mPFS) of 11.1 months versus 6.9 months) [21].

Clinical studies showed longer survival with dacomitinib than with gefitinib (mPFS of 14.7 months versus 9.2 months and median OS (mOS) of 34.1 months versus 26.8 months, respectively) [20,22]. Side effects, including skin irritation or ulceration, and gastrointestinal toxicity (diarrhea, constipation, severe nausea, and vomiting) are more frequently severe with afatinib and dacomitinib.

The most common mechanism of resistance to these drugs is a secondary mutation of EGFR kinase domain. Therefore, a third generation EGFR-RTKI, osimertinib, was designed to have more affinity for mutated receptors. Compared to first generation EGFR RTKI, osimertinib significantly improved PFS (18.9 months versus 10.2 months), with a favorable tolerability profile [20,23,24].

The current recommendation of the European Society for Medical Oncology (ESMO) for NSCLCs with an EGFR-activating mutation is the treatment with erlotinib, gefitinib, and afatinib or osimertinib as first-line therapy [25]. Combination of gefinitib with chemotherapy (carboplatin/pemetrexed) is also recommended in the first line therapy for NSCLC. Other options are under investigation but not recommended yet, such as the combination of erlotinib with bevacizumab or ramucirumab (anti-angiogenic antibodies targeting the vascular endothelial growth factor receptor (VEGFR)). Indeed, the drug combination targeting EGFR and VEGFR appears to be synergistic, probably because of the crosstalk between their signaling pathways and vascular normalization induced by anti-angiogenic therapy, which can in turn increase intra-tumor concentration of RTKI [26]. After systemic progression, the recommended second-line treatment is osimertinib in the case of a T790M mutation in exon 20 [25]. In the absence of this mutation, the guidelines recommend chemotherapy (platinum-based) with or without bevacizumab, or immunotherapy (atezolizumab) [25].

Many early phase clinical studies are investigating new combination therapies. For example, some ongoing clinical trials are investigating the combination of a first generation EGFR RTKI (gefitinib) with osimertinib as a first line treatment [27]. In addition, chidamide, an histone deacetylase (HDAC) inhibitor, is tested in combination with several RTKIs of EGFR, after promising pre-clinical results showing a synergistic action (chidamide notably prevents the activation of pathways such as RAS/MAPK and Pi3K/AKT) [28]. Further investigations are evaluating the efficacy of new third generation EGFR RTKIs (nazartinib, rociletinib, avitinib), non-selective RTKIs targeting several RTKs, including EGF and VEGF (sorafenib, anlotinib, momelotinib), or RTKIs which target the c-MET hepatocyte growth factor (capmatinib, tepotinib), the AXL receptor tyrosine kinase (gilteritinib), and Janus kinase 2 (JAK2) (pacritinib, momelotinib). While positive results are expected from theses ongoing studies, it should be noted that in the recent years, most strategies combining RTKIs have failed in clinical phases for lack of efficiency or tolerability [29].

2.2. Current Indications of Receptor Tyrosine Kinase Inhibitors in Other Types of Cancer

NSCLC with mutated EGFR is an example that can summarize the evolution of RTKIs that showed limited efficacy during the last twenty years. The situation is the same for other tumors, with the exception of chronic myeloid leukemia, which can be "cured" with one or more RTKIs.

For renal cell carcinoma (RCC), anti-angiogenic RTKIs, such as sunitinib or pazopanib, are recommended by the ESMO as first-line therapy in patients with favorable prognosis. In case of relapse after treatment with RTKI, the second line treatment is either immunotherapy (nivolumab) or another RTKI (cabozantinib or axitinib) [30]. Effectiveness of the second line is explained by dual inhibitory effects on VEGFR2, and on MET or MAPK, which are activated in cancer cells resistant to first line RTKIs [31,32].

In metastatic HER+ breast cancer, lapatinib can be used as a first line in addition to trastuzumab in selected patients due to the high toxicity of this treatment. In the second line therapy, lapatinib seems less effective than the antibody-dug conjugate trastuzumab emtansine, T-DM1 [33].

Systemic therapy for hepatocellular carcinoma relies mainly on multitarget kinase inhibitors. In the first line treatment, sorafenib (VEGFRi, PDGFRi) or lenvatinib (targeting VEGFRi, FGFRi, PDGFRi) are recommended, whereas cabozantinib (RETi, growth arrest-specific 6 (GAS6)i), regorafenib (VEGFRi, FGFRi and PDGFRi), or immunotherapy were used in second line [34].

In metastatic colorectal cancer, regorafenib, a multitarget kinase inhibitor (EGFRi, PDGFRi, FGFRi), is the first RTKI that demonstrated a modest benefit in survival (6.4 versus 5 months) in the third line after failure of antibodies targeting EGFR and VEGFR and chemotherapy [35]. Imatinib (breakpoint cluster region (BCR)-Abelson (ABL) inhibitor) revolutionized the prognosis of gastrointestinal stromal tumors expressing the RTK, KIT (CD117), with a mOS longer than 5 years [36], and is the current first line therapy. After relapse, sunitinib and regorafenib can be used [37].

Lenvatinib (VEGFRi) and sorafenib are considered as first line therapy for differentiated thyroid cancers resistant to radioactive therapy with a significant improvement of PFS (10.8 months with sorafenib versus 5.8 months with placebo, mPFS 18.3 months with lenvatinib versus 3.6 months with placebo) [38,39]. For progressive metastatic medullar thyroid carcinoma, cabozantinib and vandetanib (EGFRi, RETi) are the first-line systemic treatments (PFS are 30.5 months with vandetanib versus 19.3 months with placebo, and 11.2 months with cabozantinib versus 4.0 months with placebo) [40].

First line standard treatment for unresectable stage III/IV BRAF V600 mutated melanoma is BRAF RTKI (vemurafenib, dabrafenib, encorafenib) combined with MEK RTKI (cobimetinib, trametinib, binimetinib) with an mPFS of the order of one year. Second line treatment is based on immunotherapy alone [41].

To conclude, the best achievement of RTKIs in cancer treatment concerns chronic myeloid leukemia (CML), since the survival rate of patients treated with imatinib at 10 years is 83.3% [42]. There are some evolutionary explanations to CML exception. Cell population of CML is homogenous and is therefore not subjected to an allopatric speciation process. One dominant oncogene is present throughout the population, and clonal changes are progressive and orderly during the chronic phase of the disease. These elements explain why the CML evolves in a clonal and stepwise manner, in contrast to the dynamic and stochastic evolution of solid tumors [43]. Pre-clinical studies have identified other causes of resistance, such as compensatory hyperactivation of anti-apoptotic pathways (e.g., CRS), the involvement of efflux proteins (e.g., P-glycoprotein or the human organic cation transporter 1 (hOCT1)) [43]. In the case of low-risk chronic CML, first generation RTKIs (imatinib) or second generation RTKIs (nilotinib, dasatinib and bosutinib) are recommended, whereas only second generation RTKIs are indicated for CML in chronic phase with high risk, and panotinib and other third-generation RTKIs are reserved for the second line of treatment. [44].

2.3. Mechanisms of Resistance to Receptor Tyrosine Kinase Inhibitors

Generally, RTKI resistance can be intrinsic (primary), when the tumor does not respond to treatment, or acquired (secondary), when resistance occurs after an initial response to RTKI treatment and a progressive selection of resistant tumor cells.

Most of the mechanisms of resistance to RTKIs are mainly attributed to mutations occurring within RTK itself. Several mutations were found in key residues (e.g., gatekeeper residue) in their catalytic domains, which prevents RTKI-binding to ATP-pocket of RTK by steric hindrance [14]. Clinical studies have revealed around fifty different mutations of BCR-ABL responsible for imatinib resistance, as well as the involvement of other elements of intracellular signaling; such as the forkhead box protein O1 (FOXO1), β-catenin, STAT3, the nuclear factor-kappa B (NF-κB), and AXL in RTKI resistance [45]. In gastrointestinal stromal tumors expressing KIT, genomic analysis of tumors have highlighted mutations in gatekeeper residues in BCR-ABL and EGFR, or activating mutations in BRAF, or insulin-like growth factor 1 receptor (IGF1R) amplifications were reported in imatinib resistance [46]. Some pre-clinical studies highlight other mechanisms, such as KIT mutations of the ATP-binding pocket of the kinase domain or the kinase activation loop [47,48].

Another way to circumvent the effect of RTKI is to activate a kinase located downstream or in parallel of the targeted signaling pathway, or on a parallel pathway. This latter is the most frequently described mechanism of resistance to RTKIs. This is particularly due to the emergence of compensatory signaling pathways when the major one is blocked, and to the existence of naturally occurring crosstalks and connections between different signaling pathways [49]. For instance, changes in signaling pathways are common with activation of EGFR or loss of PTEN (phosphatase and tensin homolog), but also with alternative activation of AKT/mTOR, of STAT3, and of vascular endothelial growth factor (VEGF) by RTKI-induced autocrine secretions of interleukins IL6 and IL8, and resistance [50]. KRAS mutation in NSCLC is a well-known mechanism of resistance to anti-EGFR RTKIs in clinic [51] and in pre-clinical studies. Thus, resistance of hepatocellular carcinoma (HCC) to sorafenib is linked with activation of EGFR. In addition, by promoting cell survival, Pi3K/AKT and autophagy are involved in therapeutic resistance of HCC. Furthermore, hypoxia induced by sorafenib treatment leads to the activation of extracellular signal-regulated kinases (ERK)/MAPK and JAK/STAT, and the up-regulation of hypoxy-inducible factor 2-alpha (HIF-2α), which in turn activates the transforming growth factor alpha (TGF-α) and EGFR [52]. Resistance of thyroid cancer to RTKIs involve RET mutations [53]. Frequent resistance mechanisms to BRAF inhibitors validated on patients' tumors imply phosphorylation of EGFR, loss of PTEN, or activating mutations of MAPK, NRAS, or Pi3K-AKT [54].

Phenotypic transformation can lead to resistance to RTKIs. The most frequent example is the epithelial-mesenchymal transition (EMT) during which tumor cells lose their epithelial characteristics, such as cell-cell adhesion and polarity, in favor of mesenchymal characteristics and of the acquisition of an invasive phenotype. Thus, in NSCLC, translational studies have highlighted EMT as a mechanism of resistance to RTKIs of EGFR via the activation of EMT-specific signaling pathways (AXL and Hedgehog). Another rare transformation involved in the resistance of NSCLC to RTKIs is the histological transformation of a pulmonary adenocarcinoma into small cell lung cancer. These resistance mechanisms seem to be independent of the class of EGFR inhibitor used [23].

Another important mechanism of resistance is the selection of cancer cells expressing efflux pumps able to transport drugs. For example, in RCC, pre-clinical data showed that sorafenib and sunitinib can be sequestrated in the lysosome by ATP-binding cassette (ABC) transporter, P-glycoprotein [50]. Other mechanisms of resistance linked to the interaction of neoplastic cells with their microenvironment will be discussed in Section 3.3.

3. Improving the Use of Receptor Tyrosine Kinase Inhibitors: Combinatorial Treatment without Increasing Toxicity

As previously explained, the combination of RTKIs is ideal from a theoretical point of view, but is not easily achievable in clinical practice because of the toxicity. Therefore, combining a RTKI with another class of drug can be an interesting avenue. This section explains the rational bases for drug combinations in the light of pre-clinical analyzes of neoplastic cells and their microenvironment.

3.1. Receptor Tyrosine Kinase Inhibitor Combinations

In theory, combination of RTKIs is considered as an attractive option because it can prevent primary and secondary therapeutic resistance. The first strategy, called vertical pathway inhibition, aims to doubly inhibit the same signaling pathway. It consists in limiting the impact of a possible mutation of the targeted RTK or in activating downstream effectors. The choice of inhibiting the same target in two different ways was tested in a clinical trial with NSCLC patients treated with the first and third-generation anti-EGFR inhibitors. Currently, the only example of targeting an RTK and one of its downstream effectors is currently the double BRAF-MEK inhibition recommended in melanoma, but other combinations are still under investigation in clinical trial [27,55,56]. It should be noted that double inhibitions can be established on the basis of two selective RTKIs of a target or of a single RTKI with a double inhibitory action. For example, RO5126766, the first selective dual BRAF/CRAF and MEK inhibitor was investigated in a phase-1 dose-escalation clinical study [57].

A new strategy, called horizontal inhibition, is under development. It consists in a crosstalk inhibition to prevent the over-activation of a second pathway in response to the inhibition of the first one. Many pre-clinical data are encouraging and have given rise to phase-1 clinical trial in melanoma, combining an anti-BRAF or MEK RTKI with an anti-Pi3K. Other phase-1 agnostic clinical trials have investigated the combination of inhibitors of MEK and AKT. All these clinical trials illustrate very well the difficulty of combinations of RTKIs, since none has really resulted in a positive balance between increased toxicity and survival gain [57], as often seen in trials for combinations of RTKIs [15].

Toxicity of RTK inhibitors is therefore an integral part of the therapeutic challenge. Large part of their toxicity is attributable to their off-target effects. It should be prevented by a better determination of RTKI affinity for other targets, in order to select the most specific RTKIs [58]. Another approach consisting in reducing the distribution of RTKIs in healthy tissues using nanoparticles or pegylated liposomes is under intense research, while their clinical benefits remain to be proven [59].

3.2. Receptor Tyrosine Kinase Inhibitors and Synthetic Lethality

A combination of treatment leads to synthetic lethality when the single treatment did not cause cell death, unlike their combination. One of the first successes in synthetic lethality was the poly-adenosine diphosphate ribose polymerase (PARP) inhibitor, which is currently used in clinic to achieve synthetic lethality in breast cancer with mutated (BRCA)1 or 2. Recently, Maifrede et al. have reported that in acute myeloid leukemia, inhibition of Fms-like tyrosine kinase 3 (FLT3) by an RTKI appears to downregulate key proteins in DNA double-strand break (DSB) repair; such as BRCA1, BRCA2; and RAD51. In this study, combination of RTKI of FLT3 with a PARP inhibitor has shown very encouraging results in mouse models [60].

This concept can be extended to other therapeutic classes such as metabolic inhibitors. Ding et al. thus identified by clustered regularly interspaced short palindromic repeats (CRISPR) knock-out screening that transaldolase, an enzyme of the non-oxidative pentose phosphate pathway, was essential for the survival of tumor cells treated with lapatinib. Inactivation of this enzyme combined with inhibition of HER2 reduced the level of nicotinamide adenine dinucleotide phosphate (NADPH), and thus increased the production of reactive oxygen species (ROS) while reducing the synthesis of lipids and nucleotides [61].

The regulatory pathways of apoptosis could also be involved in drug resistance. Arsenic trioxide (ATO) is successfully used in a rare form of leukemia, acute promyelocytic leukemia, as it induces the differentiation of tumor cells. Wang et al. have noticed that ATO produces numerous apoptotic signals without succeeding in the induction of apoptosis, because it causes phosphorylation and therefore inactivation of glycogen synthase kinase (GSK)3β, one of the key pro-apoptotic enzymes. Then, they successfully tested sorafenib, which activated GSK3β, increased the rate of apoptosis, and significantly prolonged the survival rate of mouse tumor models [62].

3.3. Impact of the Non-Immune Microenvironment on Receptor Tyrosine Kinase Inhibitor Efficacy

RTKIs targeting tumor cells also act on cellular components of TME. This latter is indeed also influenced by chemotherapy, immunotherapy, and radiotherapy, and in turn influences the response to treatment [63].

Stromal cells in TME exposed to RTKIs produce cytokines, hormones, or growth factors that modulate the response of the tumor to RTKIs. Thus, RTKIs targeting focal adhesion kinase (FAK), FGFR, c-MET, and VEGFR decrease the number of fibroblasts or their activation, and therefore their role in supporting growth of various tumors [64,65].

Interestingly, the TME can itself modify the signaling of neoplastic cells and drive resistance to RTKIs. In thyroid carcinoma, pericytes lead to vemurafenib resistance through secretion of thrombospondine 1 (TSP-1) and transforming growth factor beta-1 (TGFβ1), which increase expression of protein kinase R (PKR)-like endoplasmic reticulum kinase (pERK1/2), phosphorylated AKT (pAKT), and phosphorylated mothers against decapentaplegic homolog 3 (pSMAD3) levels [66]. Similarly, stromal cells can secrete hepatocyte growth factor (HGF) which activates MET that in turn stimulates MAPK and Pi3K/AKT/mTOR, leading to BRAFi resistance of melanoma cells [67,68]. Resistance to RTKI therapy targeting HER2 could be mediated by cancer-associated fibroblasts (CAFs) through the secretion of neuregulin-1 beta (NRG1β), which is an HER3 ligand [69].

PDGFR and VEGFR inhibitors administered in small doses induce vascular normalization which improves drug distribution within the tumor. The depletion of pericytes and hypoxia caused by sunitinib treatment may increase the metastatic spread of tumor cells [64].

Few studies have looked at the effects of RTKIs on the extracellular matrix (ECM), but there is an inverse correlation between the efficacy of lapatinib in HER2+ breast cancer and the elastic modulus of ECM, which means that the more effective lapatinib, the more easily the ECM deforms [70].

3.4. Impact of the Immune Microenvironment on Receptor Tyrosine Kinase Inhibitor Efficacy

Immune microenvironment is also modulated by RTKIs. For example, dasatinib, sorafenib, and imatinib decrease T-regulator cells (Tregs) and increase anti-tumor T-cell response. Similarly, sunitinib decreases the survival and expansion of myeloid-derived suppressor cells (MDSCs) and M2 macrophages, promoting the establishment of a permissive immune-competent TME [64,71]. Cabozantinib stimulates neutrophil-mediated anticancer innate immune response [72]. Treatment with BRAF inhibitors alone or with MEK inhibitors increases the level of tumor associated CD8 + lymphocytes and melanoma antigens expression [73]. For example, RTKIs targeting FGFR, in addition to their action on neoplastic cells, reduce the number of immunosuppressive MDSCs in the tumor and induce senescence of cancer-associated fibroblasts (CAFs) [65]. VEGFR1 inhibitors, in addition to their anti-angiogenic actions, can normalize tumor microvasculature and decrease the infiltration of MDSCS, Treg lymphocytes, and some populations of immunosuppressive tumor-associated macrophages (TAMs) [71,74].

Furthermore, establishment of an immunosuppressive TME was observed during the acquisition of resistance to RTKIs. Thus, resistance of BRAF tumors to RTKIs is concomitant with an increase in MDSCs. Additionally, the resistance of glioblastoma to axitinib led to an increased number of Treg lymphocytes and the expression of the programmed cell death protein-1 (PD-1) inhibitory checkpoint. A shift in TAMs towards a phenotype promoting tumor growth was observed in gastro-intestinal stromal tumors (GISTs) becoming resistant to imatinib [64]. In addition, the RTKIs targeting EGFRs seem less effective in patients with a tumor highly infiltrated by CD8+ lymphocytes and associated with a high level of programmed death-ligand 1 (PD-L1) [75]. Taken together, these results indicate that an anti-tumor activity of immune TME seems important in the effectiveness of RTKIs [75]. In addition, the immune cells of the microenvironment can act through other mechanisms than immunity. Thus, MDSCs recruited under treatment can produce pro-angiogenic factors and stimulate VEGF-independent angiogenesis [76].

There is therefore a rational for developing combinations with RTKIs and immunotherapies. Few clinical studies have already been published on the subject and the toxicity of these combinations often seems to be very high. However, a phase-3 trial combining atezolizumab (anti-PD-L1) with sunitinib (VEGFR inhibitor) in metastatic RCC, and a phase-2 trial combining pembrolizumab (anti-PD1) with dabrafenib (BRAF inhibitor) and trametinib (MEK inhibitor) in BRAF-mutant melanoma patients have shown encouraging results with moderate toxicity [64]. Similar results were obtained with the combination of lenvatinib and pembrolizumab in a phase-2 clinical study in endometrial and kidney cancer [77], as well as with the combination of nivolumab and regorafenib, evaluated in a phase-2 clinical study in advanced gastric or colorectal cancers [78].

Tyrosine kinase receptors expressed by non-neoplastic cells may also become an attractive therapeutic target, such as AXL, the RTK expressed by TAMs, which is considered as an emerging class of innate immune checkpoints [79]. In view of all these elements, some early clinical studies are currently studying some RTKI and checkpoint inhibitor combinations (e.g., nivolumab combined with pazopanib or sunitinib, axitinib combined with pembrolizumab) [80–82]. The relationships between RTKIs and immune cells, as well as clinical trials combining RTKIs with immune checkpoints inhibitors are summarized in Table 2.

Table 2. Relationship between anti-tumor immunity and RTKIs [64,65,71,73,74,76–82].

RTKI actions in favor of an anti-tumor immune response		
RTKIs	Effects on immune cells	Characteristics of carried-out studies
BRAF inhibitors +/- MEK inhibitors	↑ CD8+ TIL and melanoma antigen expression	Patient biopsies and in vivo pre-clinical study, BRAF mutated melanoma
Cabozantinib	↑ neutrophil-mediated antitumor innate immunity	In vivo pre-clinical study, murine prostate cancer
Dasatinib	↓ MDSCs	Patient biopsies and in vivo pre-clinical study, CML
Sorafenib	↓ MDSCs	Patient biopsies and in vivo pre-clinical study, HCC
FGFR inhibitors	↓ MDSCs	In vivo pre-clinical study, murine breast cancer
Sunitinib	↓ MDSCs and M2 macrophages	In vivo pre-clinical study, RCC
VEGFR1 inhibitors	↓ MDSCs, Tregs and M2 macrophages	In vivo pre-clinical studies on RCC and NSCLC
Tumor immune tolerance observed during the acquisition of resistance to RTKI		
RTKI	Effects on immune cells	Characteristics of studies carried out
Axitinib	↑ Tregs, ↑ and PD-1 expression	In vivo pre-clinical study, glioblastoma
BRAF inhibitors	↑ MDSCs	In vivo pre-clinical study, BRAF mutated melanoma
Imatinib	↑ M2 macrophages	In vivo pre-clinical study, GIST
Combinations of RTKI and checkpoint inhibitors under investigation		
RTKI	Checkpoint inhibitors	Clinical trial
Dabrafenib	Pembrolizumab (anti-PD1)	Phase-2 trial, B-ref mutated melanoma
Lenvatinib	Pembrolizumab (anti-PD1)	Phase-2 trial, endometrial cancer and RCC
Regorafenib	Nivolumab	Phase-2 trial, gastric or colorectal cancer
Sunitinib	Atezolizumab (anti-PD-L1)	Phase-3 trial, metastatic RCC

CML: chronic myeloid leukemia; GIST: gastro intestinal stromal tumor; HCC: hepatocellular carcinoma; MDSCs: myeloid-derived suppressor cell; MEK: mitogen-activated protein kinase; NSCLC: non-small-cell lung cancer; PD1: progammed cell death protein 1; PD-L1: programmed death-ligand 1; RCC: renal cell carcinoma; TILs: tumor-infiltrating lymphocytes; Tregs: regulatory T cells.

4. Conclusions

RTKIs have revolutionized the practice of oncology and hematology other the past 20 years with over 40 compounds approved by the FDA (Figure 3). However, apart from rare exceptions, such as some cases of chronic myeloid leukemia, no patient can currently be cured by the use of RTKI as single agent in therapy. The problems of the emergence of resistance to treatment and toxicity, leading to the reduction of the given dose or to RTKI treatment discontinuation, are the main challenges for their use in cancer patients. With the current growth in the cost of treatment that discourages access to care, reduction of development costs should also be considered as a priority.

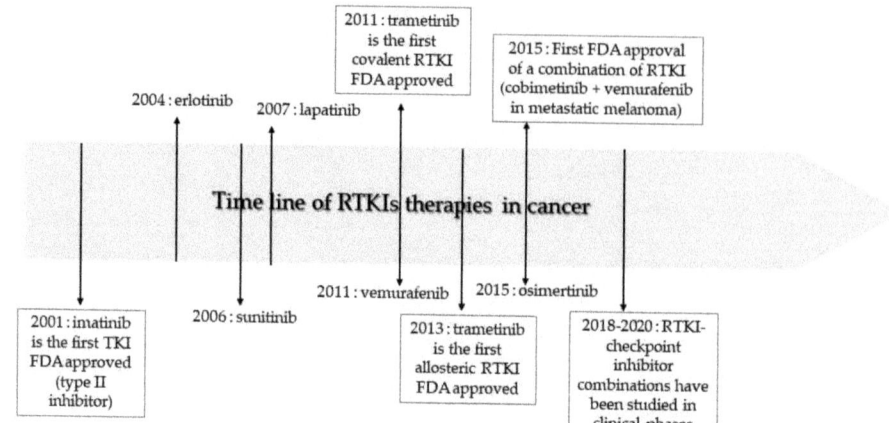

Figure 3. Time line of receptor tyrosine kinase inhibitor (RTKI) development and approval for the treatment of cancer.

Production of new RTKIs with different mechanisms of action, such as covalent inhibitors, inhibitors resistant to the most frequent tumor mutations, or inhibitors inducing RTK degradation or internalization, is a promising approach. Reducing side effects due to "off-target" effects by improving the selectivity of RTKIs is another major aspect to consider. The time for the new RTKI development, and therefore their cost, may be reduced by the use of artificial intelligence (AI). Indeed, machine learning also offers new possibilities to predict the 3D structure of a protein from the sequence of its amino acids, interactions and binding between molecules of interest, and finally to design new potential drugs [83,84]. A first example of discovery of RTKI by artificial intelligence was given by Zhavoronkov et al. in 2019. A system of deep learning made it possible to discover several candidate inhibitors of the discoidin domain receptor 1 in 21 days. Among them, two were effective in vitro and one showed interesting results in mouse models [85]. After a design of the new molecules assisted by AI, their initial development can be made more efficient by new microfluidic techniques. Desai et al, for example, produced new ABL inhibitors. Compounds selected as the most promising by algorithms are synthesized automatically in microarrays or microfluidic platforms and then screened by the determination of the IC50 and other parameters. The best candidates can then directly be integrated in pre-clinical studies [86–88].

Research for an effective and low-toxic combination is very complex. So far, apart from the BRAF-MEK combination in melanoma, few combinations of two RTKIs have been used clinically. Production of more selective RTKIs may increase the tolerance of their combination.

Another promising approach is the combination of RTKIs with another class of inhibitors. Analysis of such combinations must take into account the effects of synthetic lethality type and the effects on TME. This involves analysis of large databases, which can be performed by various AI techniques, and new in vitro models as organs-on-chips. These systems include microchannels continuously perfused by a culture medium and containing different cell types organized in organ-specific, tissue-tissue interfaces [89]. Large screening of additives or synergistic properties of an RTKI with another or with other drugs, taking into account the effect of RTKIs on the immune and nonimmune microenvironment will likely help in the development of effective therapeutics with low toxicity and cost for a better care of cancer patients.

Author Contributions: C.P., M.F. and R.L. drafted the first version of the manuscript. N.E.S. and R.L. supervised and edited the paper. All authors contributed to the elaboration of further and the final versions of the manuscript. All authors have read and agreed to the published version of the manuscript.

Funding: This research received no external funding.

Acknowledgments: This work was supported by the Research grant (CDR) from the national fund for scientific research (FRS-FNRS) # 31247715, by the PDR-TLV, FRS-FNRS # 32801162. The figures were designed on Microsoft Powerpoint and Biorender.

Conflicts of Interest: The authors declare no conflict of interest.

References

1. Lemmon, M.A.; Schlessinger, J. Cell signaling by receptor tyrosine kinases. *Cell* **2010**, *141*, 1117–1134. [CrossRef]
2. Oda, K.; Matsuoka, Y.; Funahashi, A.; Kitano, H. A comprehensive pathway map of epidermal growth factor receptor signaling. *Mol. Syst. Biol.* **2005**, *1*, 2005.0010. [CrossRef]
3. Schlessinger, J. Cell signaling by receptor tyrosine kinases. *Cell* **2000**, *103*, 211–225. [CrossRef]
4. Yu, J.S.; Cui, W. Proliferation, survival and metabolism: The role of PI3K/AKT/mTOR signalling in pluripotency and cell fate determination. *Development* **2016**, *143*, 3050–3060. [CrossRef]
5. Cooke, M.; Magimaidas, A.; Casado-Medrano, V.; Kazanietz, M.G. Protein kinase C in cancer: The top five unanswered questions. *Mol. Carcinog.* **2017**, *56*, 1531–1542. [CrossRef]
6. Aksamitiene, E.; Kiyatkin, A.; Kholodenko, B.N. Cross-talk between mitogenic Ras/MAPK and survival PI3K/Akt pathways: A fine balance. *Biochem. Soc. Trans.* **2012**, *40*, 139–146. [CrossRef]
7. Liang, F.; Ren, C.; Wang, J.; Wang, S.; Yang, L.; Han, X.; Chen, Y.; Tong, G.; Yang, G. The crosstalk between STAT3 and p53/RAS signaling controls cancer cell metastasis and cisplatin resistance via the Slug/MAPK/PI3K/AKT-mediated regulation of EMT and autophagy. *Oncogenesis* **2019**, *8*, 59. [CrossRef]
8. Liebmann, C. Regulation of MAP kinase activity by peptide receptor signalling pathway: Paradigms of multiplicity. *Cell Signal.* **2001**, *13*, 777–785. [CrossRef]
9. Offin, M.; Liu, D.; Drilon, A. Tumor-Agnostic Drug Development. *Am. Soc. Clin. Oncol. Educ. Book* **2018**, *38*, 184–187. [CrossRef]
10. Fouad, Y.A.; Aanei, C. Revisiting the hallmarks of cancer. *Am. J. Cancer Res.* **2017**, *7*, 1016–1036.
11. Yamaoka, T.; Kusumoto, S.; Ando, K.; Ohba, M.; Ohmori, T. Receptor Tyrosine Kinase-Targeted Cancer Therapy. *Int. J. Mol. Sci.* **2018**, *19*, 3491. [CrossRef] [PubMed]
12. Crisci, S.; Amitrano, F.; Saggese, M.; Muto, T.; Sarno, S.; Mele, S.; Vitale, P.; Ronga, G.; Berretta, M.; Di Francia, R. Overview of Current Targeted Anti-Cancer Drugs for Therapy in Onco-Hematology. *Medicina* **2019**, *55*, 414. [CrossRef] [PubMed]
13. Roskoski, R., Jr. Properties of FDA-approved small molecule protein kinase inhibitors. *Pharmacol. Res.* **2019**, *144*, 19–50. [CrossRef] [PubMed]
14. Fabbro, D.; Cowan-Jacob, S.W.; Moebitz, H. Ten things you should know about protein kinases: IUPHAR Review 14. *Br. J. Pharmacol.* **2015**, *172*, 2675–2700. [CrossRef] [PubMed]
15. Bhullar, K.S.; Lagaron, N.O.; McGowan, E.M.; Parmar, I.; Jha, A.; Hubbard, B.P.; Rupasinghe, H.P.V. Kinase-targeted cancer therapies: Progress, challenges and future directions. *Mol. Cancer* **2018**, *17*, 48. [CrossRef]
16. Panicker, R.C.; Chattopadhaya, S.; Coyne, A.G.; Srinivasan, R. Allosteric Small-Molecule Serine/Threonine Kinase Inhibitors. *Adv. Exp. Med. Biol* **2019**, *1163*, 253–278. [CrossRef]
17. Pacenta, H.L.; Macy, M.E. Entrectinib and other ALK/TRK inhibitors for the treatment of neuroblastoma. *Drug Des. Dev. Ther.* **2018**, *12*, 3549–3561. [CrossRef]
18. Collins, D.M.; Conlon, N.T.; Kannan, S.; Verma, C.S.; Eli, L.D.; Lalani, A.S.; Crown, J. Preclinical Characteristics of the Irreversible Pan-HER Kinase Inhibitor Neratinib Compared with Lapatinib: Implications for the Treatment of HER2-Positive and HER2-Mutated Breast Cancer. *Cancers* **2019**, *11*, 737. [CrossRef]
19. Ryu, S.; Youn, C.; Moon, A.R.; Howland, A.; Armstrong, C.A.; Song, P.I. Therapeutic Inhibitors against Mutated BRAF and MEK for the Treatment of Metastatic Melanoma. *Chonnam. Med. J.* **2017**, *53*, 173–177. [CrossRef]
20. Planchard, D.; Popat, S.; Kerr, K.; Novello, S.; Smit, E.F.; Faivre-Finn, C.; Mok, T.S.; Reck, M.; Van Schil, P.E.; Hellmann, M.D.; et al. Metastatic non-small cell lung cancer: ESMO Clinical Practice Guidelines for diagnosis, treatment and follow-up. *Ann. Oncol.* **2018**, *29*, iv192–iv237. [CrossRef]

21. Sequist, L.V.; Yang, J.C.; Yamamoto, N.; O'Byrne, K.; Hirsh, V.; Mok, T.; Geater, S.L.; Orlov, S.; Tsai, C.M.; Boyer, M.; et al. Phase III study of afatinib or cisplatin plus pemetrexed in patients with metastatic lung adenocarcinoma with EGFR mutations. *J. Clin. Oncol.* **2013**, *31*, 3327–3334. [CrossRef] [PubMed]
22. Wu, Y.L.; Cheng, Y.; Zhou, X.; Lee, K.H.; Nakagawa, K.; Niho, S.; Tsuji, F.; Linke, R.; Rosell, R.; Corral, J.; et al. Dacomitinib versus gefitinib as first-line treatment for patients with EGFR-mutation-positive non-small-cell lung cancer (ARCHER 1050): A randomised, open-label, phase 3 trial. *Lancet Oncol.* **2017**, *18*, 1454–1466. [CrossRef]
23. Morgillo, F.; Della Corte, C.M.; Fasano, M.; Ciardiello, F. Mechanisms of resistance to EGFR-targeted drugs: Lung cancer. *ESMO Open* **2016**, *1*, e000060. [CrossRef]
24. Hochmair, M.J.; Morabito, A.; Hao, D.; Yang, C.T.; Soo, R.A.; Yang, J.C.; Gucalp, R.; Halmos, B.; Wang, L.; Marten, A.; et al. Sequential afatinib and osimertinib in patients with EGFR mutation-positive non-small-cell lung cancer: Updated analysis of the observational GioTag study. *Future Oncol.* **2019**, *15*, 2905–2914. [CrossRef]
25. Planchard, D.; Popat, S.; Kerr, K.; Novello, S.; Smit, E.F.; Faivre-Finn, C.; Mok, T.S.; Reck, M.; Van Schil, P.E.; Hellmann, M.D.; et al. Correction to: "Metastatic non-small cell lung cancer: ESMO Clinical Practice Guidelines for diagnosis, treatment and follow-up". *Ann. Oncol.* **2019**, *30*, 863–870. [CrossRef]
26. Pennell, N.A.; Lynch, T.J., Jr. Combined inhibition of the VEGFR and EGFR signaling pathways in the treatment of NSCLC. *Oncologist* **2009**, *14*, 399–411. [CrossRef]
27. NIH. Clinical Trials. Available online: https://clinicaltrials.gov/ct2/show/NCT03122717 (accessed on 17 March 2020).
28. Zhang, N.; Liang, C.; Song, W.; Tao, D.; Yao, J.; Wang, S.; Ma, L.; Shi, Y.; Han, X. Antitumor activity of histone deacetylase inhibitor chidamide alone or in combination with epidermal growth factor receptor tyrosine kinase inhibitor icotinib in NSCLC. *J. Cancer* **2019**, *10*, 1275–1287. [CrossRef]
29. Yang, Z.; Tam, K.Y. Combination Strategies Using EGFR-TKi in NSCLC Therapy: Learning from the Gap between Pre-Clinical Results and Clinical Outcomes. *Int. J. Biol. Sci.* **2018**, *14*, 204–216. [CrossRef]
30. Escudier, B.; Porta, C.; Schmidinger, M.; Rioux-Leclercq, N.; Bex, A.; Khoo, V.; Grunwald, V.; Gillessen, S.; Horwich, A.; Committee, E.G. Renal cell carcinoma: ESMO Clinical Practice Guidelines for diagnosis, treatment and follow-updagger. *Ann. Oncol.* **2019**, *30*, 706–720. [CrossRef]
31. Miyazaki, A.; Miyake, H.; Fujisawa, M. Molecular mechanism mediating cytotoxic activity of axitinib in sunitinib-resistant human renal cell carcinoma cells. *Clin. Transl. Oncol.* **2016**, *18*, 893–900. [CrossRef]
32. Yu, S.S.; Quinn, D.I.; Dorff, T.B. Clinical use of cabozantinib in the treatment of advanced kidney cancer: Efficacy, safety, and patient selection. *Onco Targets Ther.* **2016**, *9*, 5825–5837. [CrossRef] [PubMed]
33. Cardoso, F.; Senkus, E.; Costa, A.; Papadopoulos, E.; Aapro, M.; Andre, F.; Harbeck, N.; Aguilar Lopez, B.; Barrios, C.H.; Bergh, J.; et al. 4th ESO-ESMO International Consensus Guidelines for Advanced Breast Cancer (ABC 4)dagger. *Ann. Oncol.* **2018**, *29*, 1634–1657. [CrossRef] [PubMed]
34. Vogel, A.; Cervantes, A.; Chau, I.; Daniele, B.; Llovet, J.M.; Meyer, T.; Nault, J.C.; Neumann, U.; Ricke, J.; Sangro, B.; et al. Hepatocellular carcinoma: ESMO Clinical Practice Guidelines for diagnosis, treatment and follow-up. *Ann. Oncol.* **2019**, *30*, 871–873. [CrossRef] [PubMed]
35. Grothey, A.; Van Cutsem, E.; Sobrero, A.; Siena, S.; Falcone, A.; Ychou, M.; Humblet, Y.; Bouche, O.; Mineur, L.; Barone, C.; et al. Regorafenib monotherapy for previously treated metastatic colorectal cancer (CORRECT): An international, multicentre, randomised, placebo-controlled, phase 3 trial. *Lancet* **2013**, *381*, 303–312. [CrossRef]
36. Blanke, C.D.; Demetri, G.D.; von Mehren, M.; Heinrich, M.C.; Eisenberg, B.; Fletcher, J.A.; Corless, C.L.; Fletcher, C.D.; Roberts, P.J.; Heinz, D.; et al. Long-term results from a randomized phase II trial of standard- versus higher-dose imatinib mesylate for patients with unresectable or metastatic gastrointestinal stromal tumors expressing KIT. *J. Clin. Oncol.* **2008**, *26*, 620–625. [CrossRef]
37. Casali, P.G.; Abecassis, N.; Aro, H.T.; Bauer, S.; Biagini, R.; Bielack, S.; Bonvalot, S.; Boukovinas, I.; Bovee, J.; Brodowicz, T.; et al. Gastrointestinal stromal tumours: ESMO-EURACAN Clinical Practice Guidelines for diagnosis, treatment and follow-up. *Ann. Oncol.* **2018**, *29*, iv68–iv78. [CrossRef]
38. Brose, M.S.; Nutting, C.M.; Jarzab, B.; Elisei, R.; Siena, S.; Bastholt, L.; de la Fouchardiere, C.; Pacini, F.; Paschke, R.; Shong, Y.K.; et al. Sorafenib in radioactive iodine-refractory, locally advanced or metastatic differentiated thyroid cancer: A randomised, double-blind, phase 3 trial. *Lancet* **2014**, *384*, 319–328. [CrossRef]

39. Schlumberger, M.; Tahara, M.; Wirth, L.J.; Robinson, B.; Brose, M.S.; Elisei, R.; Habra, M.A.; Newbold, K.; Shah, M.H.; Hoff, A.O.; et al. Lenvatinib versus placebo in radioiodine-refractory thyroid cancer. *N. Engl. J. Med.* **2015**, *372*, 621–630. [CrossRef]
40. Filetti, S.; Durante, C.; Hartl, D.; Leboulleux, S.; Locati, L.D.; Newbold, K.; Papotti, M.G.; Berruti, A.; Committee, E.G. Thyroid cancer: ESMO Clinical Practice Guidelines for diagnosis, treatment and follow-updagger. *Ann. Oncol.* **2019**, *30*, 1856–1883. [CrossRef]
41. Michielin, O.; van Akkooi, A.C.J.; Ascierto, P.A.; Dummer, R.; Keilholz, U.; Committee, E.G. Cutaneous melanoma: ESMO Clinical Practice Guidelines for diagnosis, treatment and follow-updagger. *Ann. Oncol.* **2019**, *30*, 1884–1901. [CrossRef]
42. Hochhaus, A.; Larson, R.A.; Guilhot, F.; Radich, J.P.; Branford, S.; Hughes, T.P.; Baccarani, M.; Deininger, M.W.; Cervantes, F.; Fujihara, S.; et al. Long-Term Outcomes of Imatinib Treatment for Chronic Myeloid Leukemia. *N. Engl. J. Med.* **2017**, *376*, 917–927. [CrossRef] [PubMed]
43. Horne, S.D.; Stevens, J.B.; Abdallah, B.Y.; Liu, G.; Bremer, S.W.; Ye, C.J.; Heng, H.H. Why imatinib remains an exception of cancer research. *J. Cell Physiol.* **2013**, *228*, 665–670. [CrossRef] [PubMed]
44. Hochhaus, A.; Saussele, S.; Rosti, G.; Mahon, F.X.; Janssen, J.; Hjorth-Hansen, H.; Richter, J.; Buske, C.; Committee, E.G. Chronic myeloid leukaemia: ESMO Clinical Practice Guidelines for diagnosis, treatment and follow-up. *Ann. Oncol.* **2017**, *28*, iv41–iv51. [CrossRef]
45. Soverini, S.; Mancini, M.; Bavaro, L.; Cavo, M.; Martinelli, G. Chronic myeloid leukemia: The paradigm of targeting oncogenic tyrosine kinase signaling and counteracting resistance for successful cancer therapy. *Mol. Cancer* **2018**, *17*, 49. [CrossRef] [PubMed]
46. Gramza, A.W.; Corless, C.L.; Heinrich, M.C. Resistance to Tyrosine Kinase Inhibitors in Gastrointestinal Stromal Tumors. *Clin. Cancer Res.* **2009**, *15*, 7510–7518. [CrossRef]
47. Foster, R.; Griffith, R.; Ferrao, P.; Ashman, L. Molecular basis of the constitutive activity and STI571 resistance of Asp816Val mutant KIT receptor tyrosine kinase. *J. Mol. Graph. Model.* **2004**, *23*, 139–152. [CrossRef]
48. Roberts, K.G.; Odell, A.F.; Byrnes, E.M.; Baleato, R.M.; Griffith, R.; Lyons, A.B.; Ashman, L.K. Resistance to c-KIT kinase inhibitors conferred by V654A mutation. *Mol. Cancer Ther.* **2007**, *6*, 1159–1166. [CrossRef]
49. Alexander, P.B.; Wang, X.F. Resistance to receptor tyrosine kinase inhibition in cancer: Molecular mechanisms and therapeutic strategies. *Front. Med.* **2015**, *9*, 134–138. [CrossRef]
50. Makhov, P.; Joshi, S.; Ghatalia, P.; Kutikov, A.; Uzzo, R.G.; Kolenko, V.M. Resistance to Systemic Therapies in Clear Cell Renal Cell Carcinoma: Mechanisms and Management Strategies. *Mol. Cancer Ther.* **2018**, *17*, 1355–1364. [CrossRef]
51. Del Re, M.; Rofi, E.; Restante, G.; Crucitta, S.; Arrigoni, E.; Fogli, S.; Di Maio, M.; Petrini, I.; Danesi, R. Implications of KRAS mutations in acquired resistance to treatment in NSCLC. *Oncotarget* **2018**, *9*, 6630–6643. [CrossRef]
52. Zhu, Y.J.; Zheng, B.; Wang, H.Y.; Chen, L. New knowledge of the mechanisms of sorafenib resistance in liver cancer. *Acta Pharmacol. Sin.* **2017**, *38*, 614–622. [CrossRef] [PubMed]
53. Liu, X.; Shen, T.; Mooers, B.H.M.; Hilberg, F.; Wu, J. Drug resistance profiles of mutations in the RET kinase domain. *Br. J. Pharmacol.* **2018**, *175*, 3504–3515. [CrossRef] [PubMed]
54. Kakadia, S.; Yarlagadda, N.; Awad, R.; Kundranda, M.; Niu, J.; Naraev, B.; Mina, L.; Dragovich, T.; Gimbel, M.; Mahmoud, F. Mechanisms of resistance to BRAF and MEK inhibitors and clinical update of US Food and Drug Administration-approved targeted therapy in advanced melanoma. *Onco Targets Ther.* **2018**, *11*, 7095–7107. [CrossRef] [PubMed]
55. Robert, C.; Karaszewska, B.; Schachter, J.; Rutkowski, P.; Mackiewicz, A.; Stroiakovski, D.; Lichinitser, M.; Dummer, R.; Grange, F.; Mortier, L.; et al. Improved overall survival in melanoma with combined dabrafenib and trametinib. *N. Engl. J. Med.* **2015**, *372*, 30–39. [CrossRef] [PubMed]
56. Dummer, R.; Hauschild, A.; Lindenblatt, N.; Pentheroudakis, G.; Keilholz, U.; Committee, E.G. Cutaneous melanoma: ESMO Clinical Practice Guidelines for diagnosis, treatment and follow-up. *Ann. Oncol.* **2015**, *26* (Suppl. 5), v126–v132. [CrossRef]
57. Tolcher, A.W.; Peng, W.; Calvo, E. Rational Approaches for Combination Therapy Strategies Targeting the MAP Kinase Pathway in Solid Tumors. *Mol. Cancer Ther.* **2018**, *17*, 3–16. [CrossRef]
58. Broekman, F.; Giovannetti, E.; Peters, G.J. Tyrosine kinase inhibitors: Multi-targeted or single-targeted? *World J. Clin. Oncol.* **2011**, *2*, 80–93. [CrossRef]

59. Moradpour, Z.; Barghi, L. Novel Approaches for Efficient Delivery of Tyrosine Kinase Inhibitors. *J. Pharm. Pharm. Sci.* **2019**, *22*, 37–48. [CrossRef]
60. Maifrede, S.; Nieborowska-Skorska, M.; Sullivan-Reed, K.; Dasgupta, Y.; Podszywalow-Bartnicka, P.; Le, B.V.; Solecka, M.; Lian, Z.; Belyaeva, E.A.; Nersesyan, A.; et al. Tyrosine kinase inhibitor-induced defects in DNA repair sensitize FLT3(ITD)-positive leukemia cells to PARP1 inhibitors. *Blood* **2018**, *132*, 67–77. [CrossRef]
61. Ding, Y.; Gong, C.; Huang, D.; Chen, R.; Sui, P.; Lin, K.H.; Liang, G.; Yuan, L.; Xiang, H.; Chen, J.; et al. Synthetic lethality between HER2 and transaldolase in intrinsically resistant HER2-positive breast cancers. *Nat. Commun.* **2018**, *9*, 4274. [CrossRef]
62. Wang, R.; Li, Y.; Gong, P.; Gabrilove, J.; Waxman, S.; Jing, Y. Arsenic Trioxide and Sorafenib Induce Synthetic Lethality of FLT3-ITD Acute Myeloid Leukemia Cells. *Mol. Cancer Ther.* **2018**, *17*, 1871–1880. [CrossRef] [PubMed]
63. Pottier, C.; Wheatherspoon, A.; Roncarati, P.; Longuespee, R.; Herfs, M.; Duray, A.; Delvenne, P.; Quatresooz, P. The importance of the tumor microenvironment in the therapeutic management of cancer. *Expert Rev. Anticancer Ther.* **2015**, *15*, 943–954. [CrossRef] [PubMed]
64. Tan, H.Y.; Wang, N.; Lam, W.; Guo, W.; Feng, Y.; Cheng, Y.C. Targeting tumour microenvironment by tyrosine kinase inhibitor. *Mol. Cancer* **2018**, *17*, 43. [CrossRef] [PubMed]
65. Katoh, M. FGFR inhibitors: Effects on cancer cells, tumor microenvironment and whole-body homeostasis (Review). *Int. J. Mol. Med.* **2016**, *38*, 3–15. [CrossRef]
66. Prete, A.; Lo, A.S.; Sadow, P.M.; Bhasin, S.S.; Antonello, Z.A.; Vodopivec, D.M.; Ullas, S.; Sims, J.N.; Clohessy, J.; Dvorak, A.M.; et al. Pericytes Elicit Resistance to Vemurafenib and Sorafenib Therapy in Thyroid Carcinoma via the TSP-1/TGFbeta1 Axis. *Clin. Cancer Res.* **2018**, *24*, 6078–6097. [CrossRef] [PubMed]
67. Chan, X.Y.; Singh, A.; Osman, N.; Piva, T.J. Role Played by Signalling Pathways in Overcoming BRAF Inhibitor Resistance in Melanoma. *Int. J. Mol. Sci.* **2017**, *18*, 1527. [CrossRef] [PubMed]
68. Straussman, R.; Morikawa, T.; Shee, K.; Barzily-Rokni, M.; Qian, Z.R.; Du, J.; Davis, A.; Mongare, M.M.; Gould, J.; Frederick, D.T.; et al. Tumour micro-environment elicits innate resistance to RAF inhibitors through HGF secretion. *Nature* **2012**, *487*, 500–504. [CrossRef]
69. Watson, S.S.; Dane, M.; Chin, K.; Tatarova, Z.; Liu, M.; Liby, T.; Thompson, W.; Smith, R.; Nederlof, M.; Bucher, E.; et al. Microenvironment-Mediated Mechanisms of Resistance to HER2 Inhibitors Differ between HER2+ Breast Cancer Subtypes. *Cell Syst.* **2018**, *6*, 329–342. [CrossRef]
70. Lin, C.H.; Pelissier, F.A.; Zhang, H.; Lakins, J.; Weaver, V.M.; Park, C.; LaBarge, M.A. Microenvironment rigidity modulates responses to the HER2 receptor tyrosine kinase inhibitor lapatinib via YAP and TAZ transcription factors. *Mol. Biol. Cell* **2015**, *26*, 3946–3953. [CrossRef]
71. Lacal, P.M.; Graziani, G. Therapeutic implication of vascular endothelial growth factor receptor-1 (VEGFR-1) targeting in cancer cells and tumor microenvironment by competitive and non-competitive inhibitors. *Pharmacol. Res.* **2018**, *136*, 97–107. [CrossRef]
72. Patnaik, A.; Swanson, K.D.; Csizmadia, E.; Solanki, A.; Landon-Brace, N.; Gehring, M.P.; Helenius, K.; Olson, B.M.; Pyzer, A.R.; Wang, L.C.; et al. Cabozantinib Eradicates Advanced Murine Prostate Cancer by Activating Antitumor Innate Immunity. *Cancer Discov.* **2017**, *7*, 750–765. [CrossRef] [PubMed]
73. Frederick, D.T.; Piris, A.; Cogdill, A.P.; Cooper, Z.A.; Lezcano, C.; Ferrone, C.R.; Mitra, D.; Boni, A.; Newton, L.P.; Liu, C.; et al. BRAF inhibition is associated with enhanced melanoma antigen expression and a more favorable tumor microenvironment in patients with metastatic melanoma. *Clin. Cancer Res.* **2013**, *19*, 1225–1231. [CrossRef] [PubMed]
74. Aparicio, L.M.A.; Fernandez, I.P.; Cassinello, J. Tyrosine kinase inhibitors reprogramming immunity in renal cell carcinoma: Rethinking cancer immunotherapy. *Clin. Transl. Oncol.* **2017**, *19*, 1175–1182. [CrossRef] [PubMed]
75. Matsumoto, Y.; Sawa, K.; Fukui, M.; Oyanagi, J.; Izumi, M.; Ogawa, K.; Suzumura, T.; Watanabe, T.; Kaneda, H.; Mitsuoka, S.; et al. Impact of tumor microenvironment on the efficacy of epidermal growth factor receptor-tyrosine kinase inhibitors in patients with EGFR-mutant non-small cell lung cancer. *Cancer Sci.* **2019**, *110*, 3244–3254. [CrossRef] [PubMed]
76. Shojaei, F.; Wu, X.; Qu, X.; Kowanetz, M.; Yu, L.; Tan, M.; Meng, Y.G.; Ferrara, N. G-CSF-initiated myeloid cell mobilization and angiogenesis mediate tumor refractoriness to anti-VEGF therapy in mouse models. *Proc. Natl. Acad. Sci. USA* **2009**, *106*, 6742–6747. [CrossRef]

77. Taylor, M.H.; Lee, C.H.; Makker, V.; Rasco, D.; Dutcus, C.E.; Wu, J.; Stepan, D.E.; Shumaker, R.C.; Motzer, R.J. Phase IB/II Trial of Lenvatinib Plus Pembrolizumab in Patients With Advanced Renal Cell Carcinoma, Endometrial Cancer, and Other Selected Advanced Solid Tumors. *J. Clin. Oncol.* **2020**. [CrossRef]
78. Hara, H.; Fukuoka, S.; Takahashi, N.; Kojima, T.; Kawazoe, A.; Asayama, M.; Yoshii, T.; Kotani, D.; Tamura, H.; Mikamoto, Y.; et al. Regorafenib plus nivolumab in patients with advanced colorectal or gastric cancer: An open-label, dose-finding, and dose-expansion phase 1b trial (REGONIVO, EPOC1603). *Ann. Oncol.* **2019**, *30* (Suppl. 4), iv124. [CrossRef]
79. Akalu, Y.T.; Rothlin, C.V.; Ghosh, S. TAM receptor tyrosine kinases as emerging targets of innate immune checkpoint blockade for cancer therapy. *Immunol. Rev.* **2017**, *276*, 165–177. [CrossRef]
80. Joshi, S.; Durden, D.L. Combinatorial Approach to Improve Cancer Immunotherapy: Rational Drug Design Strategy to Simultaneously Hit Multiple Targets to Kill Tumor Cells and to Activate the Immune System. *J. Oncol.* **2019**, *2019*, 5245034. [CrossRef]
81. Atkins, M.B.; Plimack, E.R.; Puzanov, I.; Fishman, M.N.; McDermott, D.F.; Cho, D.C.; Vaishampayan, U.; George, S.; Olencki, T.E.; Tarazi, J.C.; et al. Axitinib in combination with pembrolizumab in patients with advanced renal cell cancer: A non-randomised, open-label, dose-finding, and dose-expansion phase 1b trial. *Lancet Oncol.* **2018**, *19*, 405–415. [CrossRef]
82. Amin, A.; Plimack, E.R.; Ernstoff, M.S.; Lewis, L.D.; Bauer, T.M.; McDermott, D.F.; Carducci, M.; Kollmannsberger, C.; Rini, B.I.; Heng, D.Y.C.; et al. Safety and efficacy of nivolumab in combination with sunitinib or pazopanib in advanced or metastatic renal cell carcinoma: The CheckMate 016 study. *J. Immunother. Cancer* **2018**, *6*, 109. [CrossRef] [PubMed]
83. Jones, D.; Bopaiah, J.; Alghamedy, F.; Jacobs, N.; Weiss, H.L.; de Jong, W.A.; Ellingson, S.R. Polypharmacology Within the Full Kinome: A Machine Learning Approach. *AMIA Jt. Summits Transl. Sci. Proc.* **2018**, *2017*, 98–107. [PubMed]
84. Ching, T.; Himmelstein, D.S.; Beaulieu-Jones, B.K.; Kalinin, A.A.; Do, B.T.; Way, G.P.; Ferrero, E.; Agapow, P.M.; Zietz, M.; Hoffman, M.M.; et al. Opportunities and obstacles for deep learning in biology and medicine. *J. R. Soc. Interface* **2018**, *15*. [CrossRef] [PubMed]
85. Zhavoronkov, A.; Ivanenkov, Y.A.; Aliper, A.; Veselov, M.S.; Aladinskiy, V.A.; Aladinskaya, A.V.; Terentiev, V.A.; Polykovskiy, D.A.; Kuznetsov, M.D.; Asadulaev, A.; et al. Deep learning enables rapid identification of potent DDR1 kinase inhibitors. *Nat. Biotechnol.* **2019**, *37*, 1038–1040. [CrossRef] [PubMed]
86. Desai, B.; Dixon, K.; Farrant, E.; Feng, Q.; Gibson, K.R.; van Hoorn, W.P.; Mills, J.; Morgan, T.; Parry, D.M.; Ramjee, M.K.; et al. Rapid discovery of a novel series of Abl kinase inhibitors by application of an integrated microfluidic synthesis and screening platform. *J. Med. Chem.* **2013**, *56*, 3033–3047. [CrossRef] [PubMed]
87. Benz, M.; Molla, M.R.; Boser, A.; Rosenfeld, A.; Levkin, P.A. Marrying chemistry with biology by combining on-chip solution-based combinatorial synthesis and cellular screening. *Nat. Commun.* **2019**, *10*, 2879. [CrossRef]
88. Wong, Y.H.; Chiu, C.C.; Lin, C.L.; Chen, T.S.; Jheng, B.R.; Lee, Y.C.; Chen, J.; Chen, B.S. A New Era for Cancer Target Therapies: Applying Systems Biology and Computer-Aided Drug Design to Cancer Therapies. *Curr. Pharm. Biotechnol.* **2016**, *17*, 1246–1267. [CrossRef]
89. Sontheimer-Phelps, A.; Hassell, B.A.; Ingber, D.E. Modelling cancer in microfluidic human organs-on-chips. *Nat. Rev. Cancer* **2019**, *19*, 65–81. [CrossRef]

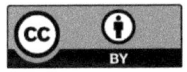

© 2020 by the authors. Licensee MDPI, Basel, Switzerland. This article is an open access article distributed under the terms and conditions of the Creative Commons Attribution (CC BY) license (http://creativecommons.org/licenses/by/4.0/).

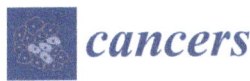

Review

The DYRK Family of Kinases in Cancer: Molecular Functions and Therapeutic Opportunities

Jacopo Boni [1,2], Carlota Rubio-Perez [3], Nuria López-Bigas [3,4], Cristina Fillat [2,5] and Susana de la Luna [1,2,4,6,*]

1. Centre for Genomic Regulation (CRG), The Barcelona Institute of Science and Technology (BIST), Dr Aiguader 88, 08003 Barcelona, Spain; jacopo.boni@crg.eu
2. Centro de Investigación Biomédica en Red en Enfermedades Raras (CIBERER), 28029 Madrid, Spain
3. Cancer Science Programme, Institute for Research in Biomedicine (IRB), The Barcelona Institute of Science and Technology (BIST), Baldiri Reixac 10, 08028 Barcelona, Spain; carlotarp@gmail.com (C.R.-P.); nuria.lopez@irbbarcelona.org (N.L.-B.)
4. Institució Catalana de Recerca i Estudis Avançats (ICREA), Passeig Lluís Companys 23, 08010 Barcelona, Spain
5. Institut d'Investigacions Biomèdiques August Pi i Sunyer (IDIBAPS), Rosselló 149-153, 08036 Barcelona, Spain; cfillat@clinic.cat
6. Universitat Pompeu Fabra (UPF), Dr Aiguader 88, 08003 Barcelona, Spain
* Correspondence: susana.luna@crg.eu; Tel.: +34-933-160-144

Received: 6 July 2020; Accepted: 27 July 2020; Published: 29 July 2020

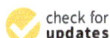

Abstract: DYRK (dual-specificity tyrosine-regulated kinases) are an evolutionary conserved family of protein kinases with members from yeast to humans. In humans, DYRKs are pleiotropic factors that phosphorylate a broad set of proteins involved in many different cellular processes. These include factors that have been associated with all the hallmarks of cancer, from genomic instability to increased proliferation and resistance, programmed cell death, or signaling pathways whose dysfunction is relevant to tumor onset and progression. In accordance with an involvement of DYRK kinases in the regulation of tumorigenic processes, an increasing number of research studies have been published in recent years showing either alterations of DYRK gene expression in tumor samples and/or providing evidence of DYRK-dependent mechanisms that contribute to tumor initiation and/or progression. In the present article, we will review the current understanding of the role of DYRK family members in cancer initiation and progression, providing an overview of the small molecules that act as DYRK inhibitors and discussing the clinical implications and therapeutic opportunities currently available.

Keywords: DYRK kinases; cellular signaling; expression dysregulation; cell cycle; cell survival; tumor progression; kinase inhibitors

1. Background

The first cancer gene identified, the proto-oncogene *c-Src*, was found to encode a protein kinase [1]. Yet, since then, almost a hundred kinase genes have been attributed a tumor suppressor or oncogenic role, and they represent the most abundant class of cancer driver genes known to date [2]. Dual-specificity tyrosine-regulated kinases (DYRKs) belong to the CMGC group of kinases, which includes cyclin-dependent kinases (CDKs), mitogen-activated protein kinases (MAPKs), CDK-like kinases, the serine-arginine-rich protein kinase, Cdc2-like kinases (CLKs) and members of the RCK family [3]. The DYRK family is formed by three subfamilies: the DYRK subfamily, the homeodomain-interacting kinases (HIPKs), and the pre-messenger RNA-processing protein 4 kinases (PRP4Ks) [3]. Here, we will use "DYRK" to refer specifically to the DYRK subfamily, which contains five members in humans that are clustered into two classes based on their phylogenetic relationships [4]:

class I DYRKs, DYRK1A and DYRK1B (also known as Mirk from minibrain-related kinase) and class II DYRKs, DYRK2, DYRK3 (also known as REDK from regulatory erythroid kinase) and DYRK4 (Figure 1A).

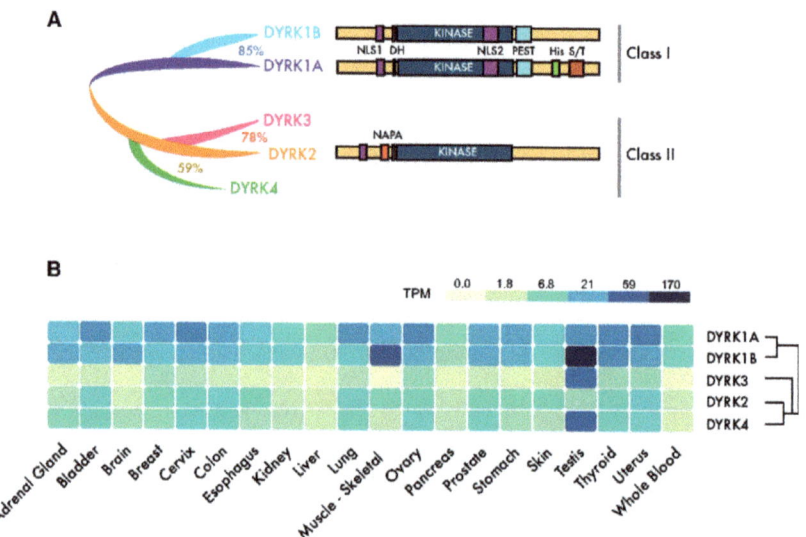

Figure 1. Dual-specificity tyrosine-regulated kinase (DYRK) protein kinases: primary structure and expression. (**A**) Scheme of the mammalian family of DYRKs, indicating their phylogenic relationships, degree of homology and protein domains. The catalytic domain (KINASE) and the DYRK homology box (DH) are common to all members of the family. Class I DYRKs have two nuclear localization signals (NLSs) (NLS1 and NLS2) and a proline-, glutamic acid-, serine- and threonine-rich (PEST) motif. DYRK1A also includes a tract of 13 consecutive histidine residues (His) and a region enriched in serine/threonine residues (S/T) at the C-terminus. Class II DYRKs have a common structure, with the characteristic N-terminal autophosphorylation accessory (NAPA) domain at the N-terminus. In the case of DYRK2 and DYRK4, functional NLSs have been described within the noncatalytic N-terminus. (**B**) The expression of human DYRKs based on the Genotype-Tissue Expression (GTEx) data represented as the median TPMs (transcripts per million: GTEx Analysis Release V8, www.gtexportal.org/home, dbGaP Accession phs000424.v8.p2). Tissues represented in the tumor data in Table S1 were chosen (brain: cortex; cervix: ectocervix; colon: sigmoid colon; esophagus: mucosa, kidney: cortex; skin: suprapubic—not sun-exposed).

DYRK kinases phosphorylate a broad set of substrates that are involved in a wide range of cellular processes, and they are thought to fulfill essential biological functions both during development and in maintaining homeostasis during the adult life. Consequently, the aberrant regulation or expression of DYRK kinases has been associated with several human pathologies, including cancer. In the present article, we will review our understanding of the role of DYRK family members in cancer initiation and progression, providing an overview of the small molecules that act as DYRK inhibitors and discussing the clinical implications and therapeutic opportunities currently available.

2. The DYRK Family of Kinases

The members of the DYRK family all share a highly conserved catalytic domain with special features within the CMGC group [5] and the so-called DYRK homology (DH) box motif located upstream of it (Figure 1A). In addition, DYRK kinases present class-specific domains: DYRK1A and DYRK1B harbor a proline-, glutamic acid-, serine- and threonine-rich (PEST) motif in the noncatalytic

C-terminal region and equally positioned nuclear localization signals (NLS) (Figure 1A). On the other hand, class II DYRKs present a N-terminal autophosphorylation accessory region (NAPA) domain, essential for catalytic activation [6] (Figure 1A). All human DYRKs accumulate in the cytosol of cells, and DYRK1A, DYRK2 and DYRK4 can be imported into the nucleus by means of dedicated NLSs [7–9]. DYRK1A translocation to the nucleus acquires special biological significance, since it has been described as a chromatin-associated kinase capable of regulating the gene expression [10,11], and it is functionally linked to the DNA damage response (DDR) [12–14]. Chromatin association in the DDR context has also been recently described for DYRK1B [15]. Moreover, a DYRK1A-specific run of histidine residues targets this family member to the subnuclear splicing compartment [7], and the noncatalytic N-terminal domain of DYRK3 serves to localize it to stress granules [16]. Both the histidine run in DYRK1A and the N-terminus of DYRK3 participate in the generation of phase-separated subcellular compartments [17,18]. Changes in the subcellular localization of DYRK proteins have been observed in response to different signals, such as that of DYRK2 in response to DNA damage or proinflammatory signals [19,20] or DYRK1A in response to Wnt signaling [21]. However, how the subcellular localization of DYRKs is regulated or how it contributes to their activity is still not well-understood.

A high-throughput transcript data analysis indicates that DYRK1A and DYRK1B are expressed ubiquitously in human tissues, whereas class II DYRKs are generally expressed more weakly and in a more tissue-restricted pattern (Figure 1B). The expression of DYRKs is regulated through alternative promoters that generate transcripts with distinct 5′-untranslated regions and/or encoding different N-terminal regions [4]. In addition, alternative splicing generates multiple protein isoforms of unclear functional significance [4,8,22–24]. DYRKs are also subject to other post-transcriptional events, such as microRNAs (miR)-mediated gene silencing [25–27] or local translation [28].

DYRK kinases are "dual specificity" kinases, as they can phosphorylate both tyrosine (Y) and serine/threonine (S/T) residues, although Y-phosphorylation is limited to their autophosphorylation activity [29]. These kinases are activated by the phosphorylation of residues within the activation loop, which drives a conformational switch from the inactive to active state [30,31]. Unlike other kinase families, this key event in DYRKs is an autocatalytic reaction that occurs during protein synthesis and that generates a constitutively active kinase [32]. As DYRK activation does not depend on upstream kinases, other regulatory mechanisms are thought to operate. These include: the dephosphorylation of residues in the activation loop, although no phosphatase has been attributed this role to date, allosteric phosphorylation performed by other kinases [9,33–36], interactions with scaffolding proteins [37–39] or accessibility to substrates due to changes in the subcellular localization. In this regard, and given the constitutive nature of DYRK kinase activity, the regulation of their intracellular levels becomes crucial to modulate their functions, and thus, altering the DYRK expression acquires additional importance in terms of their impact on normal cell fitness.

3. The Role of DYRKS in Cancer

DYRKs phosphorylate a wide range of substrates, including factors associated with one or several of the hallmarks of cancer [40] (Figure 2). Of all the DYRKs, only DYRK1A has been identified in high-throughput cancer studies, initially as a potential tumor suppressor using Tumor Suppressor and Oncogene Explorer (TUSON), a method developed to predict the potential of a given gene to act as a tumor suppressor, or oncogene, by computing somatic mutation profiles and copy number alterations (CNAs) [41]. Subsequently, it was proposed as a driver in liver cancer through a study that identified such drivers according to mutations in unusual nucleotide contexts [42]. Although these results would suggest that DYRKs are not major drivers of cancer, further evidence that they play a role in oncogenic processes has emerged over the past two decades. In the following sections, we will discuss the evidence indicating that each member of the DYRK family is involved in cancer by considering two main aspects: (i) alterations to the DYRK expression in tumor tissues, either based on published reports or on our own analysis of The Cancer Genome Atlas (TCGA: see Table S1; only cancer type cohorts with at least 10 paired samples, matched tumor-healthy tissue, were considered in the analysis), and (ii) the impact of DYRK-dependent phosphorylation on substrates involved in cancer-related events.

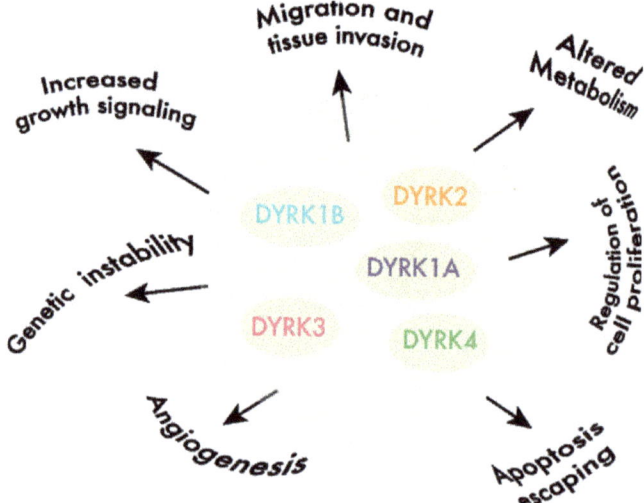

Figure 2. DYRKs are involved in cancer-associated processes. DYRK kinases participate in the regulation of crucial cell events, the perturbation of which is responsible for producing important features in cancer cells or the hallmarks of cancer.

4. DYRK1A

The *DYRK1A* gene maps to chromosome 21, and it is the most extensively studied member of the family, mainly due to its key role in neurogenesis and in the etiology of some of the pathological traits associated to Down syndrome (DS: recently reviewed in [43]). In fact, *DYRK1A* is a dosage-sensitive gene, since small variations in the amount of its protein produce clinical phenotypes. On the one hand, DYRK1A is overexpressed 1.5-fold in DS individuals [22], and indeed, some of the morphological and cognitive defects of DS are reproduced when it is overexpressed in mouse models [43]. On the other hand, DYRK1A haploinsufficiency caused by de novo truncation or by missense-inactivating mutations was recently seen to underlie a rare, severe disorder, the DYRK1A haploinsufficiency syndrome (also known as MRD7 or Mental Retardation, Autosomal Dominant 7: OMIM#614104 and ORPHA:464311 and 268261; [44,45] and references therein).

DYRK1A is a pleiotropic factor that phosphorylates a broad set of proteins involved in many different cellular processes. These include factors that have been associated with all the hallmarks of cancer, from genomic instability to increased proliferation and resistance to programmed cell death or signaling pathways whose dysfunction is relevant to tumor onset and progression (e.g., Wnt, Notch and Hedgehog (Hh); Figure 3 and Table 1). Notably, the role of DYRK1A in specific cell responses has contrasting outputs, suggesting that it can act as a bimodal signaling regulator. For instance, DYRK1A stimulates the transcriptional activity of the Hh-signaling effector GLI1 through direct phosphorylation (Figure 3), although it also represses the Hh pathway through an indirect mechanism involving regulators of the actin cytoskeleton [46,47]. Likewise, DYRK1A negatively regulates the nuclear factor of activated T-cell (NFAT) transcription factors by inducing their phosphorylation-dependent nuclear export [48], yet it serves as a positive modulator of NFAT signaling in primary endothelial cells stimulated by vascular endothelial growth factor (VEGF) [49] (Figure 3). DYRK1A bimodal activity has also been reported in Wnt signaling, where DYRK1A acts as a positive regulator of the activated pathway, but it represses basal Wnt-signaling activity [21]. Finally, DYRK1A may induce cells to either enter or exit the cell cycle by controlling the Cyclin D1-to-p21 ratio [50]. All these observations may reflect the different experimental systems used by different groups, and specifically, the ectopic expression might produce confounding effects, since dramatic changes in the DYRK1A protein might be transiently induced in these cells over and above the endogenous levels. Alternatively, these findings might actually support the bimodal activity of DYRK1A in vivo, with the different outcomes depending on specific conditions such as cell identity, subcellular localization or the levels of kinase expression. Along similar lines, several studies have ascribed opposite functions to DYRK1A in cancer, reflecting a very complex scenario. Therefore, as will become evident below, it remains unclear as to whether DYRK1A acts as a tumor suppressor or a tumor promoter or, more probably, as either, depending on the tumor context.

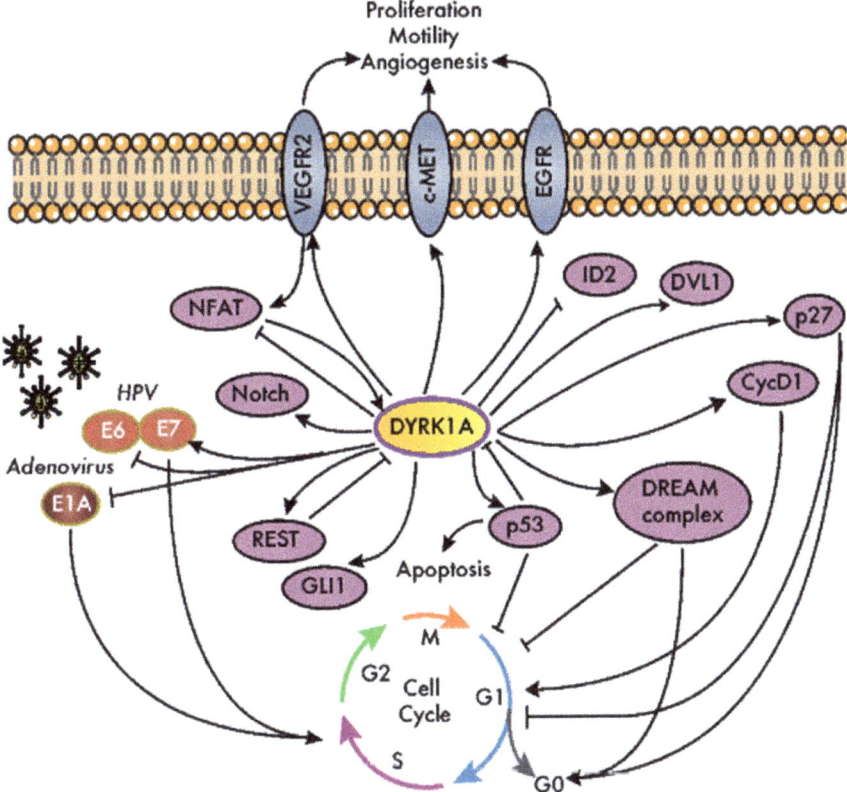

Figure 3. DYRK1A modulates the cellular factors involved in oncogenic processes. An overview of the DYRK1A interactions with the cellular factors involved neoplastic transformation and cancer-related pathways. CycD1: cyclin D1; DVL1: dishevelled 1; DREAM: dimerization partner (DP), RB-like, E2F and multi-vulval class B (MuvB); EGFR: epidermal growth factor receptor; HPV: human papilloma virus; ID2: inhibitor of DNA binding 2; NFAT: nuclear factor of activated T-cells; REST: RE1 silencing transcription factor; VEGFR2: vascular endothelial growth factor receptor 2.

Table 1. Signaling molecules targeted by DYRK1A and other dual-specificity tyrosine-regulated kinases (DYRKs).

Signaling Pathway	Target	Role	Reference	Other DYRKs	Role	Reference
Ca2+–NFAT	NFAT	Negative regulation of nuclear accumulation	[48]	DYRK2	same	[51]
Cell cycle	Cyclin D1	Negative regulation of protein levels	[50]	DYRK1B	same	[52]
	Cyclin D2	Negative regulation of protein levels	[53]	n.d.	n.d.	-
	Cyclin D3	Negative regulation of protein levels	[53]	n.d.	n.d.	-
	Lin52	Positive regulation of DREAM complex assembly	[54]	DYRK1B	same	[54]
	Myc	Negative regulation of protein levels	[55]	DYRK2	same	[56]
	p21	n.d.	-	DYRK1B	Negative regulation of protein accumulation	[57]
	p27	Positive regulation of protein levels	[58]	DYRK1B	same	[59]
	p53	Positive regulation of transcriptional activity	[60]	DYRK2	same	[19]
Hedgehog	ABLIM1	Negative regulation of F-actin formation	[47]	n.d.	n.d.	-
	GLI1	Positive regulation of nuclear accumulation and transcriptional activation	[46,47]	DYRK1B	Positive regulation of protein accumulation	[61]
	GLI2/3	n.d	-	DYRK2	Negative regulation of protein accumulation	[34]
Hypoxia	ID2	DYRK1A-mediated phosphorylation of ID2 leads to HIF2α destabilization	[62]	DYRK1B	same	[62]
	EGLN2/PHD1 *	Interaction enhances DYRK1A phosphorylation of ID2	[62]	DYRK1B	same	[62]
Notch	Notch1	Negative regulation of transcriptional activity	[63]	DYRK2	same	[64]
	Notch1	Negative regulation of protein levels	[64]	DYRK1B, DYRK2	same	[64]
RTKs	EGFR *	Positive regulation of protein levels	[65-67]	DYRK2	n.d.	-
	c-MET *	Positive regulation of protein levels	[67,68]	DYRK1B	same	[68]
	VEGFR2 *	Positive regulation of protein levels	[49]	n.d.	n.d.	-
Wnt	β-catenin	Regulation of binding to co-activators p300 or CBP	[69]	n.d.	n.d.	-
	Catenin-p120	Positive regulation of Wnt signaling	[70]	n.d.	n.d.	-
	DKK3	n.d	[21]	n.d.	n.d.	-
	DVL1	Positive regulation of DVL1-dependent induction of a TOP-FLASH reporter	[21]	n.d.	n.d.	-

* Not a direct phosphorylation target. ABLIM1: actin binding LIM protein 1; CBP: CREB binding protein; DKK3: dickkopf WNT signaling pathway inhibitor 3; DVL1: dishevelled 1; EGFR: epidermal growth factor receptor; EGLN2/PHD1: egl-9 family hypoxia inducible factor 2/prolyl hydroxylase 1; HIF2α: hypoxia-inducible factor 2-alpha; ID2: inhibitor of DNA binding 2; NFAT: nuclear factor of activated T-cells; RTKs: receptor tyrosine kinases and VEGFR2: vascular endothelial growth factor receptor 2. n.d.: not determined.

4.1. DYRK1A and Cell Cycle Regulation

The first indications of a role for DYRK1A in cell immortalization were obtained in studies on oncogenic viruses, indicating that DYRK1A potentially affects cell transformation in oncovirus-associated cancer models. Both DYRK1A and DYRK1B interact with the adenovirus oncoprotein E1A, a feature conserved in the *Saccharomyces cerevisiae* DYRK Yak1p [71,72] (Figure 3). Mutations in E1A that interfere with DYRK1A binding produce hyper-transformation in conjunction with G12V HRAS proto-oncogene [72]. Moreover, the interaction between DYRK1A and E1A is dependent on the DCAF7 scaffold protein, which favors E1A phosphorylation at S89 [39] and contributes to the ability of the adenovirus to regulate the interferon response [73]. DYRK1A also interacts functionally with human papilloma virus (HPV), and *Dyrk1a* mRNA levels increase when primary mouse keratinocytes are immortalized by HPV infection (HPV high risk strain 16) [74]. Indeed, there is more DYRK1A protein in cervical lesions from HPV-derived patient samples than in the respective normal tissues. Alterations to the DYRK1A expression might involve the miR-1246 known to target DYRK1A [26], which is significantly downregulated in lesions from cervical cancer patients in a manner associated with HPV infection [75]. DYRK1A interacts and phosphorylates HPV16 E7, stabilizing E7 and thereby potentially promoting E7-dependent cell proliferation [76] (Figure 3). Moreover, DYRK1A interacts with beta-HPV E6 proteins (Figure 3), and this DYRK1A interaction is defective in HPV E6 variants found in invasive cervical carcinoma [77].

The link between DYRK1A and cell proliferation is based on its ability to phosphorylate crucial cell cycle regulators, like Cyclin D proteins or p27 (Figure 3 and Table 1), modulating their stability and, hence, their cellular levels [50,53,58,78]. It should be noted that these regulatory mechanisms have mainly been observed in nontransformed cells, and as mentioned above, the effect of DYRK1A on the cell cycle is not straightforward, as it depends on the Cyclin D-induced stabilization of the CDK inhibitor p21, at least for Cyclin D1 [50]. In addition, DYRK1A is a kinase in the DREAM complex (dimerization partner (DP), RB-like, E2F and multi-vulval class B (MuvB)). DYRK1A promotes the assembly of this complex by phosphorylating the DREAM component Lin52 on S28, thereby triggering cell cycle exit [54] (Figure 3). Notably, DYRK1A-mediated DREAM complex formation was proposed to be responsible for ovarian cancer cell dormancy [79] and for the quiescence of gastrointestinal stromal tumor (GIST) cells induced by treatment with imatinib [80]. Another DYRK1A cell cycle-related target is the p53 tumor suppressor (Figure 3). DYRK1A positively regulates p53 transcriptional activity by the direct phosphorylation of S15 [60], but it also negatively regulates this factor by enhancing sirtuin (Sirt)1-dependent deacetylation [81]. The functional interaction of DYRK1A with p53 promotes cell cycle arrest in embryonic neuronal cells [60], as well as the survival of osteosarcoma and colorectal cancer (CRC) cell lines in response to genotoxic stress [81]. The cross-talk between DYRK1A and p53 also involves a negative feedback loop that engages two distinct regulatory mechanisms: (i) the p53-dependent induction of miR-1246, which suppresses DYRK1A expression [26], and (ii) the degradation of the DYRK1A protein mediated by the E3 ubiquitin ligase mouse double-minute 2 homolog (MDM2) [82].

4.2. DYRK1A and Receptor Tyrosine Kinase (RTK)-Dependent Signaling

An important aspect of the participation of DYRK1A in oncogenic processes is related to the regulation of RTK dependent signaling. This class of protein kinases is frequently altered in tumors, with almost half of them included in the list of driver kinases assembled in 2016 [2]. We found a conserved regulatory pattern that involves the positive effects of DYRK1A on the stability of several RTKs (Figure 3 and Table 1), yet it is unclear whether these effects are mediated by a shared DYRK1A target or one specific to each RTK. Thus, DYRK1A prevents epidermal growth factor receptor (EGFR) endocytosis-mediated degradation in neural stem cells [65] and indeed, DYRK1A-dependent EGFR stabilization has been described in glioblastoma (GBM) and non–small cell lung cancer (NSCLC) cell lines [66,67]. Indeed, DYRK1A and EGFR protein levels correlate in tissues from glioma patients [66]. In pancreatic ductal adenocarcinoma (PDAC) tumor tissue, a similar relationship was found between the expression of DYRK1A and c-MET, the hepatocyte growth factor receptor [68]. DYRK1A exerts a positive role on the c-MET protein levels in cell models of PDAC and NSCLC, which might contribute to the protumorigenic role of DYRK1A in these types of tumors [67,68]. Given that RTKs are common targets in cancer therapy [83], the inhibition of DYRK1A (and its paralog DYRK1B) could be considered an element in combinatorial therapies to simultaneously target several deregulated RTKs. Finally, DYRK1A depletion reduces the levels of membrane-bound VEGF receptor 2 (VEGFR2), and it causes defects in VEGFR2-dependent signaling and the downstream NFAT-dependent transcriptional response in endothelial cells [49]. These results are correlated with the defects in developmental angiogenesis in a mouse model in which the *Dyrk1a* dosage is reduced [49], although whether DYRK1A has a proangiogenic role in the tumor microenvironment needs to be further explored.

DYRK1A regulates other cell factors known to participate in malignant transformations, including the stemness-related RE1 silencing transcription factor REST [84] or key effectors of cancer-promoting signaling pathways, like the Hh, Wnt and Notch pathways (Table 1). However, whether DYRK1A is connected to alterations in these pathways during tumor initiation/progression has not yet been established.

4.3. DYRK1A in Cancer

Changes in the *DYRK1A* expression have been analyzed in tumor samples, and as such, *DYRK1A* was seen to be downregulated in breast cancer [27] and in acute myeloid leukemia (AML) tissue [55], and it is upregulated in GBM [66], lung cancer [67] and head and neck squamous cell carcinoma (HNSCC) [85], as well as in PDAC [68]. Indeed, a weaker DYRK1A expression was correlated with a worse overall survival in breast cancer patients [27] and a poorer prognosis in CRC and GBM patients [62,86], whereas more DYRK1A was associated with a reduced survival time in patients with lung cancer [67]. Our analysis of the TCGA RNA-Seq data revealed a clear trend towards *DYRK1A* downregulation in tumor tissues, with a significant downregulation of *DYRK1A* in 11 out of the 15 tumor types considered (Table S1): colon (COADREAD), esophagus (ESCA), HNSCC, kidney (KIRP and KIRC), liver (LIHC), lung (LUSC and LUAD), stomach (STAD), thyroid (THCA) and uterus (UCEC). No significant CNAs associated with changes in the gene expression were observed (Table S1), suggesting that the changes in RNA levels could be due to epigenetic, transcriptional or post-transcriptional alterations. The general trend towards a reduced *DYRK1A* expression in tumor samples would be in agreement with a more prominent tumor-suppressor role, even though the correlation between *DYRK1A* mRNA and the protein levels has not been properly evaluated in any cancer study.

A direct role for DYRK1A in tumor progression has been proposed in several studies. In cell models, DYRK1A knockdown or enzymatic inhibition reduced the proliferation of HNSCC cell lines [85], luminal/HER2 breast cancer [87] or PDAC [68], as well as impaired the self-renewal capacity of GBM cells [66] and compromised ovarian cancer spheroid cell viability [79]. The pro-oncogenic role suggested by these findings is in accordance with results obtained from xenografts in mouse models [66,68,85]. However, a tumor suppressor role was also proposed on the basis of DYRK1A overexpression experiments in AML cells [55]. The antitumor role of DYRK1A was suggested to be related to the lower incidence of cancer in DS individuals [88], deviating from that observed in the normal population. Indeed, epidemiological studies have demonstrated that individuals with DS have a markedly lower incidence of most solid tumors [89] and reduced cancer-associated mortality [90] relative to the age-adjusted non-DS population. However, childhood leukemia represents a strong exception to this trend, as DS children have a 10 to 50-fold increased risk of developing AML, as well as a 500-fold increased incidence of developing acute megakaryoblastic leukemia (AMKL) [91]. In this regard, DYRK1A was proposed to be a potent, megakaryoblastic oncogene, suggesting that NFAT-negative regulation through an imbalance in DYRK1A might perturb myeloid differentiation and promote AMKL in DS individuals [92].

In summary, the literature reflects a complex picture in which DYRK1A may fulfill opposite roles in different tumor contexts. Thus, more research is clearly required to fully understand how DYRK1A contributes to tumor initiation or progression.

5. DYRK1B

DYRK1B is the closest paralog to DYRK1A, sharing 85% homology that extends beyond the kinase domain (Figure 1A). Although both kinases share substrates (Table 1), the distinct clinical outcome of inactivating mutations indicates they are not functionally redundant, i.e., a disorder within the autism spectrum for DYRK1A and a metabolic syndrome for DYRK1B (abdominal obesity metabolic syndrome-3, OMIM#615812; [93]). A recent review of DYRK1B has offered extensive information on this kinase [94], and thus, here, we will focus on those aspects of the kinase that are related to its role in cancer, which, unlike DYRK1A, point mostly to a prosurvival and protumorigenic role for DYRK1B (Figure 4).

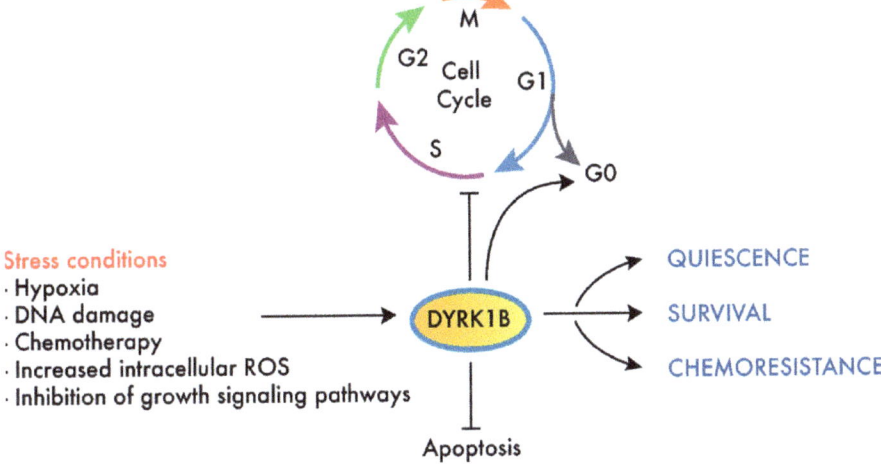

Figure 4. DYRK1B promotes survival and chemoresistance in cancer cells. Environmental stress conditions induce DYRK1B expression or activity in tumor cells, which, in turn, promotes cell cycle exit, quiescence (entry in G0) and survival. This mechanism has been proposed to mediate the resistance to chemotherapeutic agents that target dividing cells.

The first studies into the influence of DYRK1B in cancer suggested a role in the survival of cancer cells, with a stronger DYRK1B expression in CRC samples than in normal tissue [95]. Several studies extended this finding to other tumor types, included liposarcoma [96], rhabdomyosarcoma [97], osteosarcoma [98], lung [99], breast [100], ovary [101] and PDAC [68,102,103]. Indeed, a differential expression analysis using TCGA data finds *DYRK1B* to be overexpressed in several tumor types, including bladder (BLCA); breast (BRCA); kidney (KICH, KIRC and KIRP); liver (LIHC); prostate (PRAD); thyroid (THCA) and uterus (UCEC) (Table S1). Furthermore, we confirmed previous reports on the amplification of the *DYRK1B* genomic region (19q13.2) in ovarian cancer [104,105] and PDAC [102,106] (Table S1). The amplification of this region with coherent DYRK1B overexpression was observed in other tumor types (Table S1), suggesting that they may underlie the increase in *DYRK1B* expression, although this may also be provoked by transcriptional activation due to changes in the transcriptional profiles of tumor cells [107–111].

The functional interaction of DYRK1B with signaling pathways involved in cancer cell proliferation has been explored, assessing both the fluctuations in DYRK1B expression upon the perturbation of growth pathways and the output provoked by DYRK1B depletion in cancer cell lines. Several findings point to an antagonistic role of DYRK1B and MAPK signaling, with an increase in DYRK1B in response to inhibitors of the MAPK kinase (MEK) in CRC and melanoma cell lines [36,95] and a reduction following the mitogen activation of the RAS-MEK-extracellular signal-regulated kinase (ERK) pathway in skeletal myoblasts [112]. The cross-talk between DYRK1B and the MAPK pathway was further explored in ovarian cancer and NSCLC cell lines, where DYRK1B knockdown increased c-RAF and ERK activation [107]. This DYRK1B-MAPK cross-talk might be even more complex, since DYRK1B is an ERK substrate at a residue that potentiates DYRK1B activity [36], and accordingly, oncogenic KRAS mutants act as positive modulators of DYRK1B activity [113,114]. The RAS-DYRK1B axis was proposed to participate in both autocrine and paracrine Hh signaling in PDAC [114], although the role of DYRK1B in the regulation of Hh signaling in cancer remains controversial, as it has been attributed opposite functions within this signaling pathway [61,114,115]. Finally, there also appears to be cross-talk between DYRK1B and the mammalian target of rapamycin (mTOR) pathway, with DYRK1B expression upregulated upon mTOR inhibition [109] and mTOR/AKT activation induced by DYRK1B within the Hh signaling pathway in pancreatic and ovarian cancer cells [115].

Like DYRK1A, DYRK1B phosphorylates several cell cycle regulators, like Cyclin D1, p21, p27 and Lin52 [52,54,57,59] (Table 1). In this context, DYRK1B overexpression may help maintain a reversible quiescent state or inhibit cancer cell proliferation [116–118], while DYRK1B reduction can drive cell cycle entry in quiescence (by reducing the DYRK1B expression in PDAC or by DYRK1B inhibition in CRC cell lines) [119]. By contrast, the depletion of DYRK1B in HPV E7-expressing keratinocytes interferes with the induction of the S-phase promoted by E7 [120]. In addition, the depletion or inhibition of DYRK1B enhances the DNA damage, apoptosis and sensitivity to reactive oxygen species (ROS) or chemotherapeutic drugs targeting proliferating cells [15,104,121–123], as well as the sensitivity to compounds that target pathways favoring proliferation in cell lines of different tumor origins, such as mTOR and MEK inhibitors [107,109] (Figure 2).

A protumorigenic role for DYRK1B has been proven in cellular models of ovarian and pancreatic cancers. Thus, DYRK1B knockdown negatively affects different aspects of ovarian cancer cell malignancy, including viability, proliferative potential and migratory capacity [1,124,125]. Likewise, DYRK1B knockdown negatively affects PDAC cell proliferation, migration and invasion [68,102], whereas a treatment of PANC1 xenografts with a DYRK1B inhibitor impairs tumor growth [103]. In summary, and in contrast to the controversial role of DYRK1A in cancer, clear oncogenic facets have been attributed to DYRK1B, acting as a prosurvival factor that could help cancer cells survive in suboptimal growth conditions and preventing chemotherapeutic-induced DNA damage and apoptosis.

6. DYRK2

DYRK2 is a class II DYRK that has been more intensely studied in terms of its involvement in the events associated with tumor progression. The biochemistry and biology of DYRK2 was covered in recent reviews [126,127], and thus, here, we will center on the activity of this kinase in the context of tumor biology.

6.1. Altered DYRK2 Expression in Cancer

The first hints that DYRK2 may influence carcinogenesis were derived from a genomic analysis and differential gene expression studies, highlighting *DYRK2* overexpression in association with the amplification of its genomic locus in esophageal and lung adenocarcinomas [128,129], GIST [130], gastric adenocarcinoma [131] and liposarcoma [132]. Additional evidence for the involvement of DYRK2 in cancers came from a germline-somatic association study of genetic alterations in multiple cohorts of breast cancer patients [133]. Moreover, the upregulation of DYRK2 was described in triple-negative breast cancer (TNBC) and multiple myeloma [134]. Conversely, DYRK2 was downregulated in lung adenocarcinoma and squamous cell carcinoma [135], diffuse large B-cell lymphoma [136], CRC [137], hepatocellular carcinoma (HCC) [138,139] and high-grade glioma [140]. Our analysis of TCGA data found *DYRK2* to be overexpressed in eight tumor cohorts: bladder (BLCA), breast (BRCA), esophagus

(ESCA), kidney (KIRC and KIRP), liver (LIHC), lung (LUAD and LUSC) and stomach (STAD) (Table S1). An analysis of CNAs indicated that DYRK2 upregulation might be associated with gene amplification in BLCA, BRCA, LUAD, LUSC and STAD (Table S1). Moreover, a significant DYRK2 overexpression in DYRK2-amplified tumors was also observed in HNSCC, ovary (OV), melanoma (SKCM) and sarcoma (SARC) (Table S1). Notably, no correlation was observed between the DYRK2 protein and mRNA levels in breast cancer tissue when compared with healthy tissue [141]. A similar discrepancy between the DYRK2 protein and mRNA was also detected in liver and lung cancers between a published protein data analysis and our TCGA analysis of mRNA changes (Table S1). Hence, post-transcriptional mechanisms may play a crucial role in determining the levels of the DYRK2 protein in tumor cells, and these might explain, at least in part, the conflicting data obtained in relation to breast cancer (see below).

Besides the alterations to the DYRK2 expression, it has been proposed that this kinase may represent a prognostic marker for different types of cancer, based on a correlation analysis between the gene/protein expressions and distinct clinical features like the degree of malignancy, relapse, response to chemotherapy or patient survival. Thus, higher DYRK2 levels were positively correlated with a more favorable prognosis and better response to chemotherapy in lung and bladder cancer patients [142–144] and with better survival in patients with CRC liver metastases [145]. Likewise, a weaker DYRK2 expression was associated with a worse prognosis in ovarian serous adenocarcinoma [146], CRC [137,145], HCC [138,139], glioma [140] and non-Hodgkin's lymphoma [136] patients. The situation in breast cancer is less clear, with conflicting results. As mentioned above, such discordance may be due to the use of mRNA or protein to assess the DYRK2 expression. As such, DYRK2 protein levels were shown to inversely correlate with tumor invasiveness [56], and enhanced 10-year disease-free survival was evident in DYRK2-positive breast cancer patients when compared to DYRK2-negative patients [147], while a stronger DYRK2 mRNA expression was associated with a worse prognosis in another study of breast cancer patients [148]. Apart from this, and in general, it appears that the weaker the expression of DYRK2, the worse the prognosis. This model is consistent with experimental data when DYRK2 levels are manipulated in carcinoma cell lines (ovary, CRC and HCC) that are then used as xenografts in mice, whereby DYRK2 gene silencing confers an enhanced proliferative capacity and metastatic potential in vivo [139,145,146]. However, again, some discordant phenotypes have been described in vivo when studying DYRK2-depleted breast cancer cell lines.

A few works have explored the mechanisms underlying the reduction of DYRK2 levels in tumor cells. The Kruppel-like factor 4 transcription factor has been shown to repress DYRK2 expression, acting directly on the DYRK2 promoter in chronic myeloid leukemia (CML) cell lines and mouse models, thereby favoring tumor progression [149]. Moreover, the DNA-methyltransferase 1-dependent methylation of the DYRK2 promoter provokes transcriptional downregulation that may influence DYRK2 expression in CRC cells [150]. DYRK2 protein levels are also modulated by several E3 ubiquitin ligases, including seven in absentia homolog 2 (SIAH2) and MDM2 [9,151]. Interestingly, the DDR protein kinase ATM is involved in this process by phosphorylating DYRK2 and, thus, preventing DYRK2 degradation mediated by MDM2 [9,151]. This relationship could contribute to the ability of these E3 ubiquitin ligases to promote survival in states of hypoxia and in the face of DNA-damaged stress, respectively, by suppressing the proapoptotic activities of DYRK2. In particular, mutual regulation has been described for SIAH2 and DYRK2 [151]; indeed, an increase in the SIAH2 protein has been observed in lung cancer tissue and linked to DYRK2 downregulation [135]. Besides the alterations to the cellular levels of DYRK2, changes in the substrate selectivity have been seen in relation to Snail in ovarian cancer, with DYRK2 phosphorylation prevented by the prior p38-mediated phosphorylation of Snail [152].

6.2. The Molecular Mechanisms Underlying the Role of DYRK2 in Cancer Cells

Several clues have been obtained regarding the putative molecular mechanisms responsible for DYRK2-mediated tumor development/progression. Thus, DYRK2 activity appears to affect crucial processes like the cell cycle, DDR, epithelial-to-mesenchymal transition (EMT), the xenobiotic response system and cellular proteostasis [127]. The activity of DYRK2 has often been linked to its ability to negatively regulate the stability of its target proteins—in particular, through its interaction with the UBR5/EDD-DNA damage-binding protein 1 (DDB1)-DDB1- and cullin 4-associated factor homolog 1 (DCAF1/VPRBP) (EDVP) E3 ubiquitin ligase complex [38] (Figure 5A). The relevance of this interaction is highlighted by the alterations in the assembly of the EDVP complex detected in the analysis of certain DYRK2 mutants found in cancer samples [153]. In addition, it is worth noting that many of the proteins that are degraded following DYRK2 phosphorylation are targets of the tumor suppressor F-box/WD repeat-containing protein 7 (FBXW7) (Figure 5A), suggesting possible cross-talk with E3 ubiquitin ligase protein complexes made up of this factor. As previously mentioned, DYRK2 and SIAH2 cellular levels inversely correlate [151], further supporting a regulatory cross-talk between DYRK2 and several E3 ubiquitin ligases. Moreover, phosphorylation of the 19S subunit PMSC4/Rpt3 [148] might also contribute to the DYRK2-dependent modulation of protein accumulation.

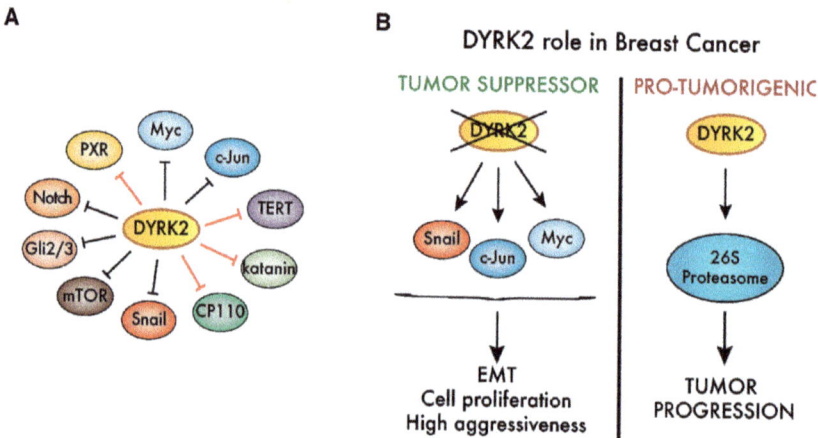

Figure 5. Cancer-associated activities of DYRK2. (**A**) DYRK2 substrates are associated with different aspects of tumorigenesis, including proliferation (Myc, c-Jun, centrosomal protein of 110 kDa (CP110) and katanin: [38,56]); transformation (TERT: [154]); invasiveness (Snail: [141]); signaling (mTOR, Notch and Gli2/3: [34,64,155]) or the xenobiotic response system (pregnane X receptor (PXR): [156]). Red lines mark those substrates that are degraded when DYRK2 associates with the multicomponent E3 ubiquitin ligase EDVP. The rest (black lines) are all targets of FBXW7, considered to be a tumor suppressor [157]. (**B**) DYRK2 has been proposed as both a protumorigenic factor, as well as a tumor suppressor, in breast cancer. On the one hand, reduced levels of DYRK2 enhance the accumulation of mitogenic transcription factors like c-Jun and Myc, as well as the epithelial-to-mesenchymal transition (EMT)-promoting factor Snail, which is correlated with tumor progression and more aggressiveness. On the other hand, DYRK2 phosphorylates and positively regulates the 26S proteasome, promoting triple-negative breast cancer (TNBC) cell growth, and thus, DYRK2 depletion or inhibition impairs tumor growth in vivo.

In conjunction with the reduced expression of DYRK2 in tumor samples, DYRK2 depletion promotes the proliferation of cell lines originating from distinct tumor types, including breast, lymphoma, osteosarcoma, CRC and HCC [56,136–139,145,158], suggesting that DYRK2 may acts as a brake on proliferation. In this regard, DYRK2 phosphorylates the oncogenic pro-proliferative transcription factors c-Jun and Myc, increasing their rate of degradation [56]. Indeed, DYRK2 levels negatively correlated with c-Jun/Myc levels in breast tumor tissues [56] (Figure 5B). Other DYRK2 targets associated with cell cycle regulation are the centrosomal proteins katanin p60 and CP110/CCP110 and the telomerase TERT (Figure 5A), although no specific link between these proteins and DYRK2-dependent tumorigenic processes has as yet been proposed [38,154,159].

Besides the cell cycle, DYRK2 also regulates cell factors involved in other processes crucial for tumor progression, such as apoptosis or DDR. The interaction between DYRK2 and the E3 ubiquitin ligase RNF8 was proposed to influence DYRK2 recruitment to the DNA repair machinery [160], and the phosphorylation of p53 by DYRK2 promotes apoptosis in response to DNA damage, with ATM acting upstream by increasing the DYRK2 nuclear accumulation [9,19]. The modulation of p53 and Myc was also proposed as a DYRK2-mediated mechanism in leukemia stem cells and CML cell lines [149]. The putative regulatory activity during DDR and/or the ability of DYRK2 to increase components of the xenobiotic response system, such as the PXR/NR1I2 nuclear receptor [156] (Figure 5A), may contribute to enhance the resistance to chemotherapy drugs observed upon DYRK2 silencing [64,138,146]. A reduction in DYRK2 has also been linked to the enhanced migration and invasion of breast, glioma and ovary cancer cell lines [56,64,140,141,146]. In this regard, DYRK2 phosphorylates the EMT transcription factor Snail, priming it for ubiquitination-mediated degradation [141] (Figure 5A), which provides additional evidence that DYRK2 prevents the activation of aggressive phenotypes in breast and ovarian cancer cells.

To date, the most controversial role for DYRK2 associated with tumors is in breast cancer (Figure 5B). Based on results from xenograft experiments using MCF-7 cells, a tumor-suppressor role was first proposed given that DYRK2 silencing favored tumor growth [56]. The enhanced expression of direct DYRK2 targets like c-Jun or Myc, and/or other proteins like CDK14, could account for this phenotype [56,158]. Similarly, DYRK2 silencing increased the invasion, metastasis [141] and breast cancer cell stemness [161]. Conversely, using a clustered regularly interspaced short palindromic repeats (CRISPR)-based approach to generate DYRK2-knock out MDA-MB-468 breast cancer cells, DYRK2 was seen to promote breast cancer cell proliferation and tumor growth in xenografts. This effect could be mediated by the DYRK2-dependent phosphorylation of the proteasomal 19S subunit PMSC4/Rpt3 [148] (Figure 5B). In this context, two DYRK2 inhibitors, the natural drug curcumin and the small-molecule LDN192960, impaired cell proliferation and invasion and induced apoptosis in multiple myeloma and TNBC cell lines [134,162]. Whether these contradictory results arise from the use of cell lines with different responsiveness to estrogen/progesterone and/or an "addiction" to proteasome activity must be further explored. In any case, the DYRK2-associated stratification of breast tumors should be properly studied before designing any DYRK2-targeting therapeutic approach.

7. DYRK3 and DYRK4

The contribution of DYRK3 and DYRK4 to tumorigenesis is less clear, with very little evidence for the participation of DYRK3 and almost no evidence for that of DYRK4. This lack of information also mirrors the limited knowledge of the biological activities of these two family members.

DYRK3 was initially described as a kinase involved in erythroid development [24,163], although its most relevant activity described to date is the ability to regulate phase-transition during mitosis, thereby mediating the formation of multiple liquid-unmixed compartments such as stress granules, an essential process for proper mitotic division [16,17]. The association of DYRK3 with the mTORC1 pathway was established through the ability of DYRK3 to phosphorylate PRAS40, thereby promoting mTORC1 activity [16].

Our analysis of the TCGA data did not reveal any specific trend for DYRK3, which is under-expressed in breast (BRCA), kidney (KIHC), lung (LUAD and LUSC), prostate (PRAD) and thyroid (THCA) tumor cohorts and overexpressed in colon (COADREAD), HNSCC, kidney (KIRC) and stomach (STAD) cancer tissues (Table S1). Likewise, no particular trend can be found in the literature. Thus, *DYRK3* mRNA was found significantly increased in highly invasive NSCLC cell lines compared with low invasive lines [164], while a strong DYRK3 expression was positively correlated with survival in glioma patients [165]. Moreover, DYRK3 was proposed as a specific early-stage tumor driver in gastric cancer [166]. Finally, a reduction in the DYRK3 protein was recently described in HCC biopsies relative to normal tissue, and low DYRK3 levels were associated with a poor prognosis in this type of cancer [167]. In addition, manipulating the DYRK3 expression in HCC cells demonstrated an inverse correlation with proliferation rates both in vitro and in tumor xenograft models, as well as with the metastatic potential of the tumor cells, further evidencing that DYRK3 fulfills a tumor-suppressor role in this type of cancer [167]. Indeed, a regulatory axis was proposed that involves the ATF4 transcription factor and its coactivator NCOA3 as a direct DYRK3 substrate, regulating the expression of key metabolic enzymes in the purine synthesis pathway that are relevant to HCC progression. However, whether this role for DYRK3 can be extrapolated to other tumors remains to be confirmed.

DYRK4 is the DYRK family member associated with the least significant alterations in the TCGA cohorts analyzed. We found that it was downregulated in lung (LUAD), prostate (PRAD) and stomach (STAD) cohorts and with different patterns of expression in the three kidney cohorts: overexpressed in KIRC and KIRP and downregulated in KIHC (Table S1). Interestingly, a recent high-throughput screen on 313 kinase-deficient cell lines revealed that DYRK4 knockout cells were among the most sensitive to agents that produce DNA damage [168], suggesting that DYRK4 might merit further exploration as a putative target to enhance chemotherapy toxicity on cancer cells.

8. DYRK Inhibitors as Antitumor Therapies

Chemical compounds that bind and functionally block protein kinases have been studied extensively and employed as antitumor agents, both in research and in clinical trials [83]. Although the role of DYRK family members in tumorigenesis and tumor progression has not been fully elucidated, pharmacological inhibitors of DYRK kinases have been tested in laboratories for their antimalignant activity, and a few of them are already undergoing clinical trials.

In the case of DYRK1A, the search for both naturally occurring and synthetic inhibitors has been extensive given that DYRK1A may be a potential pharmacological target not only in cancer but, also, in neurodegenerative diseases (reviewed in [43]), DS [169–172] and diabetes (reviewed in [173]). DYRK1A inhibitors have been comprehensively reviewed elsewhere [174–176], and so, we will only refer to the orally bioavailable archetypic DYRK1A inhibitors in tumor contexts. For instance, the anticancer properties of green tea and its derivatives have been proven in many animal models, a product that contains the natural DYRK1A inhibitor Epigallocatechin-3-gallate (EGCG). However, EGCG can potentially target many different intracellular pathways [177], making it difficult to assign particular effects to DYRK1A inhibition. Additionally, the ß-carboline alkaloid harmine selectively inhibits DYRK1A and—albeit, less efficiently—other members of the family [178,179], and it has been reported to have cytotoxic effects on cancer cell lines [66,85,180,181] and antitumor effects in vivo in glioma and in PDAC xenograft experiments [66,68], as well as synergistic effects with other chemotherapeutic agents [79,80,182]. However, the neurotoxic effects of harmine due to the targeting of monoamine oxidase A rule against its use in humans. Therefore, the search for harmine derivatives with enhanced antitumor activity and reduced neurotoxic effects has been intense in recent years [183–185]. Finally, the synthetic DYRK1A inhibitor INDY, proven to modulate the phenotypic effects of DYRK1A overexpression in vivo [186], has been shown to improve the response of ovarian cancer spheroids to carboplatin [79].

Compounds targeting DYRK1B, with either restricted or broad specificity, have been used as research tools, and they display toxicity towards several types of cancer cells or they promote the cell cycle re-entry of quiescent tumor cells (reviewed in [94]). The latter would enhance the effectiveness of other antiproliferative drugs in combinatorial approaches. For instance, the DYRK1B inhibitor AZ191 [52] increases the anticancer effects of doxorubicin in liposarcoma cell lines [96] or sensitizes the PDAC cell lines to mTOR inhibition [115]. However, AZ191 has been also shown to counteract the antitumor effects of the lysosome inhibitor Bafilomycin A1 in HCC cell lines [111]. For DYRK2, experimental data on the antitumor effects of the natural DYRK2 inhibitor curcumin and of the synthetic compound LDN192960 was obtained in both in vitro and in vivo models of TNBC and multiple myeloma, supporting the hypothesis that DYRK2 is a promising pharmaceutical target in these malignancies [134,162]. Finally, better understanding the role of DYRKs in tumor cells has proven valuable by helping to identify combinatorial therapeutic approaches, as in the cases of the DYRK1B inhibitors that enhance the inhibitory efficiency of MEK and mTOR [107,109,187] or DYRK2 inhibition sensitizing MDA-MB-468 cells to the proteasome inhibitor bortezomib [148].

Most kinase inhibitors lack complete specificity [178,188], a potentially negative property that might be exploited in multitargeting strategies, which become a familiar situation in antitumor therapies. Interestingly, the only inhibitors of the DYRK family members currently being screened in clinical trials were identified as inhibitors of other protein kinases. In particular, compound CX-4945 was initially identified as a casein kinase 2 inhibitor, but it was subsequently shown to be a potent DYRK1A and DYRK1B inhibitor [171], and it is currently in phase I and II clinical studies for medulloblastoma, cholangiocarcinoma and basal cell carcinoma (NCT02128282, NCT03904862 and NCT03897036). Recently, OTS167, a chemical initially described as a maternal embryonic leucine zipper kinase inhibitor, has been proven to have potent anti-DYRK1A activity [189]. OTS167 is currently being assessed in clinical trials for the treatment of advanced breast cancer and TNBC (phase I) and for multiple types of leukemia, including AML and advanced CML (phase II: NCT02795520). Finally, two other DYRK inhibitors have been assessed in clinical trials for non-neoplastic disorders: GSK-626616 [16] completed a phase I clinical trial to evaluate its action on anemia (NCT00443170), and lorecivivint, a potent CLK2 inhibitor that also inhibits DYRK1A [190], is being studied in a phase II trial for the treatment of moderate-to-severe symptomatic osteoarthritis (NCT03706521). Thus, they could be repurposed in trials for the treatment of specific cancer types.

9. Conclusions

In the last decade, more experimental evidence indicates that DYRK protein kinases are a novel class of "kinase-of-interest" in cancer. However, this evidence mostly comes from studies exploring DYRK expressions in tumor tissues and/or the phenotypic changes triggered by manipulating the DYRK protein in cancer cell lines. These data not only provide a partial and confusing picture of the influence of DYRKs in tumor initiation and progression, but also, they highlight the many questions that still need to be addressed. In particular, it remains unclear which molecular pathways are regulated by DYRKs in different tumor types and which of them selectively trigger cells to engage in neoplastic transformation or enhance the malignant phenotype of tumor cells. Resolving these issues will not only help understand the biology behind the activity of these kinases, but also, it will provide a basis for the rational design of therapeutic approaches based on inhibitors. In this regard, while incomplete, the currently available data provides precious information on which forthcoming therapeutic approaches may be based. Therefore, the tumor types in which downregulation of the DYRK kinase has been associated with increased tumor growth and/or invasiveness should not be considered for trials with DYRK inhibitors. Conversely, inhibitors targeting DYRK family members that are known to favor the tumorigenesis of specific tumor types should be considered for such trials. Nevertheless, putative side effects due to the inhibition of members that are essential to maintaining cellular homeostasis in normal cells, such as the dosage-sensitive DYRK1A or DYRK1B, should be carefully monitored. In this context, engineering drugs to increase their specificity, exclusively targeting proliferating cells, would be worthwhile. Finally, and considering the differential and sometimes opposite roles of distinct DYRK kinases in tumor progression, selectivity towards a specific member of the family is crucial and, at the same time, very challenging, particularly given the strong structural similarity of the catalytic domain. Smart solutions might include an allosteric drug design or other additional efforts to increase compound selectivity.

To conclude, many important advances in understanding how the dysregulation of DYRK protein kinases is associated to pathological phenotypes in humans have been made in recent years—in particular, in terms of the involvement in DYRK cancers. Still, many secrets behind the oncogenic or protective potential of DYRK kinases remain to be revealed, and we anticipate that the field will continue to grow for the foreseeable future.

Supplementary Materials: The following are available online at http://www.mdpi.com/2072-6694/12/8/2106/s1: Table S1. Differential expression of DYRK genes in TCGA tumor samples.

Author Contributions: C.R.-P. and N.L.-B. analyzed the TCGA data. J.B. created the figures and Table S1. S.D.L.L. created Table 1. J.B. and S.D.L.L. wrote the manuscript with input from C.F. All the authors have read and approved the manuscript. All authors have read and agreed to the published version of the manuscript.

Funding: J.B. is an FPI predoctoral fellow (BES-2014-069983). De la Luna's lab is supported by grants from the Spanish Ministry of Science and Innovation (BFU2016-76141-P, AEI/FEDER), the AGAUR grant from Secretaria d'Universitats i Recerca del Departament d'Empresa i Coneixement de la Generalitat de Catalunya (SGR14/674) and the CIBER de Enfermedades Raras. We thank La Marato of TV3 for its support to our research in cancer. We also acknowledge the support of the Spanish Ministry of Science and Innovation to the EMBL partnership, the Centro de Excelencia Severo Ochoa and the support of the CERCA Programme/Generalitat de Catalunya.

Acknowledgments: We are grateful to all members of Susana de la Luna's laboratory for their helpful discussions, and we thank Mark Sefton for English language editing. The authors acknowledge the efforts of the DYRK community and apologize to the investigators whose works do not appear in this review and should have been included.

Conflicts of Interest: The authors declare no conflict of interest.

References

1. Collett, M.S.; Erikson, R.L. Protein kinase activity associated with the avian sarcoma virus src gene product. *Proc. Natl. Acad. Sci. USA* **1978**, *75*, 2021–2024. [CrossRef]
2. Fleuren, E.D.; Zhang, L.; Wu, J.; Daly, R.J. The kinome 'at large' in cancer. *Nat. Rev. Cancer* **2016**, *16*, 83–98. [CrossRef]
3. Manning, G.; Whyte, D.B.; Martinez, R.; Hunter, T.; Sudarsanam, S. The protein kinase complement of the human genome. *Science* **2002**, *298*, 1912–1934. [CrossRef] [PubMed]
4. Aranda, S.; Laguna, A.; de la Luna, S. DYRK family of protein kinases: Evolutionary relationships, biochemical properties, and functional roles. *FASEB J.* **2011**, *25*, 449–462. [CrossRef] [PubMed]
5. Kannan, N.; Neuwald, A.F. Evolutionary constraints associated with functional specificity of the CMGC protein kinases MAPK, CDK, GSK, SRPK, DYRK, and CK2alpha. *Protein Sci.* **2004**, *13*, 2059–2077. [CrossRef] [PubMed]
6. Kinstrie, R.; Luebbering, N.; Miranda-Saavedra, D.; Sibbet, G.; Han, J.; Lochhead, P.A.; Cleghon, V. Characterization of a domain that transiently converts class 2 DYRKs into intramolecular tyrosine kinases. *Sci. Signal.* **2010**, *3*, ra16. [CrossRef]
7. Alvarez, M.; Estivill, X.; de la Luna, S. DYRK1A accumulates in splicing speckles through a novel targeting signal and induces speckle disassembly. *J. Cell Sci.* **2003**, *116*, 3099–3107. [CrossRef]
8. Papadopoulos, C.; Arato, K.; Lilienthal, E.; Zerweck, J.; Schutkowski, M.; Chatain, N.; Muller-Newen, G.; Becker, W.; de la Luna, S. Splice variants of the dual specificity tyrosine phosphorylation-regulated kinase 4 (DYRK4) differ in their subcellular localization and catalytic activity. *J. Biol. Chem.* **2011**, *286*, 5494–5505. [CrossRef]
9. Taira, N.; Yamamoto, H.; Yamaguchi, T.; Miki, Y.; Yoshida, K. ATM augments nuclear stabilization of DYRK2 by inhibiting MDM2 in the apoptotic response to DNA damage. *J. Biol. Chem.* **2010**, *285*, 4909–4919. [CrossRef]
10. Di Vona, C.; Bezdan, D.; Islam, A.B.; Salichs, E.; Lopez-Bigas, N.; Ossowski, S.; de la Luna, S. Chromatin-wide profiling of DYRK1A reveals a role as a gene-specific RNA polymerase II CTD kinase. *Mol. Cell* **2015**, *57*, 506–520. [CrossRef]
11. Yu, D.; Cattoglio, C.; Xue, Y.; Zhou, Q. A complex between DYRK1A and DCAF7 phosphorylates the C-terminal domain of RNA polymerase II to promote myogenesis. *Nucleic Acids Res.* **2019**, *47*, 4462–4475. [CrossRef] [PubMed]
12. Roewenstrunk, J.; Di Vona, C.; Chen, J.; Borras, E.; Dong, C.; Arato, K.; Sabido, E.; Huen, M.S.Y.; de la Luna, S. A comprehensive proteomics-based interaction screen that links DYRK1A to RNF169 and to the DNA damage response. *Sci. Rep.* **2019**, *9*, 6014. [CrossRef] [PubMed]
13. Menon, V.R.; Ananthapadmanabhan, V.; Swanson, S.; Saini, S.; Sesay, F.; Yakovlev, V.; Florens, L.; DeCaprio, J.A.; Washburn, M.P.; Dozmorov, M.; et al. DYRK1A regulates the recruitment of 53BP1 to the sites of DNA damage in part through interaction with RNF169. *Cell Cycle* **2019**, *18*, 531–551. [CrossRef] [PubMed]

14. Guard, S.E.; Poss, Z.C.; Ebmeier, C.C.; Pagratis, M.; Simpson, H.; Taatjes, D.J.; Old, W.M. The nuclear interactome of DYRK1A reveals a functional role in DNA damage repair. *Sci. Rep.* **2019**, *9*, 6539. [CrossRef] [PubMed]
15. Dong, C.; West, K.L.; Tan, X.Y.; Li, J.; Ishibashi, T.; Yu, C.H.; Sy, S.M.H.; Leung, J.W.C.; Huen, M.S.Y. Screen identifies DYRK1B network as mediator of transcription repression on damaged chromatin. *Proc. Natl. Acad. Sci. USA* **2020**. [CrossRef]
16. Wippich, F.; Bodenmiller, B.; Trajkovska, M.G.; Wanka, S.; Aebersold, R.; Pelkmans, L. Dual specificity kinase DYRK3 couples stress granule condensation/dissolution to mTORC1 signaling. *Cell* **2013**, *152*, 791–805. [CrossRef]
17. Rai, A.K.; Chen, J.X.; Selbach, M.; Pelkmans, L. Kinase-controlled phase transition of membraneless organelles in mitosis. *Nature* **2018**, *559*, 211–216. [CrossRef]
18. Lu, H.; Yu, D.; Hansen, A.S.; Ganguly, S.; Liu, R.; Heckert, A.; Darzacq, X.; Zhou, Q. Phase-separation mechanism for C-terminal hyperphosphorylation of RNA polymerase II. *Nature* **2018**, *558*, 318–323. [CrossRef]
19. Taira, N.; Nihira, K.; Yamaguchi, T.; Miki, Y.; Yoshida, K. DYRK2 is targeted to the nucleus and controls p53 via Ser46 phosphorylation in the apoptotic response to DNA damage. *Mol. Cell* **2007**, *25*, 725–738. [CrossRef]
20. Xu, L.; Sun, Y.; Li, M.; Ge, X. Dyrk2 mediated the release of proinflammatory cytokines in LPS-induced BV2 cells. *Int. J. Biol. Macromol.* **2018**, *109*, 1115–1124. [CrossRef]
21. Granno, S.; Nixon-Abell, J.; Berwick, D.C.; Tosh, J.; Heaton, G.; Almudimeegh, S.; Nagda, Z.; Rain, J.C.; Zanda, M.; Plagnol, V.; et al. Downregulated Wnt/beta-catenin signalling in the Down syndrome hippocampus. *Sci. Rep.* **2019**, *9*, 7322. [CrossRef] [PubMed]
22. Guimera, J.; Casas, C.; Estivill, X.; Pritchard, M. Human minibrain homologue (MNBH/DYRK1): Characterization, alternative splicing, differential tissue expression, and overexpression in Down syndrome. *Genomics* **1999**, *57*, 407–418. [CrossRef] [PubMed]
23. Leder, S.; Weber, Y.; Altafaj, X.; Estivill, X.; Joost, H.G.; Becker, W. Cloning and characterization of DYRK1B, a novel member of the DYRK family of protein kinases. *Biochem. Biophys. Res. Commun.* **1999**, *254*, 474–479. [CrossRef] [PubMed]
24. Lord, K.A.; Creasy, C.L.; King, A.G.; King, C.; Burns, B.M.; Lee, J.C.; Dillon, S.B. REDK, a novel human regulatory erythroid kinase. *Blood* **2000**, *95*, 2838–2846. [CrossRef]
25. da Costa Martins, P.A.; Salic, K.; Gladka, M.M.; Armand, A.S.; Leptidis, S.; el Azzouzi, H.; Hansen, A.; Coenen-de Roo, C.J.; Bierhuizen, M.F.; van der Nagel, R.; et al. MicroRNA-199b targets the nuclear kinase Dyrk1a in an auto-amplification loop promoting calcineurin/NFAT signalling. *Nat. Cell Biol.* **2010**, *12*, 1220–1227. [CrossRef]
26. Zhang, Y.; Liao, J.M.; Zeng, S.X.; Lu, H. p53 downregulates Down syndrome-associated DYRK1A through miR-1246. *EMBO Rep.* **2011**, *12*, 811–817. [CrossRef]
27. Kim, J.; Siverly, A.N.; Chen, D.; Wang, M.; Yuan, Y.; Wang, Y.; Lee, H.; Zhang, J.; Muller, W.J.; Liang, H.; et al. Ablation of miR-10b suppresses oncogene-induced mammary tumorigenesis and metastasis and reactivates tumor-suppressive pathways. *Cancer Res.* **2016**, *76*, 6424–6435. [CrossRef]
28. Vidaki, M.; Drees, F.; Saxena, T.; Lanslots, E.; Taliaferro, M.J.; Tatarakis, A.; Burge, C.B.; Wang, E.T.; Gertler, F.B. A requirement for Mena, an actin regulator, in local mRNA translation in developing neurons. *Neuron* **2017**, *95*, 608–622. [CrossRef]
29. Himpel, S.; Panzer, P.; Eirmbter, K.; Czajkowska, H.; Sayed, M.; Packman, L.C.; Blundell, T.; Kentrup, H.; Grotzinger, J.; Joost, H.G.; et al. Identification of the autophosphorylation sites and characterization of their effects in the protein kinase DYRK1A. *Biochem. J.* **2001**, *359*, 497–505. [CrossRef]
30. Kentrup, H.; Becker, W.; Heukelbach, J.; Wilmes, A.; Schurmann, A.; Huppertz, C.; Kainulainen, H.; Joost, H.G. Dyrk, a dual specificity protein kinase with unique structural features whose activity is dependent on tyrosine residues between subdomains VII and VIII. *J. Biol. Chem.* **1996**, *271*, 3488–3495. [CrossRef]
31. Soundararajan, M.; Roos, A.K.; Savitsky, P.; Filippakopoulos, P.; Kettenbach, A.N.; Olsen, J.V.; Gerber, S.A.; Eswaran, J.; Knapp, S.; Elkins, J.M. Structures of Down syndrome kinases, DYRKs, reveal mechanisms of kinase activation and substrate recognition. *Structure* **2013**, *21*, 986–996. [CrossRef]
32. Lochhead, P.A.; Sibbet, G.; Morrice, N.; Cleghon, V. Activation-loop autophosphorylation is mediated by a novel transitional intermediate form of DYRKs. *Cell* **2005**, *121*, 925–936. [CrossRef]
33. Lim, S.; Zou, Y.; Friedman, E. The transcriptional activator Mirk/Dyrk1B is sequestered by p38alpha/beta MAP kinase. *J. Biol. Chem.* **2002**, *277*, 49438–49445. [CrossRef]

34. Varjosalo, M.; Bjorklund, M.; Cheng, F.; Syvanen, H.; Kivioja, T.; Kilpinen, S.; Sun, Z.; Kallioniemi, O.; Stunnenberg, H.G.; He, W.W.; et al. Application of active and kinase-deficient kinome collection for identification of kinases regulating hedgehog signaling. *Cell* **2008**, *133*, 537–548. [CrossRef] [PubMed]
35. Tschop, K.; Conery, A.R.; Litovchick, L.; Decaprio, J.A.; Settleman, J.; Harlow, E.; Dyson, N. A kinase shRNA screen links LATS2 and the pRB tumor suppressor. *Genes Dev.* **2011**, *25*, 814–830. [CrossRef] [PubMed]
36. Ashford, A.L.; Dunkley, T.P.; Cockerill, M.; Rowlinson, R.A.; Baak, L.M.; Gallo, R.; Balmanno, K.; Goodwin, L.M.; Ward, R.A.; Lochhead, P.A.; et al. Identification of DYRK1B as a substrate of ERK1/2 and characterisation of the kinase activity of DYRK1B mutants from cancer and metabolic syndrome. *Cell Mol. Life Sci.* **2016**, *73*, 883–900. [CrossRef] [PubMed]
37. Alvarez, M.; Altafaj, X.; Aranda, S.; de la Luna, S. DYRK1A autophosphorylation on serine residue 520 modulates its kinase activity via 14-3-3 binding. *Mol. Biol. Cell* **2007**, *18*, 1167–1178. [CrossRef] [PubMed]
38. Maddika, S.; Chen, J. Protein kinase DYRK2 is a scaffold that facilitates assembly of an E3 ligase. *Nat. Cell Biol.* **2009**, *11*, 409–419. [CrossRef] [PubMed]
39. Glenewinkel, F.; Cohen, M.J.; King, C.R.; Kaspar, S.; Bamberg-Lemper, S.; Mymryk, J.S.; Becker, W. The adaptor protein DCAF7 mediates the interaction of the adenovirus E1A oncoprotein with the protein kinases DYRK1A and HIPK2. *Sci. Rep.* **2016**, *6*, 28241. [CrossRef] [PubMed]
40. Hanahan, D.; Weinberg, R.A. Hallmarks of cancer: The next generation. *Cell* **2011**, *144*, 646–674. [CrossRef] [PubMed]
41. Davoli, T.; Xu, A.W.; Mengwasser, K.E.; Sack, L.M.; Yoon, J.C.; Park, P.J.; Elledge, S.J. Cumulative haploinsufficiency and triplosensitivity drive aneuploidy patterns and shape the cancer genome. *Cell* **2013**, *155*, 948–962. [CrossRef] [PubMed]
42. Dietlein, F.; Weghorn, D.; Taylor-Weiner, A.; Richters, A.; Reardon, B.; Liu, D.; Lander, E.S.; Van Allen, E.M.; Sunyaev, S.R. Identification of cancer driver genes based on nucleotide context. *Nat. Genet.* **2020**, *52*, 208–218. [CrossRef] [PubMed]
43. Arbones, M.L.; Thomazeau, A.; Nakano-Kobayashi, A.; Hagiwara, M.; Delabar, J.M. DYRK1A and cognition: A lifelong relationship. *Pharmacol. Ther.* **2019**, *194*, 199–221. [CrossRef]
44. van Bon, B.W.; Coe, B.P.; Bernier, R.; Green, C.; Gerdts, J.; Witherspoon, K.; Kleefstra, T.; Willemsen, M.H.; Kumar, R.; Bosco, P.; et al. Disruptive de novo mutations of DYRK1A lead to a syndromic form of autism and ID. *Mol. Psychiatry* **2016**, *21*, 126–132. [CrossRef] [PubMed]
45. Arranz, J.; Balducci, E.; Arato, K.; Sanchez-Elexpuru, G.; Najas, S.; Parras, A.; Rebollo, E.; Pijuan, I.; Erb, I.; Verde, G.; et al. Impaired development of neocortical circuits contributes to the neurological alterations in DYRK1A haploinsufficiency syndrome. *Neurobiol. Dis.* **2019**, *127*, 210–222. [CrossRef] [PubMed]
46. Mao, J.; Maye, P.; Kogerman, P.; Tejedor, F.J.; Toftgard, R.; Xie, W.; Wu, G.; Wu, D. Regulation of Gli1 transcriptional activity in the nucleus by Dyrk1. *J. Biol. Chem.* **2002**, *277*, 35156–35161. [CrossRef]
47. Schneider, P.; Bayo-Fina, J.M.; Singh, R.; Kumar Dhanyamraju, P.; Holz, P.; Baier, A.; Fendrich, V.; Ramaswamy, A.; Baumeister, S.; Martinez, E.D.; et al. Identification of a novel actin-dependent signal transducing module allows for the targeted degradation of GLI1. *Nat. Commun.* **2015**, *6*. [CrossRef]
48. Arron, J.R.; Winslow, M.M.; Polleri, A.; Chang, C.P.; Wu, H.; Gao, X.; Neilson, J.R.; Chen, L.; Heit, J.J.; Kim, S.K.; et al. NFAT dysregulation by increased dosage of DSCR1 and DYRK1A on chromosome 21. *Nature* **2006**, *441*, 595–600. [CrossRef]
49. Rozen, E.J.; Roewenstrunk, J.; Barallobre, M.J.; Di Vona, C.; Jung, C.; Figueiredo, A.F.; Luna, J.; Fillat, C.; Arbones, M.L.; Graupera, M.; et al. DYRK1A kinase positively regulates angiogenic responses in endothelial cells. *Cell Rep.* **2018**, *23*, 1867–1878. [CrossRef]
50. Chen, J.Y.; Lin, J.R.; Tsai, F.C.; Meyer, T. Dosage of Dyrk1a shifts cells within a p21-cyclin D1 signaling map to control the decision to enter the cell cycle. *Mol. Cell* **2013**, *52*, 87–100. [CrossRef]
51. Gwack, Y.; Sharma, S.; Nardone, J.; Tanasa, B.; Iuga, A.; Srikanth, S.; Okamura, H.; Bolton, D.; Feske, S.; Hogan, P.G.; et al. A genome-wide Drosophila RNAi screen identifies DYRK-family kinases as regulators of NFAT. *Nature* **2006**, *441*, 646–650. [CrossRef] [PubMed]
52. Ashford, A.L.; Oxley, D.; Kettle, J.; Hudson, K.; Guichard, S.; Cook, S.J.; Lochhead, P.A. A novel DYRK1B inhibitor AZ191 demonstrates that DYRK1B acts independently of GSK3beta to phosphorylate cyclin D1 at Thr (286), not Thr (288). *Biochem. J.* **2014**, *457*, 43–56. [CrossRef] [PubMed]

53. Hille, S.; Dierck, F.; Kuhl, C.; Sosna, J.; Adam-Klages, S.; Adam, D.; Lullmann-Rauch, R.; Frey, N.; Kuhn, C. Dyrk1a regulates the cardiomyocyte cell cycle via D-cyclin-dependent Rb/E2f-signalling. *Cardiovasc. Res.* **2016**, *110*, 381–394. [CrossRef] [PubMed]
54. Litovchick, L.; Florens, L.A.; Swanson, S.K.; Washburn, M.P.; DeCaprio, J.A. DYRK1A protein kinase promotes quiescence and senescence through DREAM complex assembly. *Genes Dev.* **2011**, *25*, 801–813. [CrossRef] [PubMed]
55. Liu, Q.; Liu, N.; Zang, S.; Liu, H.; Wang, P.; Ji, C.; Sun, X. Tumor suppressor DYRK1A effects on proliferation and chemoresistance of AML cells by downregulating c-Myc. *PLoS ONE* **2014**, *9*, e98853. [CrossRef]
56. Taira, N.; Mimoto, R.; Kurata, M.; Yamaguchi, T.; Kitagawa, M.; Miki, Y.; Yoshida, K. DYRK2 priming phosphorylation of c-Jun and c-Myc modulates cell cycle progression in human cancer cells. *J. Clin. Investig.* **2012**, *122*, 859–872. [CrossRef]
57. Mercer, S.E.; Ewton, D.Z.; Deng, X.; Lim, S.; Mazur, T.R.; Friedman, E. Mirk/Dyrk1B mediates survival during the differentiation of C2C12 myoblasts. *J. Biol. Chem.* **2005**, *280*, 25788–25801. [CrossRef]
58. Soppa, U.; Schumacher, J.; Florencio Ortiz, V.; Pasqualon, T.; Tejedor, F.J.; Becker, W. The Down syndrome-related protein kinase DYRK1A phosphorylates p27 (Kip1) and Cyclin D1 and induces cell cycle exit and neuronal differentiation. *Cell Cycle* **2014**, *13*, 2084–2100. [CrossRef]
59. Deng, X.; Mercer, S.E.; Shah, S.; Ewton, D.Z.; Friedman, E. The cyclin-dependent kinase inhibitor p27Kip1 is stabilized in G (0) by Mirk/dyrk1B kinase. *J. Biol. Chem.* **2004**, *279*, 22498–22504. [CrossRef]
60. Park, J.; Oh, Y.; Yoo, L.; Jung, M.S.; Song, W.J.; Lee, S.H.; Seo, H.; Chung, K.C. Dyrk1A phosphorylates p53 and inhibits proliferation of embryonic neuronal cells. *J. Biol. Chem.* **2010**, *285*, 31895–31906. [CrossRef] [PubMed]
61. Gruber, W.; Hutzinger, M.; Elmer, D.P.; Parigger, T.; Sternberg, C.; Cegielkowski, L.; Zaja, M.; Leban, J.; Michel, S.; Hamm, S.; et al. DYRK1B as therapeutic target in Hedgehog/GLI-dependent cancer cells with Smoothened inhibitor resistance. *Oncotarget* **2016**, *7*, 7134–7148. [CrossRef] [PubMed]
62. Lee, S.B.; Frattini, V.; Bansal, M.; Castano, A.M.; Sherman, D.; Hutchinson, K.; Bruce, J.N.; Califano, A.; Liu, G.; Cardozo, T.; et al. An ID2-dependent mechanism for VHL inactivation in cancer. *Nature* **2016**, *529*, 172–177. [CrossRef] [PubMed]
63. Fernandez-Martinez, J.; Vela, E.M.; Tora-Ponsioen, M.; Ocana, O.H.; Nieto, M.A.; Galceran, J. Attenuation of Notch signalling by the Down-syndrome-associated kinase DYRK1A. *J. Cell Sci.* **2009**, *122*, 1574–1583. [CrossRef] [PubMed]
64. Morrugares, R.; Correa-Saez, A.; Moreno, R.; Garrido-Rodriguez, M.; Munoz, E.; de la Vega, L.; Calzado, M.A. Phosphorylation-dependent regulation of the NOTCH1 intracellular domain by dual-specificity tyrosine-regulated kinase 2. *Cell Mol. Life Sci.* **2019**. [CrossRef]
65. Ferron, S.R.; Pozo, N.; Laguna, A.; Aranda, S.; Porlan, E.; Moreno, M.; Fillat, C.; de la Luna, S.; Sanchez, P.; Arbones, M.L.; et al. Regulated segregation of kinase Dyrk1A during asymmetric neural stem cell division is critical for EGFR-mediated biased signaling. *Cell Stem Cell* **2010**, *7*, 367–379. [CrossRef]
66. Pozo, N.; Zahonero, C.; Fernandez, P.; Linares, J.M.; Ayuso, A.; Hagiwara, M.; Perez, A.; Ricoy, J.R.; Hernandez-Lain, A.; Sepulveda, J.M.; et al. Inhibition of DYRK1A destabilizes EGFR and reduces EGFR-dependent glioblastoma growth. *J. Clin. Investig* **2013**, *123*, 2475–2487. [CrossRef]
67. Li, Y.L.; Ding, K.; Hu, X.; Wu, L.W.; Zhou, D.M.; Rao, M.J.; Lin, N.M.; Zhang, C. DYRK1A inhibition suppresses STAT3/EGFR/Met signalling and sensitizes EGFR wild-type NSCLC cells to AZD9291. *J. Cell Mol. Med.* **2019**, *23*, 7427–7437. [CrossRef]
68. Luna, J.; Boni, J.; Cuatrecasas, M.; Bofill-De Ros, X.; Nunez-Manchon, E.; Gironella, M.; Vaquero, E.C.; Arbones, M.L.; de la Luna, S.; Fillat, C. DYRK1A modulates c-MET in pancreatic ductal adenocarcinoma to drive tumour growth. *Gut* **2019**, *68*, 1465–1476. [CrossRef]
69. Hasegawa, K.; Yasuda, S.Y.; Teo, J.L.; Nguyen, C.; McMillan, M.; Hsieh, C.L.; Suemori, H.; Nakatsuji, N.; Yamamoto, M.; Miyabayashi, T.; et al. Wnt signaling orchestration with a small molecule DYRK inhibitor provides long-term xeno-free human pluripotent cell expansion. *Stem Cells Transl. Med.* **2012**, *1*, 18–28. [CrossRef]
70. Hong, J.Y.; Park, J.I.; Lee, M.; Munoz, W.A.; Miller, R.K.; Ji, H.; Gu, D.; Ezan, J.; Sokol, S.Y.; McCrea, P.D. Down's-syndrome-related kinase Dyrk1A modulates the p120-catenin-Kaiso trajectory of the Wnt signaling pathway. *J. Cell Sci.* **2012**, *125*, 561–569. [CrossRef]

71. Zhang, Z.; Smith, M.M.; Mymryk, J.S. Interaction of the E1A oncoprotein with Yak1p, a novel regulator of yeast pseudohyphal differentiation, and related mammalian kinases. *Mol. Biol. Cell* **2001**, *12*, 699–710. [CrossRef] [PubMed]
72. Komorek, J.; Kuppuswamy, M.; Subramanian, T.; Vijayalingam, S.; Lomonosova, E.; Zhao, L.J.; Mymryk, J.S.; Schmitt, K.; Chinnadurai, G. Adenovirus type 5 E1A and E6 proteins of low-risk cutaneous beta-human papillomaviruses suppress cell transformation through interaction with FOXK1/K2 transcription factors. *J. Virol.* **2010**, *84*, 2719–2731. [CrossRef] [PubMed]
73. Zemke, N.R.; Berk, A.J. The Adenovirus E1A C-terminus suppresses a delayed antiviral response and modulates RAS signaling. *Cell Host Microbe* **2017**, *22*, 789–800. [CrossRef] [PubMed]
74. Chang, H.S.; Lin, C.H.; Yang, C.H.; Yen, M.S.; Lai, C.R.; Chen, Y.R.; Liang, Y.J.; Yu, W.C. Increased expression of Dyrk1a in HPV16 immortalized keratinocytes enable evasion of apoptosis. *Int. J. Cancer* **2007**, *120*, 2377–2385. [CrossRef]
75. Yang, Y.; Xie, Y.J.; Xu, Q.; Chen, J.X.; Shan, N.C.; Zhang, Y. Down-regulation of miR-1246 in cervical cancer tissues and its clinical significance. *Gynecol. Oncol.* **2015**, *138*, 683–688. [CrossRef]
76. Liang, Y.J.; Chang, H.S.; Wang, C.Y.; Yu, W.C. DYRK1A stabilizes HPV16E7 oncoprotein through phosphorylation of the threonine 5 and threonine 7 residues. *Int. J. Biochem. Cell Biol.* **2008**, *40*, 2431–2441. [CrossRef]
77. Kuppuswamy, M.; Subramanian, T.; Kostas-Polston, E.; Vijayalingam, S.; Zhao, L.J.; Varvares, M.; Chinnadurai, G. Functional similarity between E6 proteins of cutaneous human papillomaviruses and the adenovirus E1A tumor-restraining module. *J. Virol.* **2013**, *87*, 7781–7786. [CrossRef]
78. Thompson, B.J.; Bhansali, R.; Diebold, L.; Cook, D.E.; Stolzenburg, L.; Casagrande, A.S.; Besson, T.; Leblond, B.; Desire, L.; Malinge, S.; et al. DYRK1A controls the transition from proliferation to quiescence during lymphoid development by destabilizing Cyclin D3. *J. Exp. Med.* **2015**, *212*, 953–970. [CrossRef]
79. MacDonald, J.; Ramos-Valdes, Y.; Perampalam, P.; Litovchick, L.; DiMattia, G.E.; Dick, F.A. A systematic analysis of negative growth control implicates the DREAM complex in cancer cell dormancy. *Mol. Cancer Res.* **2017**, *15*, 371–381. [CrossRef]
80. Boichuk, S.; Parry, J.A.; Makielski, K.R.; Litovchick, L.; Baron, J.L.; Zewe, J.P.; Wozniak, A.; Mehalek, K.R.; Korzeniewski, N.; Seneviratne, D.S.; et al. The DREAM complex mediates GIST cell quiescence and is a novel therapeutic target to enhance imatinib-induced apoptosis. *Cancer Res.* **2013**, *73*, 5120–5129. [CrossRef]
81. Guo, X.; Williams, J.G.; Schug, T.T.; Li, X. DYRK1A and DYRK3 promote cell survival through phosphorylation and activation of SIRT1. *J. Biol. Chem.* **2010**, *285*, 13223–13232. [CrossRef] [PubMed]
82. Xu, X.; Liu, Q.; Zhang, C.; Ren, S.; Xu, L.; Zhao, Z.; Dou, H.; Li, P.; Zhang, X.; Gong, Y.; et al. Inhibition of DYRK1A-EGFR axis by p53-MDM2 cascade mediates the induction of cellular senescence. *Cell Death Dis.* **2019**, *10*, 282. [CrossRef] [PubMed]
83. Ferguson, F.M.; Gray, N.S. Kinase inhibitors: The road ahead. *Nat. Rev. Drug Discov.* **2018**, *17*, 353–377. [CrossRef] [PubMed]
84. Canzonetta, C.; Mulligan, C.; Deutsch, S.; Ruf, S.; O'Doherty, A.; Lyle, R.; Borel, C.; Lin-Marq, N.; Delom, F.; Groet, J.; et al. DYRK1A-dosage imbalance perturbs NRSF/REST levels, deregulating pluripotency and embryonic stem cell fate in Down syndrome. *Am. J. Hum. Genet.* **2008**, *83*, 388–400. [CrossRef] [PubMed]
85. Radhakrishnan, A.; Nanjappa, V.; Raja, R.; Sathe, G.; Puttamallesh, V.N.; Jain, A.P.; Pinto, S.M.; Balaji, S.A.; Chavan, S.; Sahasrabuddhe, N.A.; et al. A dual specificity kinase, DYRK1A, as a potential therapeutic target for head and neck squamous cell carcinoma. *Sci. Rep.* **2016**, *6*, 36132. [CrossRef] [PubMed]
86. Zou, Y.; Yao, S.; Chen, X.; Liu, D.; Wang, J.; Yuan, X.; Rao, J.; Xiong, H.; Yu, S.; Yuan, X.; et al. LncRNA OIP5-AS1 regulates radioresistance by targeting DYRK1A through miR-369-3p in colorectal cancer cells. *Eur. J. Cell Biol.* **2018**, *97*, 369–378. [CrossRef]
87. Marcotte, R.; Sayad, A.; Brown, K.R.; Sanchez-Garcia, F.; Reimand, J.; Haider, M.; Virtanen, C.; Bradner, J.E.; Bader, G.D.; Mills, G.B.; et al. Functional genomic landscape of human breast cancer drivers, vulnerabilities, and resistance. *Cell* **2016**, *164*, 293–309. [CrossRef]
88. Baek, K.H.; Zaslavsky, A.; Lynch, R.C.; Britt, C.; Okada, Y.; Siarey, R.J.; Lensch, M.W.; Park, I.H.; Yoon, S.S.; Minami, T.; et al. Down's syndrome suppression of tumour growth and the role of the calcineurin inhibitor DSCR1. *Nature* **2009**, *459*, 1126–1130. [CrossRef]
89. Hasle, H.; Clemmensen, I.H.; Mikkelsen, M. Risks of leukaemia and solid tumours in individuals with Down's syndrome. *Lancet* **2000**, *355*, 165–169. [CrossRef]

90. Hill, D.A.; Gridley, G.; Cnattingius, S.; Mellemkjaer, L.; Linet, M.; Adami, H.O.; Olsen, J.H.; Nyren, O.; Fraumeni, J.F., Jr. Mortality and cancer incidence among individuals with Down syndrome. *Arch. Intern. Med.* **2003**, *163*, 705–711. [CrossRef]
91. Lee, P.; Bhansali, R.; Izraeli, S.; Hijiya, N.; Crispino, J.D. The biology, pathogenesis and clinical aspects of acute lymphoblastic leukemia in children with Down syndrome. *Leukemia* **2016**, *30*, 1816–1823. [CrossRef]
92. Malinge, S.; Bliss-Moreau, M.; Kirsammer, G.; Diebold, L.; Chlon, T.; Gurbuxani, S.; Crispino, J.D. Increased dosage of the chromosome 21 ortholog Dyrk1a promotes megakaryoblastic leukemia in a murine model of Down syndrome. *J. Clin. Investig.* **2012**, *122*, 948–962. [CrossRef] [PubMed]
93. Keramati, A.R.; Fathzadeh, M.; Go, G.W.; Singh, R.; Choi, M.; Faramarzi, S.; Mane, S.; Kasaei, M.; Sarajzadeh-Fard, K.; Hwa, J.; et al. A form of the metabolic syndrome associated with mutations in DYRK1B. *N. Engl. J. Med.* **2014**, *370*, 1909–1919. [CrossRef] [PubMed]
94. Becker, W. A wake-up call to quiescent cancer cells—potential use of DYRK1B inhibitors in cancer therapy. *FEBS J.* **2018**, *285*, 1203–1211. [CrossRef] [PubMed]
95. Lee, K.; Deng, X.; Friedman, E. Mirk protein kinase is a mitogen-activated protein kinase substrate that mediates survival of colon cancer cells. *Cancer Res.* **2000**, *60*, 3631–3637.
96. Chen, H.; Shen, J.; Choy, E.; Hornicek, F.J.; Shan, A.; Duan, Z. Targeting DYRK1B suppresses the proliferation and migration of liposarcoma cells. *Oncotarget* **2018**, *9*, 13154–13166. [CrossRef]
97. Mercer, S.E.; Ewton, D.Z.; Shah, S.; Naqvi, A.; Friedman, E. Mirk/Dyrk1b mediates cell survival in rhabdomyosarcomas. *Cancer Res.* **2006**, *66*, 5143–5150. [CrossRef]
98. Yang, C.; Ji, D.; Weinstein, E.J.; Choy, E.; Hornicek, F.J.; Wood, K.B.; Liu, X.; Mankin, H.; Duan, Z. The kinase Mirk is a potential therapeutic target in osteosarcoma. *Carcinogenesis* **2010**, *31*, 552–558. [CrossRef]
99. Gao, J.; Zheng, Z.; Rawal, B.; Schell, M.J.; Bepler, G.; Haura, E.B. Mirk/Dyrk1B, a novel therapeutic target, mediates cell survival in non-small cell lung cancer cells. *Cancer Biol. Ther.* **2009**, *8*, 1671–1679. [CrossRef]
100. Chen, Y.; Wang, S.; He, Z.; Sun, F.; Huang, Y.; Ni, Q.; Wang, H.; Wang, Y.; Cheng, C. Dyrk1B overexpression is associated with breast cancer growth and a poor prognosis. *Hum. Pathol.* **2017**, *66*, 48–58. [CrossRef]
101. Gao, J.; Yang, X.; Yin, P.; Hu, W.; Liao, H.; Miao, Z.; Pan, C.; Li, N. The involvement of FoxO in cell survival and chemosensitivity mediated by Mirk/Dyrk1B in ovarian cancer. *Int. J. Oncol.* **2012**, *40*, 1203–1209. [CrossRef] [PubMed]
102. Deng, X.; Ewton, D.Z.; Li, S.; Naqvi, A.; Mercer, S.E.; Landas, S.; Friedman, E. The kinase Mirk/Dyrk1B mediates cell survival in pancreatic ductal adenocarcinoma. *Cancer Res.* **2006**, *66*, 4149–4158. [CrossRef] [PubMed]
103. Deng, X.; Friedman, E. Mirk kinase inhibition blocks the in vivo growth of pancreatic cancer cells. *Genes Cancer* **2014**, *5*, 337–347. [PubMed]
104. Hu, J.; Nakhla, H.; Friedman, E. Transient arrest in a quiescent state allows ovarian cancer cells to survive suboptimal growth conditions and is mediated by both Mirk/dyrk1b and p130/RB2. *Int. J. Cancer* **2011**, *129*, 307–318. [CrossRef] [PubMed]
105. Thompson, F.H.; Nelson, M.A.; Trent, J.M.; Guan, X.Y.; Liu, Y.; Yang, J.M.; Emerson, J.; Adair, L.; Wymer, J.; Balfour, C.; et al. Amplification of 19q13.1-q13.2 sequences in ovarian cancer. G-band, FISH, and molecular studies. *Cancer Genet. Cytogenet.* **1996**, *87*, 55–62. [CrossRef]
106. Kuuselo, R.; Savinainen, K.; Azorsa, D.O.; Basu, G.D.; Karhu, R.; Tuzmen, S.; Mousses, S.; Kallioniemi, A. Intersex-like (IXL) is a cell survival regulator in pancreatic cancer with 19q13 amplification. *Cancer Res.* **2007**, *67*, 1943–1949. [CrossRef] [PubMed]
107. Gao, J.; Zhao, Y.; Lv, Y.; Chen, Y.; Wei, B.; Tian, J.; Yang, Z.; Kong, F.; Pang, J.; Liu, J.L.; et al. Mirk/Dyrk1B mediates G0/G1 to S phase cell cycle progression and cell survival involving MAPK/ERK signaling in human cancer cells. *Cancer Cell Int.* **2013**, *13*, 2. [CrossRef]
108. Tang, L.; Wang, Y.; Strom, A.; Gustafsson, J.A.; Guan, X. Lapatinib induces p27 (Kip1)-dependent G (1) arrest through both transcriptional and post-translational mechanisms. *Cell Cycle* **2013**, *12*, 2665–2674. [CrossRef]
109. Deng, X.; Hu, J.; Ewton, D.Z.; Friedman, E. Mirk/dyrk1B kinase is upregulated following inhibition of mTOR. *Carcinogenesis* **2014**, *35*, 1968–1976. [CrossRef]
110. Li, Z.; Jiang, K.; Zhu, X.; Lin, G.; Song, F.; Zhao, Y.; Piao, Y.; Liu, J.; Cheng, W.; Bi, X.; et al. Encorafenib (LGX818), a potent BRAF inhibitor, induces senescence accompanied by autophagy in BRAFV600E melanoma cells. *Cancer Lett.* **2016**, *370*, 332–344. [CrossRef]

111. Yan, Y.; Jiang, K.; Liu, P.; Zhang, X.; Dong, X.; Gao, J.; Liu, Q.; Barr, M.P.; Zhang, Q.; Hou, X.; et al. Bafilomycin A1 induces caspase-independent cell death in hepatocellular carcinoma cells via targeting of autophagy and MAPK pathways. *Sci. Rep.* **2016**, *6*, 37052. [CrossRef] [PubMed]
112. Deng, X.; Ewton, D.Z.; Pawlikowski, B.; Maimone, M.; Friedman, E. Mirk/dyrk1B is a Rho-induced kinase active in skeletal muscle differentiation. *J. Biol. Chem.* **2003**, *278*, 41347–41354. [CrossRef] [PubMed]
113. Jin, K.; Park, S.; Ewton, D.Z.; Friedman, E. The survival kinase Mirk/Dyrk1B is a downstream effector of oncogenic K-ras in pancreatic cancer. *Cancer Res.* **2007**, *67*, 7247–7255. [CrossRef]
114. Lauth, M.; Bergstrom, A.; Shimokawa, T.; Tostar, U.; Jin, Q.; Fendrich, V.; Guerra, C.; Barbacid, M.; Toftgard, R. DYRK1B-dependent autocrine-to-paracrine shift of Hedgehog signaling by mutant RAS. *Nat. Struct. Mol. Biol.* **2010**, *17*, 718–725. [CrossRef] [PubMed]
115. Singh, R.; Dhanyamraju, P.K.; Lauth, M. DYRK1B blocks canonical and promotes non-canonical Hedgehog signaling through activation of the mTOR/AKT pathway. *Oncotarget* **2017**, *8*, 833–845. [CrossRef]
116. Zou, Y.; Ewton, D.Z.; Deng, X.; Mercer, S.E.; Friedman, E. Mirk/dyrk1B kinase destabilizes cyclin D1 by phosphorylation at threonine 288. *J. Biol. Chem.* **2004**, *279*, 27790–27798. [CrossRef]
117. Deng, X.; Ewton, D.Z.; Friedman, E. Mirk/Dyrk1B maintains the viability of quiescent pancreatic cancer cells by reducing levels of reactive oxygen species. *Cancer Res.* **2009**, *69*, 3317–3324. [CrossRef]
118. Jin, K.; Ewton, D.Z.; Park, S.; Hu, J.; Friedman, E. Mirk regulates the exit of colon cancer cells from quiescence. *J. Biol. Chem.* **2009**, *284*, 22916–22925. [CrossRef]
119. Ewton, D.Z.; Hu, J.; Vilenchik, M.; Deng, X.; Luk, K.C.; Polonskaia, A.; Hoffman, A.F.; Zipf, K.; Boylan, J.F.; Friedman, E.A. Inactivation of mirk/dyrk1b kinase targets quiescent pancreatic cancer cells. *Mol. Cancer Ther.* **2011**, *10*, 2104–2114. [CrossRef]
120. Zhou, N.; Yuan, S.; Wang, R.; Zhang, W.; Chen, J.J. Role of dual specificity tyrosine-phosphorylation-regulated kinase 1B (Dyrk1B) in S-phase entry of HPV E7 expressing cells from quiescence. *Oncotarget* **2015**, *6*, 30745–30761. [CrossRef]
121. Hu, J.; Friedman, E. Depleting Mirk kinase increases cisplatin toxicity in ovarian cancer cells. *Genes Cancer* **2010**, *1*, 803–811. [CrossRef] [PubMed]
122. Hu, J.; Deng, H.; Friedman, E.A. Ovarian cancer cells, not normal cells, are damaged by Mirk/Dyrk1B kinase inhibition. *Int. J. Cancer* **2013**, *132*, 2258–2269. [CrossRef] [PubMed]
123. Li, L.; Liu, Y.; Zhang, Q.; Zhou, H.; Zhang, Y.; Yan, B. Comparison of cancer cell survival triggered by microtubule damage after turning Dyrk1B kinase on and off. *ACS Chem. Biol.* **2014**, *9*, 731–742. [CrossRef] [PubMed]
124. Davis, S.J.; Sheppard, K.E.; Pearson, R.B.; Campbell, I.G.; Gorringe, K.L.; Simpson, K.J. Functional analysis of genes in regions commonly amplified in high-grade serous and endometrioid ovarian cancer. *Clin. Cancer Res.* **2013**, *19*, 1411–1421. [CrossRef]
125. Deng, X.; Hu, J.; Cunningham, M.J.; Friedman, E. Mirk kinase inhibition targets ovarian cancer ascites. *Genes Cancer* **2014**, *5*, 201–211. [CrossRef]
126. Yoshida, S.; Yoshida, K. Multiple functions of DYRK2 in cancer and tissue development. *FEBS Lett.* **2019**, *593*, 2953–2965. [CrossRef]
127. Correa-Saez, A.; Jimenez-Izquierdo, R.; Garrido-Rodriguez, M.; Morrugares, R.; Munoz, E.; Calzado, M.A. Updating dual-specificity tyrosine-phosphorylation-regulated kinase 2 (DYRK2): Molecular basis, functions and role in diseases. *Cell Mol. Life Sci.* **2020**. [CrossRef]
128. Miller, C.T.; Aggarwal, S.; Lin, T.K.; Dagenais, S.L.; Contreras, J.I.; Orringer, M.B.; Glover, T.W.; Beer, D.G.; Lin, L. Amplification and overexpression of the dual-specificity tyrosine-(Y)-phosphorylation regulated kinase 2 (DYRK2) gene in esophageal and lung adenocarcinomas. *Cancer Res.* **2003**, *63*, 4136–4143.
129. Miller, C.T.; Moy, J.R.; Lin, L.; Schipper, M.; Normolle, D.; Brenner, D.E.; Iannettoni, M.D.; Orringer, M.B.; Beer, D.G. Gene amplification in esophageal adenocarcinomas and Barrett's with high-grade dysplasia. *Clin. Cancer Res.* **2003**, *9*, 4819–4825.
130. Koon, N.; Schneider-Stock, R.; Sarlomo-Rikala, M.; Lasota, J.; Smolkin, M.; Petroni, G.; Zaika, A.; Boltze, C.; Meyer, F.; Andersson, L.; et al. Molecular targets for tumour progression in gastrointestinal stromal tumours. *Gut* **2004**, *53*, 235–240. [CrossRef]
131. Gorringe, K.L.; Boussioutas, A.; Bowtell, D.D.; Melbourne Gastric Cancer Group, P.M.M.A.F. Novel regions of chromosomal amplification at 6p21, 5p13, and 12q14 in gastric cancer identified by array comparative genomic hybridization. *Genes Chromosom. Cancer* **2005**, *42*, 247–259. [CrossRef] [PubMed]

132. Italiano, A.; Bianchini, L.; Keslair, F.; Bonnafous, S.; Cardot-Leccia, N.; Coindre, J.M.; Dumollard, J.M.; Hofman, P.; Leroux, A.; Mainguene, C.; et al. HMGA2 is the partner of MDM2 in well-differentiated and dedifferentiated liposarcomas whereas CDK4 belongs to a distinct inconsistent amplicon. *Int. J. Cancer* **2008**, *122*, 2233–2241. [CrossRef]

133. Bonifaci, N.; Gorski, B.; Masojc, B.; Wokolorczyk, D.; Jakubowska, A.; Debniak, T.; Berenguer, A.; Serra Musach, J.; Brunet, J.; Dopazo, J.; et al. Exploring the link between germline and somatic genetic alterations in breast carcinogenesis. *PLoS ONE* **2010**, *5*, e14078. [CrossRef] [PubMed]

134. Banerjee, S.; Wei, T.; Wang, J.; Lee, J.J.; Gutierrez, H.L.; Chapman, O.; Wiley, S.E.; Mayfield, J.E.; Tandon, V.; Juarez, E.F.; et al. Inhibition of dual-specificity tyrosine phosphorylation-regulated kinase 2 perturbs 26S proteasome-addicted neoplastic progression. *Proc. Natl. Acad. Sci. USA* **2019**, *116*, 24881–24891. [CrossRef]

135. Moreno, P.; Lara-Chica, M.; Soler-Torronteras, R.; Caro, T.; Medina, M.; Alvarez, A.; Salvatierra, A.; Munoz, E.; Calzado, M.A. The expression of the ubiquitin ligase SIAH2 (Seven in Absentia Homolog 2) is increased in human lung cancer. *PLoS ONE* **2015**, *10*, e0143376. [CrossRef] [PubMed]

136. Wang, Y.; Wu, Y.; Miao, X.; Zhu, X.; Miao, X.; He, Y.; Zhong, F.; Ding, L.; Liu, J.; Tang, J.; et al. Silencing of DYRK2 increases cell proliferation but reverses CAM-DR in Non-Hodgkin's Lymphoma. *Int. J. Biol. Macromol.* **2015**, *81*, 809–817. [CrossRef] [PubMed]

137. Yan, H.; Hu, K.; Wu, W.; Li, Y.; Tian, H.; Chu, Z.; Koeffler, H.P.; Yin, D. Low expression of DYRK2 (Dual Specificity Tyrosine Phosphorylation Regulated Kinase 2) correlates with poor prognosis in colorectal cancer. *PLoS ONE* **2016**, *11*, e0159954. [CrossRef]

138. Zhang, X.; Xu, P.; Ni, W.; Fan, H.; Xu, J.; Chen, Y.; Huang, W.; Lu, S.; Liang, L.; Liu, J.; et al. Downregulated DYRK2 expression is associated with poor prognosis and Oxaliplatin resistance in hepatocellular carcinoma. *Pathol. Res. Pract.* **2016**, *212*, 162–170. [CrossRef]

139. Yokoyama-Mashima, S.; Yogosawa, S.; Kanegae, Y.; Hirooka, S.; Yoshida, S.; Horiuchi, T.; Ohashi, T.; Yanaga, K.; Saruta, M.; Oikawa, T.; et al. Forced expression of DYRK2 exerts anti-tumor effects via apoptotic induction in liver cancer. *Cancer Lett.* **2019**, *451*, 100–109. [CrossRef]

140. Shen, Y.; Zhang, L.; Wang, D.; Bao, Y.; Liu, C.; Xu, Z.; Huang, W.; Cheng, C. Regulation of glioma cells migration by DYRK2. *Neurochem. Res.* **2017**, *42*, 3093–3102. [CrossRef]

141. Mimoto, R.; Taira, N.; Takahashi, H.; Yamaguchi, T.; Okabe, M.; Uchida, K.; Miki, Y.; Yoshida, K. DYRK2 controls the epithelial-mesenchymal transition in breast cancer by degrading Snail. *Cancer Lett.* **2013**, *339*, 214–225. [CrossRef] [PubMed]

142. Yamashita, S.; Chujo, M.; Tokuishi, K.; Anami, K.; Miyawaki, M.; Yamamoto, S.; Kawahara, K. Expression of dual-specificity tyrosine-(Y)-phosphorylation-regulated kinase 2 (DYRK2) can be a favorable prognostic marker in pulmonary adenocarcinoma. *J. Thorac. Cardiovasc. Surg.* **2009**, *138*, 1303–1308. [CrossRef] [PubMed]

143. Yamashita, S.; Chujo, M.; Moroga, T.; Anami, K.; Tokuishi, K.; Miyawaki, M.; Kawano, Y.; Takeno, S.; Yamamoto, S.; Kawahara, K. DYRK2 expression may be a predictive marker for chemotherapy in non-small cell lung cancer. *Anticancer Res.* **2009**, *29*, 2753–2757.

144. Nomura, S.; Suzuki, Y.; Takahashi, R.; Terasaki, M.; Kimata, R.; Terasaki, Y.; Hamasaki, T.; Kimura, G.; Shimizu, A.; Kondo, Y. Dual-specificity tyrosine phosphorylation-regulated kinase 2 (DYRK2) as a novel marker in T1 high-grade and T2 bladder cancer patients receiving neoadjuvant chemotherapy. *BMC Urol.* **2015**, *15*, 53. [CrossRef] [PubMed]

145. Ito, D.; Yogosawa, S.; Mimoto, R.; Hirooka, S.; Horiuchi, T.; Eto, K.; Yanaga, K.; Yoshida, K. Dual-specificity tyrosine-regulated kinase 2 is a suppressor and potential prognostic marker for liver metastasis of colorectal cancer. *Cancer Sci.* **2017**, *108*, 1565–1573. [CrossRef]

146. Yamaguchi, N.; Mimoto, R.; Yanaihara, N.; Imawari, Y.; Hirooka, S.; Okamoto, A.; Yoshida, K. DYRK2 regulates epithelial-mesenchymal-transition and chemosensitivity through Snail degradation in ovarian serous adenocarcinoma. *Tumour Biol.* **2015**, *36*, 5913–5923. [CrossRef] [PubMed]

147. Enomoto, Y.; Yamashita, S.; Yoshinaga, Y.; Fukami, Y.; Miyahara, S.; Nabeshima, K.; Iwasaki, A. Downregulation of DYRK2 can be a predictor of recurrence in early stage breast cancer. *Tumour Biol.* **2014**, *35*, 11021–11025. [CrossRef]

148. Guo, X.; Wang, X.; Wang, Z.; Banerjee, S.; Yang, J.; Huang, L.; Dixon, J.E. Site-specific proteasome phosphorylation controls cell proliferation and tumorigenesis. *Nat. Cell Biol.* **2016**, *18*, 202–212. [CrossRef]

149. Park, C.S.; Lewis, A.H.; Chen, T.J.; Bridges, C.S.; Shen, Y.; Suppipat, K.; Puppi, M.; Tomolonis, J.A.; Pang, P.D.; Mistretta, T.A.; et al. A KLF4-DYRK2-mediated pathway regulating self-renewal in CML stem cells. *Blood* **2019**, *134*, 1960–1972. [CrossRef]
150. Kumamoto, T.; Yamada, K.; Yoshida, S.; Aoki, K.; Hirooka, S.; Eto, K.; Yanaga, K.; Yoshida, K. Impairment of DYRK2 by DNMT1mediated transcription augments carcinogenesis in human colorectal cancer. *Int. J. Oncol.* **2020**, *56*, 1529–1539. [CrossRef]
151. Perez, M.; Garcia-Limones, C.; Zapico, I.; Marina, A.; Schmitz, M.L.; Munoz, E.; Calzado, M.A. Mutual regulation between SIAH2 and DYRK2 controls hypoxic and genotoxic signaling pathways. *J. Mol. Cell Biol.* **2012**, *4*, 316–330. [CrossRef] [PubMed]
152. Ryu, K.J.; Park, S.M.; Park, S.H.; Kim, I.K.; Han, H.; Kim, H.J.; Kim, S.H.; Hong, K.S.; Kim, H.; Kim, M.; et al. p38 stabilizes Snail by suppressing DYRK2-mediated phosphorylation that is required for GSK3beta-betaTrCP-induced Snail degradation. *Cancer Res.* **2019**, *79*, 4135–4148. [CrossRef] [PubMed]
153. Mehnert, M.; Ciuffa, R.; Frommelt, F.; Uliana, F.; van Drogen, A.; Ruminski, K.; Gstaiger, M.; Aebersold, R. Multi-layered proteomic analyses decode compositional and functional effects of cancer mutations on kinase complexes. *Nat. Commun.* **2020**, *11*, 3563. [CrossRef] [PubMed]
154. Jung, H.Y.; Wang, X.; Jun, S.; Park, J.I. Dyrk2-associated EDD-DDB1-VprBP E3 ligase inhibits telomerase by TERT degradation. *J. Biol. Chem.* **2013**, *288*, 7252–7262. [CrossRef] [PubMed]
155. Mimoto, R.; Nihira, N.T.; Hirooka, S.; Takeyama, H.; Yoshida, K. Diminished DYRK2 sensitizes hormone receptor-positive breast cancer to everolimus by the escape from degrading mTOR. *Cancer Lett.* **2017**, *384*, 27–38. [CrossRef] [PubMed]
156. Ong, S.S.; Goktug, A.N.; Elias, A.; Wu, J.; Saunders, D.; Chen, T. Stability of the human pregnane X receptor is regulated by E3 ligase UBR5 and serine/threonine kinase DYRK2. *Biochem. J.* **2014**, *459*, 193–203. [CrossRef]
157. Yeh, C.H.; Bellon, M.; Nicot, C. FBXW7: A critical tumor suppressor of human cancers. *Mol. Cancer* **2018**, *17*, 115. [CrossRef]
158. Imawari, Y.; Mimoto, R.; Hirooka, S.; Morikawa, T.; Takeyama, H.; Yoshida, K. Downregulation of dual-specificity tyrosine-regulated kinase 2 promotes tumor cell proliferation and invasion by enhancing cyclin-dependent kinase 14 expression in breast cancer. *Cancer Sci.* **2018**, *109*, 363–372. [CrossRef]
159. Hossain, D.; Javadi Esfehani, Y.; Das, A.; Tsang, W.Y. Cep78 controls centrosome homeostasis by inhibiting EDD-DYRK2-DDB1 (Vpr) (BP). *EMBO Rep.* **2017**, *18*, 632–644. [CrossRef]
160. Yamamoto, T.; Taira Nihira, N.; Yogosawa, S.; Aoki, K.; Takeda, H.; Sawasaki, T.; Yoshida, K. Interaction between RNF8 and DYRK2 is required for the recruitment of DNA repair molecules to DNA double-strand breaks. *FEBS Lett.* **2017**, *591*, 842–853. [CrossRef]
161. Mimoto, R.; Imawari, Y.; Hirooka, S.; Takeyama, H.; Yoshida, K. Impairment of DYRK2 augments stem-like traits by promoting KLF4 expression in breast cancer. *Oncogene* **2017**, *36*, 1862–1872. [CrossRef] [PubMed]
162. Banerjee, S.; Ji, C.; Mayfield, J.E.; Goel, A.; Xiao, J.; Dixon, J.E.; Guo, X. Ancient drug curcumin impedes 26S proteasome activity by direct inhibition of dual-specificity tyrosine-regulated kinase 2. *Proc. Natl. Acad. Sci. USA* **2018**, *115*, 8155–8160. [CrossRef] [PubMed]
163. Geiger, J.N.; Knudsen, G.T.; Panek, L.; Pandit, A.K.; Yoder, M.D.; Lord, K.A.; Creasy, C.L.; Burns, B.M.; Gaines, P.; Dillon, S.B.; et al. mDYRK3 kinase is expressed selectively in late erythroid progenitor cells and attenuates colony-forming unit-erythroid development. *Blood* **2001**, *97*, 901–910. [CrossRef] [PubMed]
164. Sargent, L.M.; Ensell, M.X.; Ostvold, A.C.; Baldwin, K.T.; Kashon, M.L.; Lowry, D.T.; Senft, J.R.; Jefferson, A.M.; Johnson, R.C.; Li, Z.; et al. Chromosomal changes in high- and low-invasive mouse lung adenocarcinoma cell strains derived from early passage mouse lung adenocarcinoma cell strains. *Toxicol. Appl. Pharmacol.* **2008**, *233*, 81–91. [CrossRef]
165. Yamanaka, R.; Arao, T.; Yajima, N.; Tsuchiya, N.; Homma, J.; Tanaka, R.; Sano, M.; Oide, A.; Sekijima, M.; Nishio, K. Identification of expressed genes characterizing long-term survival in malignant glioma patients. *Oncogene* **2006**, *25*, 5994–6002. [CrossRef]
166. Kang, G.; Hwang, W.C.; Do, I.G.; Wang, K.; Kang, S.Y.; Lee, J.; Park, S.H.; Park, J.O.; Kang, W.K.; Jang, J.; et al. Exome sequencing identifies early gastric carcinoma as an early stage of advanced gastric cancer. *PLoS ONE* **2013**, *8*, e82770. [CrossRef]
167. Ma, F.; Zhu, Y.; Liu, X.; Zhou, Q.; Hong, X.; Qu, C.; Feng, X.; Zhang, Y.; Ding, Q.; Zhao, J.; et al. Dual-Specificity Tyrosine Phosphorylation-Regulated Kinase 3 loss activates purine metabolism and promotes hepatocellular carcinoma progression. *Hepatology* **2019**, *70*, 1785–1803. [CrossRef]

168. Owusu, M.; Bannauer, P.; Ferreira da Silva, J.; Mourikis, T.P.; Jones, A.; Majek, P.; Caldera, M.; Wiedner, M.; Lardeau, C.H.; Mueller, A.C.; et al. Mapping the human kinome in response to DNA damage. *Cell Rep.* **2019**, *26*, 555–563. [CrossRef]
169. Nguyen, T.L.; Duchon, A.; Manousopoulou, A.; Loaec, N.; Villiers, B.; Pani, G.; Karatas, M.; Mechling, A.E.; Harsan, L.A.; Limanton, E.; et al. Correction of cognitive deficits in mouse models of Down syndrome by a pharmacological inhibitor of DYRK1A. *Dis. Model. Mech.* **2018**, *11*. [CrossRef]
170. Neumann, F.; Gourdain, S.; Albac, C.; Dekker, A.D.; Bui, L.C.; Dairou, J.; Schmitz-Afonso, I.; Hue, N.; Rodrigues-Lima, F.; Delabar, J.M.; et al. DYRK1A inhibition and cognitive rescue in a Down syndrome mouse model are induced by new fluoro-DANDY derivatives. *Sci. Rep.* **2018**, *8*, 2859. [CrossRef]
171. Kim, H.; Lee, K.S.; Kim, A.K.; Choi, M.; Choi, K.; Kang, M.; Chi, S.W.; Lee, M.S.; Lee, J.S.; Lee, S.Y.; et al. A chemical with proven clinical safety rescues Down-syndrome-related phenotypes in through DYRK1A inhibition. *Dis. Model. Mech.* **2016**, *9*, 839–848. [CrossRef] [PubMed]
172. de la Torre, R.; de Sola, S.; Hernandez, G.; Farre, M.; Pujol, J.; Rodriguez, J.; Espadaler, J.M.; Langohr, K.; Cuenca-Royo, A.; Principe, A.; et al. Safety and efficacy of cognitive training plus epigallocatechin-3-gallate in young adults with Down's syndrome (TESDAD): A double-blind, randomised, placebo-controlled, phase 2 trial. *Lancet Neurol.* **2016**, *15*, 801–810. [CrossRef]
173. Belgardt, B.F.; Lammert, E. DYRK1A: A promising drug target for islet transplant-based Diabetes therapies. *Diabetes* **2016**, *65*, 1496–1498. [CrossRef]
174. Ionescu, A.; Dufrasne, F.; Gelbcke, M.; Jabin, I.; Kiss, R.; Lamoral-Theys, D. DYRK1A kinase inhibitors with emphasis on cancer. *Mini Rev. Med. Chem.* **2012**, *12*, 1315–1329. [PubMed]
175. Jarhad, D.B.; Mashelkar, K.K.; Kim, H.R.; Noh, M.; Jeong, L.S. Dual-Specificity Tyrosine Phosphorylation-Regulated Kinase 1A (DYRK1A) inhibitors as potential therapeutics. *J. Med. Chem.* **2018**, *61*, 9791–9810. [CrossRef]
176. Nguyen, T.L.; Fruit, C.; Herault, Y.; Meijer, L.; Besson, T. Dual-specificity tyrosine phosphorylation-regulated kinase 1A (DYRK1A) inhibitors: A survey of recent patent literature. *Expert Opin. Ther. Pat.* **2017**, *27*, 1183–1199. [CrossRef]
177. Yang, C.S.; Wang, X.; Lu, G.; Picinich, S.C. Cancer prevention by tea: Animal studies, molecular mechanisms and human relevance. *Nat. Rev. Cancer* **2009**, *9*, 429–439. [CrossRef]
178. Bain, J.; Plater, L.; Elliott, M.; Shpiro, N.; Hastie, C.J.; McLauchlan, H.; Klevernic, I.; Arthur, J.S.; Alessi, D.R.; Cohen, P. The selectivity of protein kinase inhibitors: A further update. *Biochem. J.* **2007**, *408*, 297–315. [CrossRef]
179. Gockler, N.; Jofre, G.; Papadopoulos, C.; Soppa, U.; Tejedor, F.J.; Becker, W. Harmine specifically inhibits protein kinase DYRK1A and interferes with neurite formation. *FEBS J.* **2009**, *276*, 6324–6337. [CrossRef]
180. Cao, M.R.; Li, Q.; Liu, Z.L.; Liu, H.H.; Wang, W.; Liao, X.L.; Pan, Y.L.; Jiang, J.W. Harmine induces apoptosis in HepG2 cells via mitochondrial signaling pathway. *Hepatobiliary Pancreat. Dis. Int.* **2011**, *10*, 599–604. [CrossRef]
181. Uhl, K.L.; Schultz, C.R.; Geerts, D.; Bachmann, A.S. Harmine, a dual-specificity tyrosine phosphorylation-regulated kinase (DYRK) inhibitor induces caspase-mediated apoptosis in neuroblastoma. *Cancer Cell Int.* **2018**, *18*, 82. [CrossRef] [PubMed]
182. Atteya, R.; Ashour, M.E.; Ibrahim, E.E.; Farag, M.A.; El-Khamisy, S.F. Chemical screening identifies the beta-Carboline alkaloid harmine to be synergistically lethal with doxorubicin. *Mech. Ageing Dev.* **2017**, *161*, 141–148. [CrossRef] [PubMed]
183. Frederick, R.; Bruyere, C.; Vancraeynest, C.; Reniers, J.; Meinguet, C.; Pochet, L.; Backlund, A.; Masereel, B.; Kiss, R.; Wouters, J. Novel trisubstituted harmine derivatives with original in vitro anticancer activity. *J. Med. Chem.* **2012**, *55*, 6489–6501. [CrossRef]
184. Li, S.; Wang, A.; Gu, F.; Wang, Z.; Tian, C.; Qian, Z.; Tang, L.; Gu, Y. Novel harmine derivatives for tumor targeted therapy. *Oncotarget* **2015**, *6*, 8988–9001. [CrossRef] [PubMed]
185. Marx, S.; Bodart, L.; Tumanov, N.; Wouters, J. Design and synthesis of a new soluble natural beta-carboline derivative for preclinical study by intravenous injection. *Int. J. Mol. Sci.* **2019**, *20*, 1491. [CrossRef] [PubMed]
186. Ogawa, Y.; Nonaka, Y.; Goto, T.; Ohnishi, E.; Hiramatsu, T.; Kii, I.; Yoshida, M.; Ikura, T.; Onogi, H.; Shibuya, H.; et al. Development of a novel selective inhibitor of the Down syndrome-related kinase Dyrk1A. *Nat. Commun.* **2010**, *1*, 86. [CrossRef] [PubMed]

187. Kettle, J.G.; Ballard, P.; Bardelle, C.; Cockerill, M.; Colclough, N.; Critchlow, S.E.; Debreczeni, J.; Fairley, G.; Fillery, S.; Graham, M.A.; et al. Discovery and optimization of a novel series of Dyrk1B kinase inhibitors to explore a MEK resistance hypothesis. *J. Med. Chem.* **2015**, *58*, 2834–2844. [CrossRef]
188. Karaman, M.W.; Herrgard, S.; Treiber, D.K.; Gallant, P.; Atteridge, C.E.; Campbell, B.T.; Chan, K.W.; Ciceri, P.; Davis, M.I.; Edeen, P.T.; et al. A quantitative analysis of kinase inhibitor selectivity. *Nat. Biotechnol.* **2008**, *26*, 127–132. [CrossRef]
189. Allegretti, P.A.; Horton, T.M.; Abdolazimi, Y.; Moeller, H.P.; Yeh, B.; Caffet, M.; Michel, G.; Smith, M.; Annes, J.P. Generation of highly potent DYRK1A-dependent inducers of human beta-cell replication via multi-dimensional compound optimization. *Bioorg. Med. Chem.* **2019**, *28*, 115193. [CrossRef]
190. Deshmukh, V.; O'Green, A.L.; Bossard, C.; Seo, T.; Lamangan, L.; Ibanez, M.; Ghias, A.; Lai, C.; Do, L.; Cho, S.; et al. Modulation of the Wnt pathway through inhibition of CLK2 and DYRK1A by lorecivivint as a novel, potentially disease-modifying approach for knee osteoarthritis treatment. *Osteoarthr. Cartil.* **2019**, *27*, 1347–1360. [CrossRef]

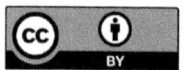

© 2020 by the authors. Licensee MDPI, Basel, Switzerland. This article is an open access article distributed under the terms and conditions of the Creative Commons Attribution (CC BY) license (http://creativecommons.org/licenses/by/4.0/).

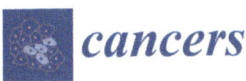

Article

The Relevance of the SH2 Domain for c-Src Functionality in Triple-Negative Breast Cancer Cells

Víctor Mayoral-Varo [1,†], María Pilar Sánchez-Bailón [1,2,†], Annarica Calcabrini [1,3,†], Marta García-Hernández [4], Valerio Frezza [4], María Elena Martín [4], Víctor M. González [4] and Jorge Martín-Pérez [1,5,*]

1. Instituto de Investigaciones Biomédicas A, Sols/Dpto. Bioquímica (CSIC/UAM), Arturo Duperier 4, 28029 Madrid, Spain; vmayoral@iib.uam.es (V.M.-V.); Pilar.Sanchez@mdc-berlin.de (M.P.S.-B.); annarica.calcabrini@iss.it (A.C.)
2. Max Delbrück Center for Molecular Medicine (MDC), Robert-Rössle-Str. 10, 13092 Berlin, Germany
3. National Center for Drug Research and Evaluation, Istituto Superiore di Sanità, Viale Regina Elena 299, 00161 Rome, Italy
4. Grupo de Aptámeros, Servicio Bioquímica-Investigación, IRYCIS-Hospital Ramón y Cajal. Ctra. Colmenar Viejo km 9100, 28034 Madrid, Spain; marta.garcia@hrc.es (M.G.-H.); valerio.frezza@hrc.es (V.F.); m.elena.martin@hrc.es (M.E.M.); victor.m.gonzalez@hrc.es (V.M.G.)
5. Instituto de Investigaciones Sanitarias del Hospital La Paz (IdiPAZ), Paseo de la Castellana 261, 28046 Madrid, Spain
* Correspondence: jorge.martin.perez@csic.es or jmartin@iib.uam.es; Tel.: +34-91-585-4416; Fax: +34-91-585-4401
† The authors have equally contributed to this work.

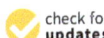

Citation: Mayoral-Varo, V.; Sánchez-Bailón, M.P.; Calcabrini, A.; García-Hernández, M.; Frezza, V.; Martín, M.E.; González, V.M.; Martín-Pérez, J. The Relevance of the SH2 Domain for c-Src Functionality in Triple-Negative Breast Cancer Cells. *Cancers* 2021, 13, 462. https://doi.org/10.3390/cancers13030462

Academic Editor: Francisco M. Vega
Received: 30 December 2020
Accepted: 19 January 2021
Published: 26 January 2021

Publisher's Note: MDPI stays neutral with regard to jurisdictional claims in published maps and institutional affiliations.

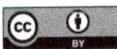

Copyright: © 2021 by the authors. Licensee MDPI, Basel, Switzerland. This article is an open access article distributed under the terms and conditions of the Creative Commons Attribution (CC BY) license (https://creativecommons.org/licenses/by/4.0/).

Simple Summary: Triple-Negative breast cancers (TNBC) have not specific therapeutic targets and are considered the most aggressive mammary tumors. c-Src controls several cellular processes: proliferation, differentiation, survival, motility, and angiogenesis. Alteration of c-Src functionality, by increasing its expression and/or its kinase activity, is associated to progression and metastasis of tumors in mammary gland, pancreas, colon, brain, and lung. However, c-Src tyrosine kinase inhibitors alone are not fully clinically effective, suggesting that c-Src adapter SH2/SH3 domains may be important. We questioned whether the SH2-c-Src domain is relevant for tumorigenicity of TNBC SUM159 and MDA-MB-231 human cell lines. Conditional expression of SH2 and SH3 inactivating mutants in these TNBC cells, or transfection of aptamers directed to SH2, allowed us to show that this domain is required for their tumorigenesis. Therefore, the SH2-c-Src domain could be a promising therapeutic target that, combined with c-Src kinase inhibitors, may represent a novel therapeutic strategy for TNBC patients.

Abstract: The role of Src family kinases (SFKs) in human tumors has been always associated with tyrosine kinase activity and much less attention has been given to the SH2 and SH3 adapter domains. Here, we studied the role of the c-Src-SH2 domain in triple-negative breast cancer (TNBC). To this end, SUM159PT and MDA-MB-231 human cell lines were employed as model systems. These cells conditionally expressed, under tetracycline control (Tet-On system), a c-Src variant with point-inactivating mutation of the SH2 adapter domain (R175L). The expression of this mutant reduced the self-renewal capability of the enriched population of breast cancer stem cells (BCSCs), demonstrating the importance of the SH2 adapter domain of c-Src in the mammary gland carcinogenesis. In addition, the analysis of anchorage-independent growth, proliferation, migration, and invasiveness, all processes associated with tumorigenesis, showed that the SH2 domain of c-Src plays a very relevant role in their regulation. Furthermore, the transfection of two different aptamers directed to SH2-c-Src in both SUM159PT and MDA-MB-231 cells induced inhibition of their proliferation, migration, and invasiveness, strengthening the hypothesis that this domain is highly involved in TNBC tumorigenesis. Therefore, the SH2 domain of c-Src could be a promising therapeutic target and combined treatments with inhibitors of c-Src kinase enzymatic activity may represent a new therapeutic strategy for patients with TNBC, whose prognosis is currently very negative.

Keywords: triple-negative breast cancer (TNBC); c-Src; SH2 domain; inactivating point mutation; aptamers

1. Introduction

The Src family of non-receptor tyrosine kinases (SFKs) is composed of nine members, and it has a modular structure, containing the SH2 and SH3 (Src homology domains 2 and 3), which are involved in protein-protein interactions with tyrosine phosphorylated proteins or with proteins containing proline rich sequences, respectively [1,2]. These two domains are also present in many other adapter and regulatory proteins, and facilitate the formation of intracellular signaling complexes [3]. While the activity of c-Src, the prototype of the SFKs, is mainly modulated by phosphorylation, the SH2 and SH3 domains are also required for the conformational changes associated with its cellular distribution, kinase activity, and cell functionality [4–7]. c-Src plays a key regulatory role of many cellular processes, including proliferation, differentiation, survival, motility, and angiogenesis. Therefore, alteration of c-Src functionality, by increasing its expression and/or its kinase activity, has been associated to progression and metastasis of tumors in the mammary gland, pancreas, colon, and lung [1,5–8].

Breast tumors are diverse, and they have been classified according to their genetic and histological characteristics [9,10]. Among them, the basal triple negative breast cancer (TNBC) does not express estrogen and progesterone receptors (ER^-, PR^-), nor overexpresses HER2, and usually has an inactive p53 mutant [10–12]. TNBCs do not have specific therapeutic targets and are considered the most aggressive mammary tumors, with a tendency to metastasize mainly into the lung, brain, and bone [13,14].

Experimentally, inhibitors of c-Src kinase activity, or its suppression, block proliferation, survival, migration, and invasion, as well as tumorigenesis in vivo [15–17]. However, inhibitors of c-Src tyrosine kinase activity alone do not appear to be fully clinically effective [8,18], suggesting that its adapter domains may play an important role for c-Src functionality in tumorigenesis. In this context, expression of c-Src with point-inactivating mutations at either SH2 or SH3 domains, which conferred stimulation of its kinase activity, blocks the prolactin-induce activation of Jak2 in MCF7 [19]. In mouse SYF fibroblasts, expression of c-Src-R175L prevents Fak auto-phosphorylation (pY397), malignant transformation, motility defects, and focal adhesion formation, indicating the relevance of the SH2 domain of c-Src [20]. The SH2 domain of c-Src interacts with the pY397-Fak facilitating the open conformation of c-Src that activates its kinase activity and, in turn, protects pY397-Fak from phosphatases [21,22]. In addition, c-Src phosphorylates Fak on several tyrosine residues, thus promoting cellular signaling and tumor progression [6,23,24].

Small molecules, such as inhibitory peptides and non-peptides, have been used to block the SH3/SH2 domains of c-Src [25–29] with a relative success. Aptamers are single stranded oligonucleotides (DNA or RNA) that bind to proteins with high affinity and specificity, blocking their functionality. They have been used for diagnosis and therapy in several infectious, inflammation, vascular diseases, as well as in other pathologies including breast cancer [30–32].

Here, we analyzed the role of the adapter domain of c-Src in the in vitro tumorigenic properties of SUM159PT (from now on SUM159) and MDA-MB-231 TNBC cell lines. We found that the conditional expression of c-Src variants with suppression of SH2 functionality caused profound effects on the behavior of these triple negative cell lines. Consistently, two different aptamers directed to SH2-c-Src inhibited proliferation, migration, and invasiveness of both SUM159 and MDA-MB-231 cells. Thus, the SH2-c-Src domain appears to play a crucial role in TNBC tumorigenesis.

2. Results

2.1. c-Src Variants of the SH2 Adapter Domain

In the studies presented here we used two different triple negative breast cancer (TNBC) cell lines, SUM159 and MDA-MB-231. Although SUM159 and MDA-MB-231 are both Basal-Mesenchymal TNBC cell lines with a spindle phenotype, they show differences in deleted and mutated genes. Furthermore, previously published data from the laboratory using both SUM159 and MDA-MB-231 cells showed that they differ in some signaling responses [16]. All together, we can conclude that even if both are representing TNBC cells, their cellular behavior could diverge.

To analyze the role of the SH2 adapter-domain of c-Src in the in vitro tumorigenic properties of SUM159 and MDA-MB-231 cell lines, we conditionally expressed (Tet-On system) chicken c-Src variants with point mutations inactivating this domain (Figure 1A). It should be pointed out that chicken c-Src could replace human c-Src functionality [16], as they have more than 94% identity at the amino acid sequence [33]. Nevertheless, the EC10 mouse monoclonal antibody (Millipore, no. 05-185) specifically recognizes chicken c-Src, making it possible to determine by Western blot (WB) the expression of c-Src variants in the presence of the endogenous human c-Src of SUM159 and MDA-MB-231 cells.

We used the R175L point mutation (SH2) affecting intra- and inter-molecular c-Src interactions, preventing c-Src from being in the close configuration, consequently, c-Src-R175L has a constitutive tyrosine-kinase activity [34]. The c-Src-SH2-SH3 double variant (c-Src-W118A-R175L) [19], which also has a constitutive tyrosine-kinase activity, was also employed to test for the impact of the SH3 domain in SH2 functionality. To avoid undesirable effects due to the insertion of the c-Src variants in the genome of the cells upon transfection, each cell line was made of a pool of, at least, three positive independent clones. Since we are studying the role of SH2 domain in TNBCs SUM159 and MDA-MB-231, we expressed the wild type c-Src (c-Src-wt) to compare the results obtained with the SH2 mutant. As observed in Figure 1B, the chicken c-Src variants were induced by the addition of Doxy to culture media (0.2 µg/mL, 72 h) at similar levels in SUM159 and MDA-MB-231. Analyses of the degree of activation of c-Src chicken variants by determining the autophosphorylation at Y418 showed that the expression of c-Src-wt slightly increased the levels of phosphorylation at Y418 in both cell lines. In contrast and consistent with the scheme presented in Figure 1A, expression of both c-Src-R175L and c-Src-W118A/R175L showed a high degree of phosphorylation at Y418, which agrees with the stimulated tyrosine kinase activity of these mutants (Figure 1B).

SFKs expression is associated with a different outcome in breast cancer patients [35]. Thus, we decided to determine the protein levels of several SFKs members in both cell models by WB. Expression of c-Src and Fyn was higher in SUM159 than in MDA-MB-231 cells, while the contrary was observed for c-Yes. Regarding Lyn protein, SUM159 cells showed higher Lyn A levels than MDA-MB-231, whereas the opposite situation was observed for Lyn B expression (Figure 1C). Expression of c-Src variants did not alter that of endogenous Src-kinases (data not shown). Therefore, we used two TNBC cell lines that exhibit a different expression pattern of SFKs, which better represent the variability of TNBC.

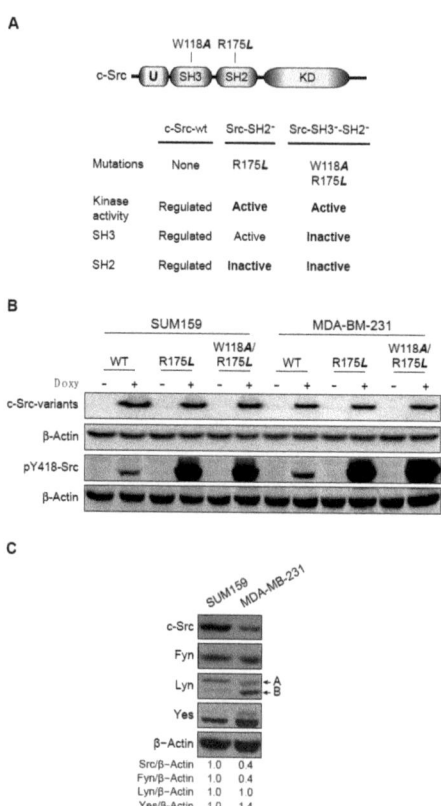

Figure 1. c-Src variants and expression of Src kinases in SUM159 and MDA-MB-231 cells. (**A**) Schematic design of c-Src and the variants employed in this study, which were conditionally expressed (Tet-On system) upon addition of doxycycline (Doxy, 0.2 µg/mL) to the cell culture. The R175L mutation inhibits both intra- and inter-molecular interactions of the SH2 domain of c-Src. The W118A/R175L double mutation inhibits both the SH2 and SH3 domains. (**B**) Induction of chicken c-Src variants by Doxy was detected by Western blot (WB) using the EC10 mouse monoclonal antibody that specifically recognizes chicken c-Src and β-Actin as a loading control. (**C**) Comparative expression of Src kinases in SUM159 versus MDA-MB-231 cells determined by WB. Actin was used as a loading control and the ratio of kinase/actin in SUM159 was considered as 1.

2.2. SH2 Domain of c-Src Is Important for In Vitro Breast Cancer Stem Cell-Renewal

Within a tumor, there is a small portion of the tumor-mass (1–2%) derived from the stem-cell population that by mutations acquired tumorigenic properties. These breast cancer stem cells (BCSCs) are slow dividing and capable of regenerating a tumor upon transplantation in nude mice [35]. To determine the self-renewal capacity of the enriched population of BCSCs, we performed the mammosphere formation assay during three generations to define, at the third generation, the sphere formation efficiency (SFE, see Materials and Methods) [36–38]. We observed that SFE increased in all SUM159 and MDA-MB-231 cells expressing c-Src variants, indicating the enrichment of BCSCs population (Figures S1 and S2). Nevertheless, it should be noticed that SUM159 contained higher numbers of mammospheres than MDA-MB-231. We then analyzed the effect of c-Src variants described above (Figure 1A) on the BCSCs renewal ability of each cell line SUM159 or MDA-MB-231 expressing c-Src-mutants and compared it with the c-Src-wt. The functionality of SH2 and SH3 adapter domains appeared to be relevant for SFE, as both c-Src-R175L and c-Src-W11A/R175L significantly reduced the self-renewal of the enriched population of MDA-MB-231 and SUM159-BCSCs (Figure 2A).

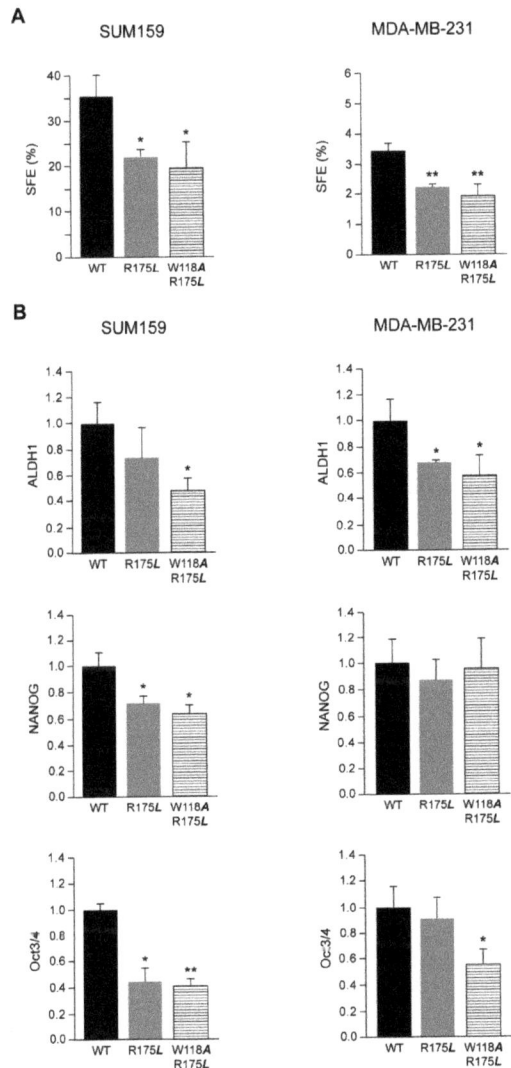

Figure 2. Role of c-Src variants in the self-renewal of breast cancer stem cells (BCSCs) derived from SUM159 and MDA-MB-231. The evaluation of self-renewal was determined by the sphere formation efficiency (SFE) in the enriched subpopulation of BCSCs derived from SUM159 and MDA-MB-231 (**A**). The SFE was measured at the third generation of mammospheres (see Materials and Methods). Each experiment was measured in triplicates ($n = 3$) and repeated three times. Results were expressed as a percentage of the mean ± standard deviation (SD). The statistical significance is referred to those obtained from c-Src-wt, * $p < 0.5$, ** $p < 0.01$. Quantitative analyses of stem cell markers ALDH1, NANOG, and Oct3/4 expression by WB in SUM159 and MDA-MB-231 cells conditionally expressing c-Src variants (**B**). Results represented data obtained from three independent WB ($n = 3$) using β-Actin as a loading control expressed as a percentage of the mean ± SD, and were referred to those obtained from cells expressing c-Src-wt considered as 1. The statistical significance is referred to cells expressing c-Src-wt, * $p < 0.5$, ** $p < 0.01$.

We have also found that the induction of SrcDN (c-Src-K295M/Y527F, which is devoid of catalytic activity but with functional SH2 and SH3 domains), a functional mirror image of c-Src-W118A/R175L, significantly reduced SFE in both SUM159 and MDA-MB-231. Furthermore, the endogenous c-Src function is required for SFE in MDA-MB-231 cells, as its conditional suppression [16] inhibited SFE (Figure S3).

Altogether, the findings indicate that the three domains are necessary for self-renewal, as the alteration of only one of them reduced the sphere formation ability of both TNBC cells.

Consistent with the reduction of the enriched population of BCSCs induced by the expression of c-Src-R175L and c-Src-W118A/R175L c-Src mutants in both SUM159 and MDA-MB-231 cells, we analyzed the expression of ALDH1 by WB, a stem cell marker [36–39]. The results showed that in the MDA-MB-231 disruption of the functionality of c-Src SH2 domain by R175L mutation inhibited the ALDH1 level as compared to c-Src-wt (Figure 2B and Figure S4). Disruption of the functionality of c-Src SH2 and SH3 domains by the double mutant c-Src-W118A/R175L clearly reduced ALDH1 levels in either SUM159 or MDA-MB-231 (Figure 2B and Figure S4). Expression of NANOG and Oct3/4 was reduced in SUM159 cells expressing c-Src-R175L and c-Src-W118A/R175L mutants as compared to the expression of c-Src-wt (Figure 2B and Figure S4). In contrast, in MDA-MB-231, only the induction of c-Src-W118A/R175L mutant reduced the levels of Oct3/4, while none of the c-Src mutants altered the expression of NANOG (Figure 2B and Figure S4). Furthermore, the levels of NANOG and Oct3/4 were reduced in SUM159 and MDA-MB-231 cells following SrcDN expression or suppression of the endogenous c-Src (Figure S3).

Collectively, these results indicate that the SH2-c-Src domain is relevant for renewal of the enriched population of BCSCs in SUM159 and MDA-MB-231 cells.

2.3. Role of Adapter Domains in Anchorage-Independent Growth

Anchorage-independent growth correlates with cellular tumorigenic and metastatic potential, a typical feature of in vivo TNBC aggressive phenotype. Thus, we analyzed the role of the SH2 adapter domain of c-Src in this event by determining cellular growth in soft agar. In SUM159 cells, induction of the c-Src-R175L mutant did not alter the colony formation as compared to the wild type. In contrast, mutation of the SH2 and SH3 domains together appeared to be relevant for colony formation in soft agar, as expression of c-Src-W118A/R175L significantly reduced the number of colonies in the agar (Figure 3A and Figure S5). In MDA-MB-231 cells, Doxy induction of either c-Src-R175L or c-Src-W118A/R175L mutants significantly inhibited soft-agar colony formation, as compared to c-Src-wt (Figure 3A and Figure S5). Concurrently, these results support the role of the SH2-c-Src domain in anchorage-independent growth.

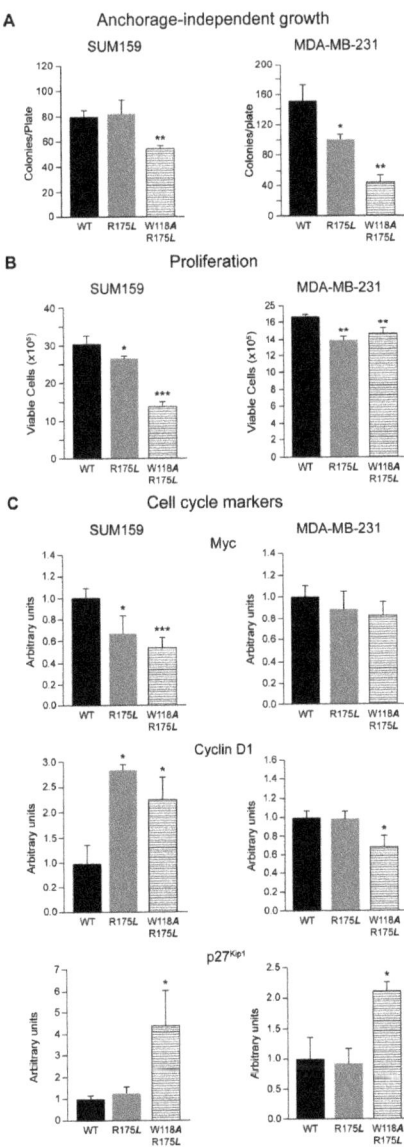

Figure 3. Modulation of anchorage-independent growth and cell proliferation by expression of c-Src variants in SUM159 and MDA-MB-231 cells. (**A**) Colony formation in soft-agar was employed to determine the effect of c-Src variants expression in SUM159 and MDA-MB-231 cells in anchorage-independent growth (see Materials and Methods). Each experiment was measured in triplicates ($n = 3$) and repeated three times. Results were expressed as the mean ± SD of the number of colonies/plate, * $p < 0.5$, ** $p < 0.01$. (**B**) Cell proliferation of SUM159 and MDA-MB-231 expressing c-Src variants was determined by the trypan blue exclusion assay (see Materials and Methods), * $p < 0.5$, ** $p < 0.01$, *** $p < 0.001$. (**C**) Quantitative analyses of cell proliferation markers Myc, cyclin D1, and p27 expression by WB in SUM159 and MDA-MB-231 cells conditionally expressing c-Src variants. Results represented data obtained from three independent WB ($n = 3$) using either β-Actin, α-Tubulin, or GAPDH as a loading control expressed as a percentage of the mean ± SD, and were referred to those obtained from cells expressing c-Src-wt considered as 1. The statistical significance is referred to cells expressing c-Src-wt, * $p < 0.5$, *** $p < 0.001$.

2.4. c-Src-SH2 Domain Modulates Cellular Proliferation

Several data show the relevance of c-Src in cell proliferation and survival [1]. Therefore, we evaluated the effect of c-Src variants in SUM159 and MDA-MB-231 cell proliferation. In SUM159, induction of the c-Src-R175L and c-Src-W118A/R175L significantly reduced cell proliferation compared to c-Src-wt (Figure 3B). Similar results were obtained in MDA-MB-231 cells. Nevertheless, the reduction of cell proliferation observed in SUM159 was higher than in MDA-MB-231, which was modest (Figure 3B). When proliferation was analyzed considering cells without Doxy-induction as the control (Figure S6), since c-Src-wt expression did not alter proliferation, we observed similar results to those obtained considering c-Src-wt as the control. Cell cycle analyses by propidium iodide showed that in these mutants the number of cells in "Sub-G1" increased, and "G2-M" was reduced (Figure S7), which may help in understanding the proliferation differences. Analyses of cell cycle by pulse/chase with BrdU and propidium iodide in SUM159-Tet-On-c-Src-W118A/R175L showed an increased number of cells in the G1 phase upon induction of this mutant versus control (Doxy), a reduction of "S", as well as in "G2/M". MTT analyses of these cells showed a 45% reduction of metabolic active cells, which may be related to the number of viable and proliferating cells [40]. These results agree with those observed here (Figure 3B). Together, these results suggest that both c-Src-R175L and c-Src-W118A/R175L variants reduced proliferation with no signs of toxic effects.

We then analyzed by WB the levels of Myc, cyclin D1, and $p27^{kip1}$ cell cycle makers (Figure 3C). The functionality of SH2-c-Src domain appeared relevant as induction of c-Src-R175L and c-Src-W118A/R175L in SUM159 reduced Myc expression. In contrast, in MDA-MB-231, no significant variations were detected upon induction of c-Src variants (Figure 3C). Interestingly, in SUM159 cells, expression of c-Src-R175L and c-Src-W118A/R715L variants highly induced cyclin D1 (Figure 3C). In MDA-MB-231 cells, while c-Src-R175L did not modify cyclin D1 levels, the double mutant c-Src-W118A/R175L significantly reduced them. When the data were analyzed considering cells without Doxy induction as the control, the results showed the same tendency (Figure S6). The cyclin D1 gene regulation is complex and it varies between cell lines and experimental conditions. In rodent cells, it has been reported that Myc induces D1 in some cases while in others, Myc does not induce or even repress D1 (for review see [41]). Therefore, the downregulation of Myc observed in SUM159 cells may contribute to the upregulation of cyclin D1.

Furthermore, regarding the cell cycle inhibitor $p27^{Kip1}$, induction of both c-Src-R175L and c-Src-W118A/R175L mutants significantly increased its expression in SUM159 and in MDA-MB-231 (Figure 3C and Figure S6).

These results showed that SUM159 cells seemed to be more sensitive than MDA-MB-231 to the alteration of SH2-SH3 adapter domain functionality, as demonstrated by the effects induced by the expression of mutants on cell proliferation and cell cycle marker levels. Therefore, the kinase activity has an essential role in cell proliferation as the SH2 domain just partially modulates cell proliferation.

2.5. Regulation of Cellular Migration and Invasion by c-Src Adapter Domains

Cell migration is one of the essential steps of the metastatic cascade. We analyzed by wound-healing assays the effect of c-Src variants expression in SUM159 and MDA-MB-231 cell migration. In SUM159, Doxy induction of either c-Src -R175L or -W118A/R175L did not significantly alter migration as compared to c-Src-wt expression, and as shown by the lack of significant difference in the remaining wound-healing area after 13 h of migration between the control and the two variants (Figure 4A and Figure S9). When the analyses were made considering unstimulated c-Src variants (Doxy) as the control, it was observed that c-Src-wt inhibited cell migration in SUM159, while induced it in MDA-MB-231 (Figures S8–S10). Nevertheless, the results showed the same tendency as observed when the c-Src-wt expression was used as the control. However, looking at the recording videos of migration, we observed abnormal movements of SUM159 cells expressing the c-Src-W118A/R175L variant. Thus, we further analyzed the migration pattern of individual cells at the migration border by tracking the path of single cells. We found that only the expression of c-Src-W118A/R175L variant in SUM159 cells caused random migration, as the ratio of Euclidean/Accumulated distances was significantly reduced, while the velocity of cell migration was increased, as compared to the control (Figure 4A and Figure S9). Consequently, SUM159 cells expressing the c-Src-W118A/R175L variant did not close the wound-healing area more or faster than cells expressing c-Src-wt or c-Src-R175L (Figure 4A). Indeed, they were moving randomly, not all in the direction to close the wound area, and at higher velocity than the other cells. In MDA-MB-231 cells, mutations affecting the SH2 domain functionality (R175L and W118A/R175L) reduced migration compared to c-Src-wt (Figure 4A and Figure S9). However, none of these mutations caused random migration in MDA-MB-231 cells.

The oncogenic potential of c-Src in tumor cells is pleiotropic and controls cytoskeletal-linked events, such as extracellular matrix-adhesion, migration, and invasion. We previously showed that the catalytic activity of this proto-oncogene is involved in invasion and migration [15]. Now, we analyzed whether the SH2 adapter domain of c-Src is involved in the regulation of SUM159 and MDA-MB-231 cellular invasion. In SUM159, expression of c-Src-R175L variant inhibited the number of invading cells, while the double SH2/SH3 mutant c-Src-W118A/R175L, was unable to modify the invasiveness of SUM159 cells, as compared to the c-Src-wt (Figure 4B). In contrast to SUM159, expression of c-Src -R175L and -W118A/R175L significantly inhibited cell invasion in MDA-MB-231 in comparison to c-Src-wt (Figure 4B). When the analyses were made considering unstimulated c-Src variants (Doxy) as the control, it was observed that c-Src-wt did not alter invasiveness in SUM159, while induced it in MDA-MB-231 (Figure S8). Nevertheless, the results showed the same tendency as observed when the c-Src-wt expression was used as the control.

The growth factor or integrin stimulation induces Fak autophosphorylation on Y397, generating a high affinity binding site for the Src SH2 domain [20,21], which in turn phosphorylates Fak at several tyrosine residues allowing the activation of multiple signaling pathways [42]. The association of Src with Fak controls the turnover of focal adhesion complexes, which are involved in cell motility, migration, and invasion [39]. These processes involve the dynamic control of protein associated with focal adhesion complex, among them, Fak, Paxillin, Caveolin 1, etc., due to, at least in part, their phosphorylation/activation [16,42,43]. We then analyzed the degree of activation/phosphorylation of these proteins involved in cell migration and invasion by WB. In SUM159, expression of c-Src-W118A/R175L increased Caveolin 1 levels (Figure S11A), while only c-Src-R175L increased pY14-Caveolin 1. Paxillin expression remained constant upon induction of c-Src variants, albeit pY118-Paxillin/Paxillin augmented in c-Src-R175L expressing SUM159 cells (Figure S11A). Fak expression was constant, whereas pY397 diminished upon induction of c-Src-R175L and c-Src-W118A/R175L compared to c-Src-wt. Phosphorylation of Fak at Y576 was significantly reduced in cells expressing c-Src-R175L, while it was increased by c-Src-W118A/R175L, as compared to c-Src-wt (Figure S11A). In MDA-MB-231, expression of Caveolin 1 remained constant for all c-src variants expressing cells (Figure S11B). The mutants c-Src-R175L and c-Src-W118A/R175L have an open conformation, consequently, they highly increased the activation of Caveolin 1 (Figure S11B). Expression of c-Src mutants did not alter the levels of Paxillin protein, while the activation of Paxillin (ratio p118Y-Paxillin/Paxillin) was surprisingly inhibited in MDA-MB-231 expressing c-Src -R175L and -W118A/R175L, as compared to c-Src-wt (Figure S11B). Fak protein levels were unaltered in any of the MDA-MB-231 cell lines expressing c-Src variants (Figure S11B). Conversely, Fak autophosphorylation at Y397 was increased by expression of W118A/R175L. The specific activity of Fak (pY576-Fak/Fak) was not augmented in all c-Src mutants expressed in MDA-MB-231 (Figure S11B) as compared to c-Src-wt. When the results of WBs were analyzed considering non-induced conditions for c-Src variants as the control (Doxy conditions), the results showed the same tendency (Figures S12 and S13). When all the c-Src variants expressing SUM159 and MDA-MB-231 cells were analyzed together in a single WB, the results showed that expression of total c-Src was higher in SUM159 than in MDA-MB-231, supporting the data from Figure 1B, as it was observed for total Fak. Changes in pY397-Fak were not evident in any of the two cell lines. In contrast, phosphorylation of Fak by c-Src at Y576 increased upon expression of the mutants in both cell lines. However, results from triplicate experiments (Figures S11–S13) showed inhibition of pY576-Fak in SUM159 expressing c-Src-R175L. Possibly, this discrepancy is due to the fact that the analysis of Figure S14 represents a single sample, while data from Figures S11 and S12 represented the average of three different samples. Similarly, while the levels of total Akt practically unchanged in SUM159 and MDA-MB-231 cells due to the expression of c-Src variants, the extent of pS473-Akt was increased upon induction of all the c-Src variants (Figure S14).

We have also analyzed the effect of c-Src mutants in the cellular distribution of pY14-Caveolin 1 and pY418-Src in both SUM159 and MDA-MB-231 cells by confocal microscopy. In c-Src-wt or in c-Src-R175L expressing SUM159 cells, pY14-Caveolin 1 and pY418-Src co-localized at the focal adhesion sites (Figure S15), whereas in those expressing c-Src-W118A/R175L, distribution of pY418-Src did not fully co-localize with pY14-Caveolin 1 at focal adhesion sites (Figure S15 basal layer, and Figure S15 upper layer). However, if we focus at higher levels, we find that in both mutant expressing SUM159 cells pY14-Caveolin and pY418-Src decorated caveolae (spherical structures within the cellular cytoplasm) (Figure S15).

Confocal microscopy analyses at the basal layer of MDA-MB-231 overexpressing c-Sr-wt and -R175L showed a distribution of pY14-Caveolin 1/pY418-Src at the adhesion areas. The intracellular accumulation of pY418-Src was also detected at perinuclear areas. In cells expressing c-Src-W118A/R175L, the focal adhesion was not clearly displayed (Figure S15). The distribution of pY14-Caveolin 1/pY418-Src in MDA-MB-231-c-Src-R175L at the upper layer showed their co-localization at the perinuclear region, and in the cytoplasm where they decorated some vacuolar structures, as observed in SUM159. Similar to SUM159, in MDA-MB-231-c-Src-W118A/R175L, the vacuolar structures were also observed but to a much lesser extent (Figure S15).

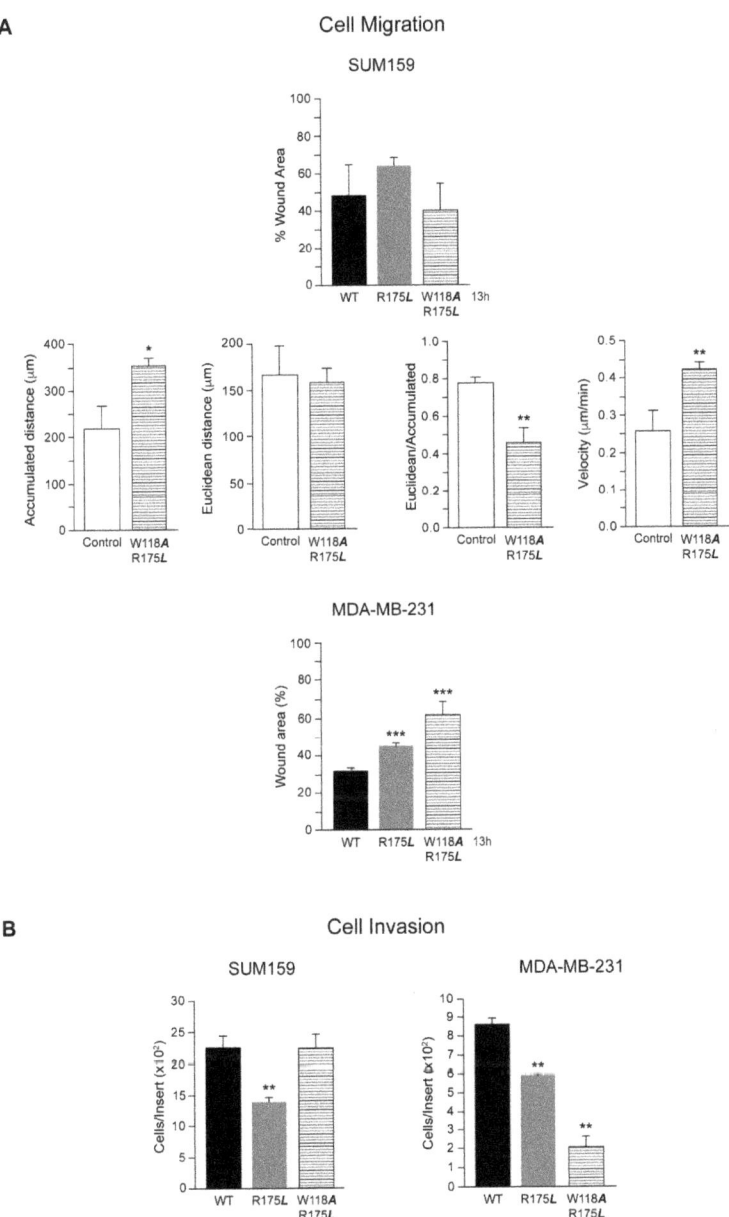

Figure 4. Effect of c-Src variants expression in SUM159 and MDA-MB-231 cellular migration and invasion. Migration of cells was analyzed by wound-healing assays, and tracking analyses ($n = 3$), as described in Materials and Methods in SUM159 and MDA-MB-231 cells (**A**). Additionally, tracking analyses of W118A/R175L to determine the cell migration of at least 100 individual cells determine the Accumulated distance, Euclidean, and the Velocity of migration to evaluate the ration of Euclidean/Accumulated distance that define random migration. (**B**) The capability of cells to migrate through a layer of Matrigel was employed to determine cell invasion (see Materials and Methods) in both SUM159 and MDA-MB-231 conditionally expressing c-Src variants. The control value is similar to that in Figure 2. Results of three independent experiments ($n = 3$) were expressed as the mean ± SD. The statistical significance is referred to cells expressing c-Src-wt, * $p < 0.5$, ** $p < 0.01$, *** $p < 0.001$.

2.6. SH2-c-Src Directed Aptamers Reduced Cell Proliferation

The 14F and 17F aptamers directed to SH2-c-Src were designed and selected as described (Materials and Methods, and in the extended methods in Supplementary Information). The analyses of aptamers have been referred to the aptamer control (containing 38xAG, see Material and Methods), as in preliminary studies no differences were detected in cell proliferation of either SUM159 or MDA-MB-231 cells when compared to the transfection of the control (38xAG) and mock (empty transfection) [40]. We then determined the IC50 concentration for each aptamer in SUM159 and MDA-MB-231 cells by considering the total number of cells after the treatment with different concentrations of the aptamers (0, 25, 50, 200, and 500 nM), taking as 0% the concentration of aptamers with no effect and as 100% the effect at the maximal concentration of the aptamers for each cell line (see Materials and Methods). The results were graphically represented (Figure 5A). The IC50 values for 14F (117.1 and 141.7 nM) and 17F (94.3 and 97.0 nM) for SUM159 and MD-MB-231, respectively, were slightly different. Nevertheless, we decided to perform all the experiments at 100 nM for each aptamer at both cell lines. We determined the effect of SH2-c-Src directed aptamers (100 nM) in cell proliferation using the trypan blue exclusion method, allowing us to evaluate the total number of cells, the dead cells, and the living cells 72 h after transfection. The results showed (Figure 5B) that in both cell lines the number of dead cells was similar for all aptamers control (aptamer control), 14F and 17F, indicating that at this concentration they were not cytotoxic (Figure 5B). The 14F and 17F aptamers reduced the total cell number, as well as the number of viable cells in SUM159, while in MDA-MB-231 only the 14F caused a significant reduction of total and viable cells, as there is no significant reduction in viable cells in the MDA-MB-231 cell line with the 17F aptamer.

Then, we analyzed the levels of Myc, cyclin D1, and p27^{Kip1} in SUM159 and MDA-MB-231 cells treated with 14F and 17F aptamers. As compared to the aptamer control considered as 1, these aptamers reduced the expression of Myc and cyclin D1, while they increased those of p27^{Kip1} in both SUM159 and MDA-MB-231 cells (Figure S18).

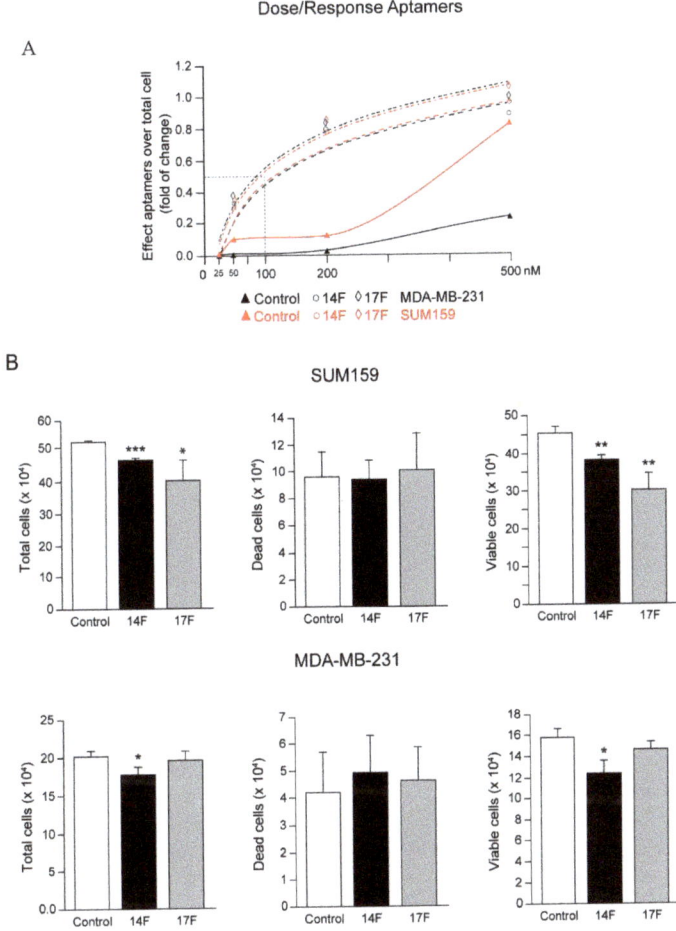

Figure 5. Dose/response of SH2-c-Src directed aptamers in SUM159 and MDA-MB-231 cells and evaluation of cell proliferation. (**A**) Control aptamer (38xAG) and SH2-c-Src directed aptamers 14F and 17F were transfected at 25, 50, 200, and 500 nM to SUM159 and MDA-MB-231and the IC50 values were determined as described in Material and Methods ($n = 3$). (**B**) Control and SH2-c-Src directed aptamers 14F and 17F were transfected at 100 nM to either SUM159 or MDA-MB-231 and, 72 h later, the number of total, dead, and viable cells were determined by the trypan blue exclusion method (see Materials and Methods). Each experiment was measured in triplicates ($n = 3$) and repeated three times. Results were expressed as a percentage of the mean ± SD, * $p < 0.5$, ** $p < 0.01$, *** $p < 0.001$.

2.7. Role of 14F and 17F in Cell Migration and Invasion

As cell migration and invasion are steps required for TNBC metastasis, we evaluated the relevance of the SH2 -c-Src domain in the regulation of these events by blocking its functionality in SUM159 and MDA-MB-231. We first observed that MDA-MB-231 cells migrated significantly less than SUM159, as the wound area after 13 h of migration was bigger. In either of the cell lines, the aptamers significantly reduced migration, as both 14F and 17F had a bigger wound area at the end of the experiments compared to the control (Figure 6A, Figures S16 and S17).

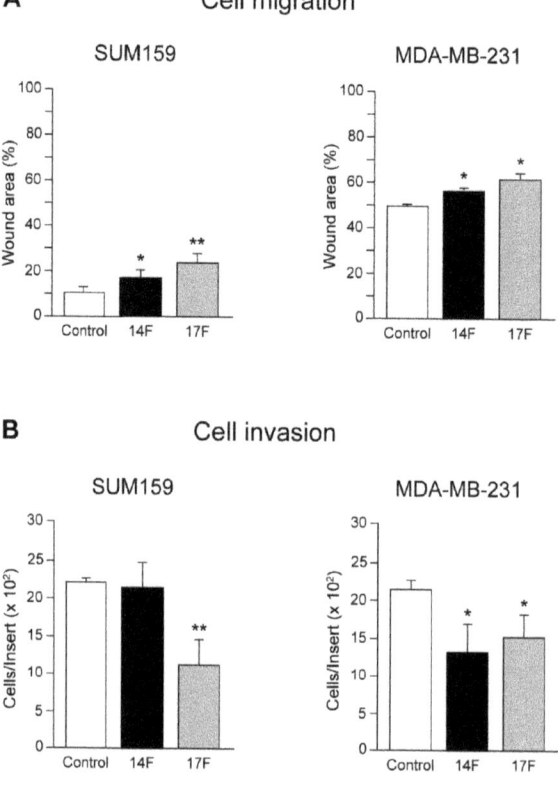

Figure 6. Role of SH2-c-Src directed aptamers in SUM159 and MDA-MB-231 cells to evaluate cellular migration and invasion. Wild type SUM159 and MDA-MB-231 cells were transfected with either control, 14F or 17F aptamers at 100 nM and cell migration (**A**) and invasion (**B**) were determined as described in Materials and Methods. Each experiment was measured in triplicates ($n = 3$) and repeated three times. Results were expressed as a percentage of the mean ± SD, * $p < 0.5$, ** $p < 0.01$.

As for cell invasion, while only the 17F aptamer clearly reduced invasiveness in SUM159 cells, both 14F and 17F inhibited cell invasion of MDA-MB-231 cells (Figure 6B). We analyzed the effects of 14F and 17F aptamers on the expression of c-Src, pY418-Src/C-Src, Fak, pY397-Fak, Caveolin 1, pY14-Caveolin 1/Caveolin 1, Paxillin, and pY118-Paxillin/Paxillin in both SUM159 and MDA-MB-231 cells by WB considering the aptamer control as 1. In SUM159 and MDA-MB-231 cells, expression of c-Src and the activated form were unmodified, as also observed for Fak and auto-phosphorylated (Figure S18). In contrast, Caveolin 1 levels were reduced by aptamer 14F and increased by aptamer 17F, whereas pY14-Caveolin 1/Caveolin 1 was reduced by both aptamers in SUM159, but not in MDA-MB-231. Paxillin levels were unaltered by either of these aptamers, although the pY118-Paxillin/Paxillin ratio was significantly reduced by both 14F and 17F in both SUM159 and MDA-MB-231 cells (Figure S18). These results are different to those observed in Figure S11, as employing aptamers were blocking the functionality of the SH2 domain (Figure S18), while through the other experimental approach the induction of expression of c-Src variants was achieved.

Considering that migration and invasion are required for the metastatic process, these results support the experiments carried out with the conditional expression of c-Src variants and indicated that the SH2 domain is relevant for c-Src functionality.

3. Discussion

The SFKs control many signaling pathways involved in the regulation of several cellular processes. Thus, the deregulation of their functionality is associated with tumors, including breast cancer [1,7,44]. Here, we studied the relevance of the SH2 adapter domain of c-Src in two TNBC cell lines SUM159 and MDA-MB-231. Several scientific reports showed that, even though the two cell lines share several common characteristics, as both are considered Basal-Mesenchymal TNBC cell lines with a spindle phenotype, SUM159 (primary breast adenocarcinoma) has mutations in HRAS and PIK3CA (https://web.expasy.org/cellosaurus/CVCL_5423), while MDA-MB-231 (pleural effusion) has deletions in p14ARF, p16, and CDKN2, and mutations in the KRAS, BRAF, and TERT promoter (https://web.expasy.org/cellosaurus/CVCL_0062), supporting the heterogeneity observed in TNBC [12,45–48].

Our analyses of SFKs expression in SUM159 and MDA-MB-231 cells showed that c-Src, Fyn, and Lyn A were expressed at higher levels in SUM159 than in MDA-MB-231, while the opposite occurred for Lyn B and Yes.

To determine the relevance of the SH2-c-Src domain we followed two independent and complementary approaches, the conditional expression of c-Src variants with inactivating point mutations affecting SH2 functionality (R175L, W118A/R175L), and the transfection of two different aptamers directed to the SH2-c-Src domain, that interacted and then blocked the SH2-c-Src function in SUM159 and MDA-MB-231

It is well established that c-Src increased its expression/activity as the tumor progresses [1,5,7]. Our results also indicated that the c-Src played a relevant role in the renewal of the enriched population of BCSCs. The role of Src in the maintenance of these cells was previously observed in MCF7 [38], and here in SUM159 and MDA-MB-231 cells by the conditional expression of the dominant negative form of c-Src (SrcDN), as well as in MDA-MB-231 that conditionally have c-Src suppressed. Indirectly, expression of miR205 in SUM159, which inhibits SFKs members expression, suppressed SUM159 BCSCs renewal and stem cell markers [37]. Moreover, selective inhibitors of SFKs tyrosine-kinase activity also have an inhibitory effect in BCSCs renewal. In SUM159, resistant to paclitaxel, Dasatinib causes epithelial differentiation and enhances sensitization to paclitaxel, and a combination of both compounds reduces stem cell renewal and synergizes to diminish the viability of paclitaxel-resistant SUM159 cells [49]. In high-grade serous ovarian cancer cells, co-treatment of Saracatinib (SFKs inhibitor, AZD0530) and selumetinib (MEK inhibitor, AZD6244) reduced SFE and ALDH1 positive cells and, in vivo the loss of tumor-initiating cells following serial tumor xenografting [50]. Our results showed that the inactivating mutation of the SH2 and SH3 domains R175L and W118A/R175L significantly reduced BCSCs renewal in both cell lines, supporting the relevance of the adapter domains in the renewal of the tumor initiating cells. In primary PDAC cultures, established from patient-derived xenografts with Dasatinib or PP2 reduced the clonogenic, self-renewal, and tumor-initiating capacity of PaCSCs, which we attribute to the downregulation of key signaling factors such as p-FAK, p-ERK1-2, and p-AKT [51].

The anchorage-independent growth, which characterized tumor cells, showed the discrepancy between SUM159 and MDA-MB-231 cells. While in SUM159 cells only the suppression of both SH2 and SH3 functionality reduced it, in MDA-MB-231 cells, both c-Src-R175L and c-Src-W188A/R175L diminished colony formation in soft-agar as compared to c-Src-wt. Suppression of endogenous c-Src in MDA-MB-231 cells significantly reduced anchorage-independent growth [16]. Likewise, specifically silencing c-Src and not Yes or Fyn inhibited soft-agar colony formation in MDA-MB-231, MDA-MB-436, and SKBR3 [52]. Furthermore, SFKs catalytic activity inhibition or stable transfection of catalytically inactive c-Src into MDAMB-468 and MCF7 reduced the colony formation ability [53]. In addition, inhibition of SFKs expression by miR205 in SUM159 significantly diminished the anchorage-independent growth [37]. Inhibitors of SFKs catalytic activity such as Dasatinib inhibits soft-agar colony formation in BxPC3 and PANC1 pancreatic cancer cells [54]. Therefore, the

SH2-c-Src domain appeared relevant for MDA-MB-231 breast cancer cells in the anchorage-independent growth.

Cell proliferation was also influenced by SH2 functionality, as it was reduced upon induced expression of c-Src-R175L and c-Src-W118A/R175L variants as compared to c-Src-wt, as it was Myc expression in SUM159. On the contrary, we observed that in MDA-MB-231, inhibition of cell proliferation was not linked to alteration in the levels of Myc. Inhibition of SFKs tyrosine-kinase activity clearly blocks cell proliferation in MDA-MB-231 cells [15]. Interestingly, while Myc expression was reduced, cyclin D1 increased in response to the expression of c-Src-R175L and c-src-W118A/R175L in SUM159 cells. In this context, in rodent cells, it has been reported that Myc induces D1 in some cases, while in others, Myc does not induce or even repress D1, supporting the concept of the complex regulation of cyclin D1 gene (for review see [41]). Thus, the downregulation of Myc observed in SUM159 cells may contribute to the upregulation of cyclin D1.

Numerous studies show that the catalytic activity of SFKs is important for migration and invasion of tumor cells [6,15,16,22,55–57]. Induction of Fak autophosphorylation by the growth factor or by integrins facilitates its interaction with the SH2 domain of c-Src, opening c-Src conformation and, consequently, increasing its tyrosine kinase activity. Then, c-Src phosphorylates Fak at other sides, and facilitates the interaction/activation of other signaling molecules [1,7,20,21]. The complex Src/Fak phosphorylates/activates several focal adhesion proteins involved in migration and invasion [16,39,42,43]. In addition, our results showed that the SH2-c-Src domain was also relevant for modulation of invasion in both TNBC cell lines. Interestingly, they also revealed in SUM159 cells that altering the functionality of both SH2 and SH3 c-Src domains (c-Src-W118A/R175L variant) caused migration to occur in a random manner, as cells had high motility but they did not close the wound healing area. In HT1080 fibrosarcoma, overexpression of PEAK1 kinase, which is phosphorylated/activated at Y665 by SFKs, causes random migration and elevates cell invasion [58]. Consistently, in SUM159 cells, increased migration was associated with the activation of focal adhesion proteins caveolin1, paxillin, and Fak which were increased by overexpression of c-Src-W118A/R175L variant. In contrast, the c-Src-R175L reduced pY576-Fak/Fak. Confocal-microscopy analyses of the cellular distribution of activated Src (pY418-Src) and caveolin 1 (pY14-Caveolin 1) in SUM159 cells expressing the c-Src-R175L mutant at the basal layer showed their colocalization at the focal adhesion sites, as observed in SUM159-c-Src-wt. Interestingly, at the upper layer of analyses both c-Src -R175L and -W118A/R175L variants showed co-decoration of caveolae-like structures as compared to c-Src-wt. As mentioned above, SUM159 and MDA-MB-231 cells though they share a good number of common properties, also show some differences. Nevertheless, results showed that the SH2-c-Src domain played an important functional role in SUM159 and MDA-MB-231 TNBC cells.

To support these data, we approached this study by a different and complementary method. We designed two different aptamers directed to interact with the SH2-c-Src domain. The results showed that at a dose around the IC50 concentration both aptamers significantly inhibited the proliferation of SUM159 and MDA-MB-231, without inducing apoptosis, as the number of dead cells was unaltered. In agreement with these observations, the expression of Myc and cyclin D1 were reduced, while p27Kip1 levels were augmented. As observed for cells expressing c-Src-R175L, these aptamers inhibited migration and invasion in both TNBC cells. The aptamers design to bind to MNK1, which controls the eIF4E function by phosphorylation, significantly inhibits proliferation and migration of MDA-MB-231 [30]. The AS1411 aptamer directed to nucleolin induces blc-2 mRNA instability, reduces cell growth by causing cytotoxicity in MCF7 and MDA-MB-231 [59]. This aptamer has been tested in different tumors including glioma, renal cell carcinoma [31].

The results obtained indicated that the functionality of SH2-c-Src domain is important for the potential tumorigenicity of SUM159 and MDA-MB-231 cells as the inactivating point-mutation of this domain inhibited the biological functions required for the TNBC cell. Similarly, aptamers directed to the SH2-c-Src domain also significantly reduced the performance of these TNBC cells.

4. Materials and Methods

4.1. Antibodies and Reagents

Table S1 contains the antibody information. The chemical reagents and enzymes used were of analytical grade and purchased from Thermo-Fisher (Waltham, MA, USA), Roche (Basel, Switzerland), Corning (Merck, Darmstadt, Germany), PeproTech (London, UK), PAA Laboratories GmbH (Cölbe, Germany), Bio-Rad (Hercules, CA, USA), GE Healthcare and Sigma-Aldrich/Merck (Merck, Darmstadt, Germany).

4.2. Cell Lines and Culture

MDA-MB-231 (HTB-26) was from ATCC, and SUM159PT (CVCL-5423) [60] was provided by Dr. G. Dontu [61]. Cell lines were mycoplasma free and authenticated by the short-tandem-repeat analysis (GenePrintR 10 System from Promega (Madison, WI, USA), and GeneMapper v3.7 STR profile analysis software, Life Technologies, Carlsbad, CA, USA) (see Supplementary Information). Profiles were checked against public databases ATCC and DSMZ. MDA-MB-231 was maintained in DMEM, 5% FCS, 2 mM glutamine, 100 IU/mL penicillin, and 100 µg/mL streptomycin. SUM159 was cultured in Ham's F12, 5% FCS, 5 µg/mL insulin, 1 µg/mL hydrocortisone, 2 mM glutamine, 100 IU/mL penicillin, and 100 µg/mL streptomycin.

Generation of SUM159PT-Tet-On-c-Src- and MDA-MB-231-Tet-On-c-Src -wt, -R175L, - and -W118A/R175L, was carried out as described [16], and grown in the presence of 3 µg/mL blasticidin, 100 µg/mL zeocin to maintain the plasmid selection of cells expressing c-Src-wt and c-Src-R175L or with 3 µg/mL blasticidin, 3 µg/mL hygromycin for the selection of cell expressing c-Src-W118A/R175L.

The wild type (wt) and c-Src variants used in these experiments were from a chicken origin [1,4,19]. The BLASTp comparative analysis of c-Src protein sequences between *Homo Sapiens* (Protein Accession Number: P12931.3) and *Gallus-Gallus* (Protein Accession: P00523.4) resulted in over 94% identity at the amino acid sequences [33]. Since the EC10 mouse monoclonal antibody (Millipore, #05-185) specifically recognizes chicken c-Src, it was possible to determine c-Src variants in the presence of the endogenous human c-Src of SUM159 and MDA-MB-231 cells.

4.3. Mammosphere Cultures

Single cell suspensions of adherent cultures were plated in 6-well ultralow attachment plates (Falcon, Corning Life Science, Merck, Darmstadt, Germany) at 2×10^3 cells/well. Mammosphere cultures were maintained in serum-free DMEM/F12 media (1:1), B27 (1:50), EGF (20 ng/mL) and bFGF (20 ng/mL), insulin (5 µg/mL), hydrocortisone (5 µg/mL). After 10 days, cells were pipetted up and down to eliminate cellular aggregates and mammospheres (sphere-like structures with diameter ≥ 50 µm) were clearly detected by the optical phase contrast microscope (Nikon-Eclipse TS100, 4× magnification). Cultures were then trypsinized to induce mammosphere dissociation to single cells, which were seeded again for mammosphere formation. The experiment ended at the third generation of mammosphere formation. Sphere forming efficiency (SFE) was then calculated as the number of spheres formed per number of seeded cells and expressed as % means ± SD, as described [37,38].

4.4. Anchorage-Independent Growth

Cells were resuspended in a warmed solution of 0.3% agarose in a complete medium and seeded at 10^5 cells/60 mm dishes with a bottom layer of 0.5% agarose. Cells were re-fed every 72 h with a complete medium (300 µL/dish). At the 10-day growth, plates were stained with 0.5 mL of 0.005% crystal violet/water for 1 h and colonies with diameter ≥ 0.1 mm from 4–5 fields/plate were counted, as described [37].

4.5. Cell Proliferation

Cell proliferation was evaluated by counting viable cells performing a Trypan blue (Sigma-Aldrich) exclusion assay. Cells were seeded at 3×10^5 cells/60 mm dishes, 72 h later they were trypsinized, cells were pelleted and resuspended in a culture medium, mixed with a 0.4% Trypan blue/PBS solution (1:1), loaded on a hemocytometer, and Trypan blue-negative (viable cells) and Trypan blue-positive cells (dead cells) were counted.

4.6. Cell Migration

Cells were seeded in a complete medium in a 6-well plate and grown to confluence. The monolayer was scratched with a 200 µL micropipette tip, and washed with a fresh medium to remove floating cells. A complete medium was added to the cultures, and photomicrographs were taken every 30 min with a Microscope Cell Observer Z1 system (Carl Zeiss AG) equipped with a controlled environment chamber and Camera Cascade 1 k to monitor the wound closure. Migration was quantified using the wound-healing tool ImageJ, as described [15,37]. Tracking of cell migration was carried out in 100 cells/assay using the "manual-tracking" from the ImageJ program together with the "chemotaxis and migration tool".

4.7. Invasion Assay

Invasiveness was determined as described [15]. Briefly, cells were seeded in a serum-free medium on the upper chamber of cell culture inserts of 24-well plates (8 µm-pore PET membranes, BD) coated with Matrigel™ (5×10^4/well/200 µL). The lower chamber was filled with 600 µL of 20% FBS; 22 h later, after removing the cells on top of the inserts, those on the lower surface were fixed with methanol, nuclei stained with DAPI, and mounted on slides with a Prolong antifade-reagent. Filters were observed with a Plan $20 \times /0.50$ objective of an axiophot fluorescence microscope (Zeiss, Oberkochen, Germany) equipped with an Olympus DP70 digital camera. DAPI-stained nuclei were counted.

4.8. Western Blot Analysis

Cell lysates preparation and Western Blot (WB) analyses were carried out, as previously described [37]. Briefly, cells were lysed at 4 °C with a lysis buffer (10 mM Tris–HCl (pH 7.6), 50 mM NaCl, 30 mM sodium pyrophosphate, 5 mM EDTA, 5 mM EGTA, 0.1% SDS, 1% Triton X-100, 50 mM NaF, 0.1 mM Na_3VO_4, 1 mM PMSF, 1 mM benzamidine, 1 mM iodoacetamide, and 1 mM phenantroline). Cell lysates were obtained by centrifugation at $21,380 \times g$ for 30 min at 4 °C; the protein concentration in the supernatant was determined by the BCA protein assay (Pierce, Rockford, IL, USA), and lysates were adjusted to equivalent concentrations with a lysis buffer. Aliquots of 30 µg of total cell lysates were then separated on SDS–PAGE. Proteins were transferred to PVDF membranes that were blocked 1 h at room temperature with 5% non-fat milk in TTBS (TBS with 0.05% Tween-20) or 5% BSA in TTBS for phosphoproteins. Incubation with primary specific antibodies was carried out overnight at 4 °C, and horseradish peroxidase-conjugated secondary antibodies in a blocking solution for 1 h at room temperature. Immunoreactive bands were visualized by the ECL kit.

4.9. Aptamers Design and Selection

The SH2 and SH3 domains of c-Src cloned into GST [62] and expressed in E. coli were purified from the soluble fraction by glutathione-resin affinity chromatography (Genescript, Piscataway, NJ, USA) as described [30]. Aptamers selection, cloning and sequencing, and secondary ssDNA structure prediction, as well as an enzyme-linked oligonucleotide assay (ELONA) methodology was previously described [30]. The aptamers employed were: 1. Control containing 38xAG, as described [30]; ApSH2.F14: GCGGATGAAGACTGGTGTAGACAATGGATACTCCCGCCACCTCCTCCCCCG CCCC-CCCGCCCTAAATACGAGCAAC; ApSH2.17F: GCGGATGAAGACTGGTGTGCGGTGGT

GGGTTGGGTGGGTGGGTTTGCGGGTTGCGTTGGCCCTAAATACGAGCAAC. Please see the extended method in the Supplementary Information for details.

4.10. Aptamers Transfection and IC50

SUM159 and MDA-MB-231 cells were seeded in 24 multi-well plates (10^4 cells/well/ 500 µL) in their corresponding culture media without antibiotics; 24 h later, cells were washed twice with their serum and antibiotic-free corresponding media. Then, the cells were incubated in 400 µL of culture media without antibiotics and 100 µL of the transfection mixture: 1. 0.25, 0.5, 2, or 5 µL of each aptamer, corresponding to 25, 50, 200, or 500 nM, in 49.75, 49.5, 48, or 45 µL of culture media; 2. 1.25 µL of DharmaFECT-4 (Thermo-Scientific) in 48.75 µL culture of media, following the manufacturer's manual; 8 h later, the cells were extensively washed with a culture media without antibiotics, then incubated for an additional 40 h and then analyzed as previously described in the cell proliferation assay section. The IC50 for each aptamer was determined considering the total number of SUM159 or MDA-MB-231 cells after the treatment with different concentrations of the aptamers. To this end, the untreated cells were considered as 0% (without effect) and 100% the effect at the maximal concentration of the aptamers for each cell line. Then, the obtained data were graphically represented employing the mathematical formula for the logarithmic trendline calculated with Excel to obtain the IC50 for each aptamer. Then, the IC50 values of each aptamer were used to determine their effects in cell proliferation, migration, and invasion of SUM159 and MDA-MB-231 cells, as previously described.

4.11. Statistical Analyses

Mean values, standard deviation, and statistical significance between data from the two different experimental conditions (±Doxy) were determined by the two-tail Student *t*-test. Data were normalized to the activity of the c-Src-wt variant for each cellular assay.

5. Conclusions

Our results conclude that the SH2-c-Src domain functionality is relevant for the potential tumorigenicity of SUM159 and MDA-MB-231, as the inducible expression of c-Src with the unfunctional SH2-c-Src domain inhibited the renewal of the enriched BCSCs cells, as well as other relevant functionalities in these TNBC cells. Similarly, the aptamers directed to the SH2-c-Src domain also significantly reduced the performance of these TNBC cells. Therefore, using a combination of SH2-c-Src functional inhibitors with those directed to the tyrosine kinase activity should be able to fully block the c-Src functionality and, consequently, could be therapeutically effective in the breast cancer treatment. Furthermore, as c-Src is also involved in other types of tumors (pancreas, colorectal, lung, etc.) [1,7,18,43,63,64], our results could eventually be extrapolated to these other pathologies.

Supplementary Materials: The following are available online at https://www.mdpi.com/2072-6694/13/3/462/s1. 1. Supplementary Materials and Methods: 1. Purification and selection of aptamers for the SH2 domain of c-Src (extended method); 2. Immunofluorescence by lasers-canning confocal microscopy; 2. Supplementary Figures: Figure S1: Analyses of sphere formation efficiency (SFE); Figure S2: Images of mammospheres of SUM159 and MDA-MB-231 cells expressing c-Src variants; Figure S3: Effect of conditional expression of SrcDN in SUM159 and MDA-MB-231 cells or suppression of endogenous c-Src in MDA-MB-231 on SFE; Figure S4: Western blot analyses of ALDH1, NANOG, and Oct3-4 from mammospheres of SUM159 and MDA-MB-231 cells expressing c-Src variants; Figure S5: Soft-agar colonies from SUM159 and MDA-MB-231 cells expressing c-Src variants; Figure S6: Analyses of cell proliferation and Myc, cyclin D1, and p27Kip1 in Sum159 and MDA-MB-231 cells expressing c-Src variants, considering—Doxy conditions as the control; Figure S7: Cell cycle analyses of SUM159 and MDA-MB-231 cells expressing c-Src variants; Figure S8: Migration and invasion data of SUM159 and MDA-MB-231 cells expressing c-Src variants; Figure S9: Kinetics curves of wound-healing assays of SUM159 and MDA-MB-231 cells expressing c-Src variants; Figure S10: Representative images of wound-healing assays of SUM159 and MDA-MB-231 cells expressing c-Src variants; Figure S11: Expression and activation of Caveolin 1, Paxillin, and Fak in SUM159 and MDA-MB-231 cells expressing c-Src variants. Referred to c-Src-wt as the control; Figure S12: Expression and activation of Caveolin 1, Paxillin, and Fak in SUM159 and MDA-MB-231 cells expressing c-Src variants. Referred to—Doxy as the control; Figure S13: Representative WB analyses of expression and activation of Caveolin 1, Paxillin, and Fak from the total cell extract from SUM159 and MDA-MB-231 cells expressing c-Src variants; Figure S14: Western Blot analyses of total c-Src, Fak, phosphorylated pY397-Fak, pY576-Fak, and Akt and phosphorylated pS473-Akt from SUM159 and MDA-MB-231 cells expressing c-Src variants; Figure S15: Confocal scanning microscopy analyses of pY14-Caveolin 1 and pY418-Src localization in SUM159 and MDA-MB-231 cells expressing c-Src variants; Figure S16: Kinetics curves of wound-healing assays of SUM159 and MDA-MB-231 cells treated with aptamers 14F and 17F; Figure S17: Representative images of wound-healing assays of SUM159 and MDA-MB-231 cells treated with aptamers 14F and 17F; Figure S18: Analyses by WB of expression of proliferation markers Myc, Cyclin D1, p27^{Kip1}, and of migration Caveolin 1, Paxillin, and Fak in SUM159 and MDA-MB-231 cells treated with aptamers; Table S1: Detailed information for antibodies used in this work. Authentication of SUM159PT and MDA-MB-231 cell lines by short-tandem-repeat analyses. Uncropped gels of Figures 1–4, S3, S7, S8, S9, S12, S13.

Author Contributions: Conceptualization, J.M.-P., V.M.-V., A.C., and M.P.S.-B.; methodology, J.M.-P., V.M.-V., A.C., M.P.S.-B., M.E.M., and V.M.G.; software: J.M.-P., V.M.-V., A.C., M.P.S.-B., M.E.M., and V.M.G.; validation: J.M.-P., V.M.-V., A.C., M.P.S.-B., M.E.M., and V.M.G.; investigation: J.M.-P., V.M.-V., A.C., M.P.S.-B., M.G.-H., V.F., M.E.M., and V.M.G.; resources: J.M.-P.; writing—original draft preparation, J.M.-P.; writing—review and editing: J.M.-P., V.M.-V., A.C., M.P.S.-B., M.E.M., and V.M.G.; funding acquisition, J.M.-P. All authors have read and agreed to the published version of the manuscript.

Funding: This work and the salary of Víctor Mayoral-Varo have been supported by grant number SAF2016-75991-R (MINECO, AEI/FEDER, UE) to Jorge Martín-Pérez.

Institutional Review Board Statement: Not applicable.

Informed Consent Statement: Not applicable.

Data Availability Statement: The data presented in this study are available in Cancers-1076808 and in its Supplementary Materials.

Acknowledgments: We are thankful to M. Izquierdo, J. León, I. Palmero, and L. Molero for their comments and support, and to Javier Pérez for his comments and suggestions in art graphics. J.M.-P. is a member of the GEICAM (Grupo Español de Investigación en Cáncer de Mama) and IdiPaz. We acknowledge support for the publication fee by the CSIC Open Access Publication Support Initiative through its Unit for Information Resources for Research (URICI).

Conflicts of Interest: The authors declare no conflict of interest.

References

1. Espada, J.; Martin-Perez, J. An Update on Src Family of Nonreceptor Tyrosine Kinases Biology. *Int. Rev. Cell Mol. Biol.* **2017**, *331*, 83–122. [CrossRef] [PubMed]
2. Shah, N.H.; Amacher, J.F.; Nocka, L.M.; Kuriyan, J. The Src module: An ancient scaffold in the evolution of cytoplasmic tyrosine kinases. *Crit. Rev. Biochem. Mol. Biol.* **2018**, *53*, 535–563. [CrossRef]
3. Pawson, T.; Raina, M.; Nash, P. Interaction domains: From simple binding events to complex cellular behavior. *FEBS Lett.* **2002**, *513*, 2–10. [CrossRef]
4. Cary, L.A.; Klinghoffer, R.A.; Sachsenmaier, C.; Cooper, J.A. SRC catalytic but not scaffolding function is needed for integrin-regulated tyrosine phosphorylation, cell migration, and cell spreading. *Mol. Cell Biol.* **2002**, *22*, 2427–2440. [CrossRef] [PubMed]
5. Avizienyte, E.; Fincham, V.J.; Brunton, V.G.; Frame, M.C. Src SH3/2 domain-mediated peripheral accumulation of Src and phospho-myosin is linked to deregulation of E-cadherin and the epithelial-mesenchymal transition. *Mol. Biol. Cell* **2004**, *15*, 2794–2803. [CrossRef]
6. Brunton, V.G.; Avizienyte, E.; Fincham, V.J.; Serrels, B.; Metcalf, C.A., 3rd; Sawyer, T.K.; Frame, M.C. Identification of Src-specific phosphorylation site on focal adhesion kinase: Dissection of the role of Src SH2 and catalytic functions and their consequences for tumor cell behavior. *Cancer Res.* **2005**, *65*, 1335–1342. [CrossRef]
7. Guarino, M. Src signaling in cancer invasion. *J. Cell Physiol.* **2010**, *223*, 14–26. [CrossRef]
8. Roskoski, R., Jr. Src protein-tyrosine kinase structure, mechanism, and small molecule inhibitors. *Pharmacol. Res.* **2015**, *94*, 9–25. [CrossRef]

9. Cheang, M.C.; Martin, M.; Nielsen, T.O.; Prat, A.; Voduc, D.; Rodriguez-Lescure, A.; Ruiz, A.; Chia, S.; Shepherd, L.; Ruiz-Borrego, M.; et al. Defining breast cancer intrinsic subtypes by quantitative receptor expression. *Oncologist* **2015**, *20*, 474–482. [CrossRef]
10. Cejalvo, J.M.; Martinez de Duenas, E.; Galvan, P.; Garcia-Recio, S.; Burgues Gasion, O.; Pare, L.; Antolin, S.; Martinello, R.; Blancas, I.; Adamo, B.; et al. Intrinsic Subtypes and Gene Expression Profiles in Primary and Metastatic Breast Cancer. *Cancer Res.* **2017**, *77*, 2213–2221. [CrossRef]
11. Holliday, D.L.; Speirs, V. Choosing the right cell line for breast cancer research. *Breast. Cancer Res.* **2011**, *13*, 215. [CrossRef]
12. Lehmann, B.D.; Jovanovic, B.; Chen, X.; Estrada, M.V.; Johnson, K.N.; Shyr, Y.; Moses, H.L.; Sanders, M.E.; Pietenpol, J.A. Refinement of Triple-Negative Breast Cancer Molecular Subtypes: Implications for Neoadjuvant Chemotherapy Selection. *PLoS ONE* **2016**, *11*, e0157368. [CrossRef] [PubMed]
13. Bayraktar, S.; Gluck, S. Molecularly targeted therapies for metastatic triple-negative breast cancer. *Breast. Cancer Res. Treat.* **2013**, *138*, 21–35. [CrossRef] [PubMed]
14. Jitariu, A.A.; Cimpean, A.M.; Ribatti, D.; Raica, M. Triple negative breast cancer: The kiss of death. *Oncotarget* **2017**, *8*, 46652–46662. [CrossRef] [PubMed]
15. Sanchez-Bailon, M.P.; Calcabrini, A.; Gomez-Dominguez, D.; Morte, B.; Martin-Forero, E.; Gomez-Lopez, G.; Molinari, A.; Wagner, K.U.; Martin-Perez, J. Src kinases catalytic activity regulates proliferation, migration and invasiveness of MDA-MB-231 breast cancer cells. *Cell Signal* **2012**, *24*, 1276–1286. [CrossRef]
16. Sanchez-Bailon, M.P.; Calcabrini, A.; Mayoral-Varo, V.; Molinari, A.; Wagner, K.U.; Losada, J.P.; Ciordia, S.; Albar, J.P.; Martin-Perez, J. Cyr61 as mediator of Src signaling in triple negative breast cancer cells. *Oncotarget* **2015**, *6*, 13520–13538. [CrossRef]
17. Adams, B.D.; Wali, V.B.; Cheng, C.J.; Inukai, S.; Booth, C.J.; Agarwal, S.; Rimm, D.L.; Gyorffy, B.; Santarpia, L.; Pusztai, L.; et al. miR-34a Silences c-SRC to Attenuate Tumor Growth in Triple-Negative Breast Cancer. *Cancer Res.* **2016**, *76*, 927–939. [CrossRef]
18. Aleshin, A.; Finn, R.S. SRC: A century of science brought to the clinic. *Neoplasia* **2010**, *12*, 599–607. [CrossRef]
19. Garcia-Martinez, J.M.; Calcabrini, A.; Gonzalez, L.; Martin-Forero, E.; Agullo-Ortuno, M.T.; Simon, V.; Watkin, H.; Anderson, S.M.; Roche, S.; Martin-Perez, J. A non-catalytic function of the Src family tyrosine kinases controls prolactin-induced Jak2 signaling. *Cell Signal* **2010**, *22*, 415–426. [CrossRef]
20. Yeo, M.G.; Partidge, M.A.; Ezratty, E.J.; Shen, Q.; Gundersen, G.G.; Marcantonio, E.E. Src SH2 arginine 175 is required for cell motility: Specific focal adhesion kinase targeting and focal adhesion assembly function. *Mol. Cell Biol.* **2006**, *24*, 4399–4409. [CrossRef]
21. Schaller, M.D.; Hildebrand, J.D.; Shannon, J.D.; Fox, J.W.; Vines, R.R.; Parsons, J.T. Autophosphorylation of the focal adhesion kinase, pp125FAK, directs SH2- dependent binding of pp60src. *Mol. Cell Biol.* **1994**, *14*, 1680–1688. [CrossRef] [PubMed]
22. Gonzalez, L.; Agullo-Ortuno, M.T.; Garcia-Martinez, J.M.; Calcabrini, A.; Gamallo, C.; Palacios, J.; Aranda, A.; Martin-Perez, J. Role of c-Src in Human MCF7 Breast Cancer Cell Tumorigenesis. *J. Biol. Chem.* **2006**, *281*, 20851–20864. [CrossRef] [PubMed]
23. Schlaepfer, D.D.; Hunter, T. Evidence for in vivo phosphorylation of the Grb2 SH2-domain binding site on focal adhesion kinase by Src-family protein-tyrosine kinases. *Mol. Cell Biol.* **1996**, *16*, 5623–5633. [CrossRef] [PubMed]
24. Wu, J.C.; Chen, Y.C.; Kuo, C.T.; Wenshin, Y.H.; Chen, Y.Q.; Chiou, A.; Kuo, J.C. Focal adhesion kinase-dependent focal adhesion recruitment of SH2 domains directs SRC into focal adhesions to regulate cell adhesion and migration. *Sci. Rep.* **2015**, *5*, 18476. [CrossRef] [PubMed]
25. Shakespeare, W.; Yang, M.; Bohacek, R.; Cerasoli, F.; Stebbins, K.; Sundaramoorthi, R.; Azimioara, M.; Vu, C.; Pradeepan, S.; Metcalf, C., 3rd; et al. Structure-based design of an osteoclast-selective, nonpeptide src homology 2 inhibitor with in vivo antiresorptive activity. *Proc. Natl. Acad. Sci. USA* **2000**, *97*, 9373–9378. [CrossRef]
26. Mandine, E.; Jean-Baptiste, V.; Vayssiere, B.; Gofflo, D.; Benard, D.; Sarubbi, E.; Deprez, P.; Baron, R.; Superti-Furga, G.; Lesuisse, D. High-affinity Src-SH2 ligands which do not activate Tyr(527)-phosphorylated Src in an experimental in vivo system. *Biochem. Biophys. Res. Commun.* **2002**, *298*, 185–192. [CrossRef]
27. Oneyama, C.; Agatsuma, T.; Kanda, Y.; Nakano, H.; Sharma, S.V.; Nakano, S.; Narazaki, F.; Tatsuta, K. Synthetic inhibitors of proline-rich ligand-mediated protein-protein interaction: Potent analogs of UCS15A. *Chem. Biol.* **2003**, *10*, 443–451. [CrossRef]
28. Lu, X.L.; Cao, X.; Liu, X.Y.; Jiao, B.H. Recent progress of Src SH2 and SH3 inhibitors as anticancer agents. *Curr. Med. Chem.* **2010**, *17*, 1117–1124. [CrossRef]
29. Moroco, J.A.; Baumgartner, M.P.; Rust, H.L.; Choi, H.G.; Hur, W.; Gray, N.S.; Camacho, C.J.; Smithgall, T.E. A Discovery Strategy for Selective Inhibitors of c-Src in Complex with the Focal Adhesion Kinase SH3/SH2-binding Region. *Chem. Biol. Drug Des.* **2015**, *86*, 144–155. [CrossRef]
30. Garcia-Recio, E.M.; Pinto-Diez, C.; Perez-Morgado, M.I.; Garcia-Hernandez, M.; Fernandez, G.; Martin, M.E.; Gonzalez, V.M. Characterization of MNK1b DNA Aptamers That Inhibit Proliferation in MDA-MB231 Breast Cancer Cells. *Mol. Ther. Nucleic. Acids* **2016**, *5*, e275. [CrossRef]
31. Nimjee, S.M.; White, R.R.; Becker, R.C.; Sullenger, B.A. Aptamers as Therapeutics. *Annu. Rev. Pharmacol. Toxicol.* **2017**, *57*, 61–79. [CrossRef] [PubMed]
32. Nuzzo, S.; Roscigno, G.; Affinito, A.; Ingenito, F.; Quintavalle, C.; Condorelli, G. Potential and Challenges of Aptamers as Specific Carriers of Therapeutic Oligonucleotides for Precision Medicine in Cancer. *Cancers (Basel)* **2019**, *11*, 1521. [CrossRef] [PubMed]

33. Anderson, S.K.; Gibbs, C.P.; Tanaka, A.; Kung, H.J.; Fujita, D.J. Human cellular src gene: Nucleotide sequence and derived amino acid sequence of the region coding for the carboxy-terminal two-thirds of pp60c-src. *Mol. Cell Biol.* **1985**, *5*, 1122–1129. [CrossRef] [PubMed]
34. Hirai, H.; Varmus, H.E. Site-directed mutagenesis of the SH2- and SH3-coding domains of c-src produces varied phenotypes, including oncogenic activation of p60c-src. *Mol. Cell Biol.* **1990**, *10*, 1307–1318. [CrossRef] [PubMed]
35. Elsberger, B.; Fullerton, R.; Zino, S.; Jordan, F.; Mitchell, T.J.; Brunton, V.G.; Mallon, E.A.; Shiels, P.G.; Edwards, J. Breast cancer patients' clinical outcome measures are associated with Src kinase family member expression. *Br. J. Cancer* **2010**, *103*, 899–909. [CrossRef] [PubMed]
36. Al-Hajj, M.; Wicha, M.S.; Benito-Hernandez, A.; Morrison, S.J.; Clarke, M.F. Prospective identification of tumorigenic breast cancer cells. *Proc. Natl. Acad. Sci. USA* **2003**, *100*, 3983–3988. [CrossRef] [PubMed]
37. Mayoral-Varo, V.; Calcabrini, A.; Sanchez-Bailon, M.P.; Martin-Perez, J. miR205 inhibits stem cell renewal in SUM159PT breast cancer cells. *PLoS ONE* **2017**, *12*, e0188637. [CrossRef]
38. Mayoral-Varo, V.; Calcabrini, A.; Sanchez-Bailon, M.P.; Martinez-Costa, O.H.; Gonzalez-Paramos, C.; Ciordia, S.; Hardisson, D.; Aragon, J.J.; Fernandez-Moreno, M.A.; Martin-Perez, J. c-Src functionality controls self-renewal and glucose metabolism in MCF7 breast cancer stem cells. *PLoS ONE* **2020**, *15*, e0235850. [CrossRef]
39. Ginestier, C.; Hur, M.H.; Charafe-Jauffret, E.; Monville, F.; Dutcher, J.; Brown, M.; Jacquemier, J.; Viens, P.; Kleer, C.G.; Liu, S.; et al. ALDH1 Is a Marker of Normal and Malignant Human Mammary Stem Cells and a Predictor of Poor Clinical Outcome. *Cell Stem. Cell* **2007**, *1*, 555–567. [CrossRef]
40. Mayoral-Varo, V.; IIBM, Madrid, Spain. IIBM Seminars Series 2018-19. Personal communication, 2018.
41. Garcia-Gutierrez, L.; Delgado, M.D.; Leon, J. MYC Oncogene Contributions to Release of Cell Cycle Brakes. *Genes (Basel)* **2019**, *10*, 244. [CrossRef]
42. Kleinschmidt, E.G.; Schlaepfer, D.D. Focal adhesion kinase signaling in unexpected places. *Curr. Opin. Cell Biol.* **2017**, *45*, 24–30. [CrossRef] [PubMed]
43. Meng, F.; Saxena, S.; Liu, Y.; Joshi, B.; Wong, T.H.; Shankar, J.; Foster, L.J.; Bernatchez, P.; Nabi, I.R. The phospho-caveolin-1 scaffolding domain dampens force fluctuations in focal adhesions and promotes cancer cell migration. *Mol. Biol. Cell* **2017**, *28*, 2190–2201. [CrossRef] [PubMed]
44. Martellucci, S.; Clementi, L.; Sabetta, S.; Mattei, V.; Botta, L.; Angelucci, A. Src Family Kinases as Therapeutic Targets in Advanced Solid Tumors: What We Have Learned so Far. *Cancers (Basel)* **2020**, *12*, 1448. [CrossRef] [PubMed]
45. Hollestelle, A.; Nagel, J.H.; Smid, M.; Lam, S.; Elstrodt, F.; Wasielewski, M.; Ng, S.S.; French, P.J.; Peeters, J.K.; Rozendaal, M.J.; et al. Distinct gene mutation profiles among luminal-type and basal-type breast cancer cell lines. *Breast. Cancer Res. Treat.* **2010**, *121*, 53–64. [CrossRef] [PubMed]
46. Perou, C.M. Molecular stratification of triple-negative breast cancers. *Oncologist* **2011**, *16*, 61–70. [CrossRef]
47. Barnabas, N.; Cohen, D. Phenotypic and Molecular Characterization of MCF10DCIS and SUM Breast Cancer Cell Lines. *Int. J. Breast. Cancer* **2013**, *2013*, 872743. [CrossRef] [PubMed]
48. Sausgruber, N.; Coissieux, M.M.; Britschgi, A.; Wyckoff, J.; Aceto, N.; Leroy, C.; Stadler, M.B.; Voshol, H.; Bonenfant, D.; Bentires-Alj, M. Tyrosine phosphatase SHP2 increases cell motility in triple-negative breast cancer through the activation of SRC-family kinases. *Oncogene* **2015**, *34*, 2272–2278. [CrossRef]
49. Tian, J.; Raffa, F.A.; Dai, M.; Moamer, A.; Khadang, B.; Hachim, I.Y.; Bakdounes, K.; Ali, S.; Jean-Claude, B.; Lebrun, J.J. Dasatinib sensitises triple negative breast cancer cells to chemotherapy by targeting breast cancer stem cells. *Br. J. Cancer* **2018**, *119*, 1495–1507. [CrossRef]
50. Simpkins, F.; Jang, K.; Yoon, H.; Hew, K.E.; Kim, M.; Azzam, D.J.; Sun, J.; Zhao, D.; Ince, T.A.; Liu, W.; et al. Dual Src and MEK Inhibition Decreases Ovarian Cancer Growth and Targets Tumor Initiating Stem-Like Cells. *Clin. Cancer Res.* **2018**, *24*, 4874–4886. [CrossRef]
51. Alcalá, S.; Mayoral-Varo, V.; Ruiz-Cañas, L.; López-Gil, J.C.; Heeschen, C.; Martín-Pérez, J.; Sainz, B., Jr. Targeting SRC Kinase Signaling in Pancreatic Cancer Stem Cells. *Int. J. Mol. Sci.* **2020**, *21*, 7437. [CrossRef]
52. Zheng, X.; Resnick, R.J.; Shalloway, D. Apoptosis of estrogen-receptor negative breast cancer and colon cancer cell lines by PTP alpha and src RNAi. *Int. J. Cancer* **2008**, *122*, 1999–2007. [CrossRef] [PubMed]
53. Ishizawar, R.C.; Miyake, T.; Parsons, S.J. c-Src modulates ErbB2 and ErbB3 heterocomplex formation and function. *Oncogene* **2007**, *26*, 3503–3510. [CrossRef] [PubMed]
54. Nagaraj, N.S.; Smith, J.J.; Revetta, F.; Washington, M.K.; Merchant, N.B. Targeted inhibition of SRC kinase signaling attenuates pancreatic tumorigenesis. *Mol. Cancer Ther.* **2010**, *9*, 2322–2332. [CrossRef] [PubMed]
55. Thomas, S.; Overdevest, J.B.; Nitz, M.D.; Williams, P.D.; Owens, C.R.; Sanchez-Carbayo, M.; Frierson, H.F.; Schwartz, M.A.; Theodorescu, D. Src and caveolin-1 reciprocally regulate metastasis via a common downstream signaling pathway in bladder cancer. *Cancer Res.* **2011**, *71*, 832–841. [CrossRef]
56. Je, D.W.; Ou, Y.M.; Ji, Y.G.; Cho, Y.; Lee, D.H. The inhibition of SRC family kinase suppresses pancreatic cancer cell proliferation, migration, and invasion. *Pancreas* **2014**, *43*, 768–776. [CrossRef]
57. Sun, L.; Xu, X.; Chen, Y.; Zhou, Y.; Tan, R.; Qiu, H.; Jin, L.; Zhang, W.; Fan, R.; Hong, W.; et al. Rab34 regulates adhesion, migration, and invasion of breast cancer cells. *Oncogene* **2018**, *37*, 3698–3714. [CrossRef]

58. Bristow, J.M.; Reno, T.A.; Jo, M.; Gonias, S.L.; Klemke, R.L. Dynamic phosphorylation of tyrosine 665 in pseudopodium-enriched atypical kinase 1 (PEAK1) is essential for the regulation of cell migration and focal adhesion turnover. *J. Biol. Chem.* **2013**, *288*, 123–131. [CrossRef]
59. Soundararajan, S.; Chen, W.; Spicer, E.K.; Courtenay-Luck, N.; Fernandes, D.J. The nucleolin targeting aptamer AS1411 destabilizes Bcl-2 messenger RNA in human breast cancer cells. *Cancer Res.* **2008**, *68*, 2358–2365. [CrossRef]
60. Flanagan, L.; Van Weelden, K.; Ammerman, C.; Ethier, S.P.; Welsh, J. SUM-159PT cells: A novel estrogen independent human breast cancer model system. *Breast. Cancer Res. Treat.* **2000**, *58*, 193–204. [CrossRef]
61. Marlow, R.; Honeth, G.; Lombardi, S.; Cariati, M.; Hessey, S.; Pipili, A.; Mariotti, V.; Buchupalli, B.; Foster, K.; Bonnet, D.; et al. A novel model of dormancy for bone metastatic breast cancer cells. *Cancer Res.* **2013**, *73*, 6886–6899. [CrossRef]
62. Bibbins, K.B.; Boeuf, H.; Varmus, H.E. Binding of the Src SH2 domain to phosphopeptides is determined by residues in both the SH2 domain and the phosphopeptides. *Mol. Cell Biol.* **1993**, *13*, 7278–7287. [CrossRef] [PubMed]
63. Wheeler, D.L.; Iida, M.; Dunn, E.F. The role of Src in solid tumors. *Oncologist* **2009**, *14*, 667–678. [CrossRef] [PubMed]
64. Sen, B.; Johnson, F.M. Regulation of SRC family kinases in human cancers. *J. Signal Transduct.* **2011**, *2011*, 865819. [CrossRef] [PubMed]

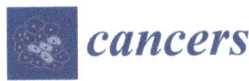

Article

Identification of VRK1 as a New Neuroblastoma Tumor Progression Marker Regulating Cell Proliferation

Ana Colmenero-Repiso [1,2], María A. Gómez-Muñoz [1,2], Ismael Rodríguez-Prieto [1,2], Aida Amador-Álvarez [1,3], Kai-Oliver Henrich [4], Diego Pascual-Vaca [5], Konstantin Okonechnikov [6], Eloy Rivas [5], Frank Westermann [4], Ricardo Pardal [1,2,*] and Francisco M. Vega [1,3,*]

[1] Instituto de Biomedicina de Sevilla (IBiS), Hospital Universitario Virgen del Rocío/CSIC/Universidad de Sevilla, 41013 Seville, Spain; acolmenero-ibis@us.es (A.C.-R.); magomez-ibis@us.es (M.A.G.-M.); ismaelropri@us.es (I.R.-P.); aaalvarez@us.es (A.A.-Á.)
[2] Departamento de Fisiología Médica y Biofísica, Universidad de Sevilla, 41013 Seville, Spain
[3] Departamento de Biología Celular, Facultad de Biología, Universidad de Sevilla, 41012 Seville, Spain
[4] German Cancer Research Center (DKFZ), Division Neuroblastoma Genomics, 69120 Heidelberg, Germany; k.henrich@kitz-heidelberg.de (K.-O.H.); f.westermann@kitz-heidelberg.de (F.W.)
[5] Departamento de Anatomía Patológica, Hospital Universitario Virgen del Rocío, 41013 Sevilla, Spain; diego.pascualvaca.sspa@juntadeandalucia.es (D.P.-V.); eloy.rivas.sspa@juntadeandalucia.es (E.R.)
[6] Pediatric Neurooncology, German Cancer Research Center (DKFZ), 69120 Heidelberg, Germany; k.okonechnikov@kitz-heidelberg.de
* Correspondence: rpardal@us.es (R.P.); fmvega@us.es (F.M.V.)

Received: 15 October 2020; Accepted: 19 November 2020; Published: 20 November 2020

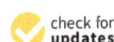

Simple Summary: Aggressive neuroblastoma (NB) is one of the most common pediatric cancers and causes a disproportionate mortality among affected children. A better knowledge about the biology of this tumor is needed to be able to provide new treatments and prognostic tools. Protein kinases are one of the best targets for molecular cancer treatment, as we are potentially able to produce inhibitors that abrogate its activity. In this study we have identified that the human protein kinase VRK1 is associated with tumor aggressiveness and patient survival in NB. We have characterized the function of VRK1 in NB tumor cells and determined that VRK1 is an essential mediator of NB cell proliferation. We also study the relationship between VRK1 and the oncogene MYCN, the best-known marker for NB progression to date. Our work suggests that VRK1 synergize with MYCN to drive NB progression and that VRK1 inhibition may constitute a novel cell-cycle-targeted strategy for anticancer therapy in neuroblastoma.

Abstract: Neuroblastoma (NB) is one of the most common pediatric cancers and presents a poor survival rate in affected children. Current pretreatment risk assessment relies on a few known molecular parameters, like the amplification of the oncogene MYCN. However, a better molecular knowledge about the aggressive progression of the disease is needed to provide new therapeutical targets and prognostic markers and to improve patients' outcomes. The human protein kinase VRK1 phosphorylates various signaling molecules and transcription factors to regulate cell cycle progression and other processes in physiological and pathological situations. Using neuroblastoma tumor expression data, tissue microarrays from fresh human samples and patient-derived xenografts (PDXs), we have determined that VRK1 kinase expression stratifies patients according to tumor aggressiveness and survival, allowing the identification of patients with worse outcome among intermediate risk. VRK1 associates with cell cycle signaling pathways in NB and its downregulation abrogates cell proliferation in vitro and in vivo. Through the analysis of ChIP-seq and methylation data from NB tumors, we show that VRK1 is a MYCN gene target, however VRK1 correlates with

NB aggressiveness independently of MYCN gene amplification, synergizing with the oncogene to drive NB progression. Our study also suggests that VRK1 inhibition may constitute a novel cell-cycle-targeted strategy for anticancer therapy in neuroblastoma.

Keywords: neuroblastoma; high-risk; VRK1; proliferation; MYCN; tumorigenesis

1. Introduction

Neuroblastoma is a pediatric solid tumor with embryonic origin derived from sympathoadrenal precursors of the neural crest [1]. It is the most common type of cancer diagnosed during the first year of life and the most frequent extracranial solid tumor in children [2]. Neuroblastoma is clinically characterized by a great heterogeneity, with patients presenting extensive metastasis and with frequent relapses. This cancer displays an event-free survival below 50% [3]. At the cellular level, intratumoral heterogeneity has emerged as a hallmark for these tumors, with presence of cell populations that differ in their differentiation status, proliferative potential and response to treatment [4,5]. Aggressive neuroblastomas are incurable to date, reflecting the pressing need for a better understanding of the cellular and molecular mechanisms that mediate aggressiveness, relapse and metastasis, in order to elucidate new and better prognostic markers and therapeutic targets.

Although neuroblastomas can occur in familial contexts, most cases arise sporadically. Few recurrent alterations in common oncogenes or tumor suppressors have been identified. Among those, the oncogene MYCN is amplified in about 20–30% of all tumors, being associated with poor prognosis [6]. Many aggressive tumors however do not harbor MYCN amplification [7]. It is believed that many of the changes leading to neuroblastoma initiation and progression are aberrant epigenetic events affecting transcriptional programs, probably linked to processes occurring during sympathoadrenal development from the neural crest [8,9].

Vaccinia-related kinase 1 (VRK1) is a member of a ser/thr kinase family that phosphorylates various molecules and transcription factors implicated in chromatin condensation, DNA repair and cell cycle progression [10–12]. VRK1 acts in some context as a chromatin remodelling enzyme, as it is known to phosphorylate several histones, affecting their acetylation and methylation status, and influencing gene transcription, DNA damage response and cell cycle [11,13]. A physiological role for VRK1 has been described in fetal tissues, for example during uterine development or embryonic development of the hematopoietic system [14,15]. VRK1 is also highly expressed in spermatogonia stem cells, being essential for spermatogonia cell maintenance [16].

VRK1 activity has been also associated with pathological situations. Genetic variants of VRK1 have been linked to diverse neurodegenerative disorders [17,18]. High VRK1 expression has been associated with poor prognosis in various cancers like head and neck [19], lung carcinomas [20] or hepatocellular carcinomas [21,22]. Furthermore, it is known that high VRK1 protein levels confer a stronger resistance to treatment in breast [23] and lung cancer [24]. The possible implication of VRK1 in neuroblastoma or other pediatric cancers is unknown. However, the *VRK1* gene has been suggested as a potential transcriptional target for the oncoprotein MYCN [25].

Given the evidence linking VRK1 to tumor progression and the connection with MYCN, we decided to analyze the contribution of this protein to neuroblastoma cell biology, focusing on its pathological significance and prognostic value. We demonstrate that VRK1 is highly expressed in high-grade neuroblastoma and is associated with proliferation and dedifferentiation in tumor cells. Functional experiments show that VRK1 is essential for NB cell proliferation and tumor progression, and thus could be a new target for neuroblastoma treatment. Despite being a target of MYCN transcription factor, VRK1 is a marker of tumor progression and malignancy independent of MYCN expression. The expression of VRK1 can serve as a prognostic factor for MYCN nonamplified tumors with malignant progression or to stratify intermediate grade patients with uncertain outcome.

2. Results

2.1. VRK1 Expression Correlates with Aggressiveness in Neuroblastoma Tumors

To elucidate the possible implication of VRK1 in NB tumors, we explored the expression of *VRK1* in several cohorts of human NB patient tumor samples, using expression data from public databases. *VRK1* is highly expressed in the International Neuroblastoma Staging System (INSS) stage 4 NB compared with normal adrenal tissue, and significant differences can be observed between more aggressive neuroblastoma stages (stages 3 and 4) and more benign ones (Stages 1, 2 and 4S) (Figure 1a and Figure S1a).

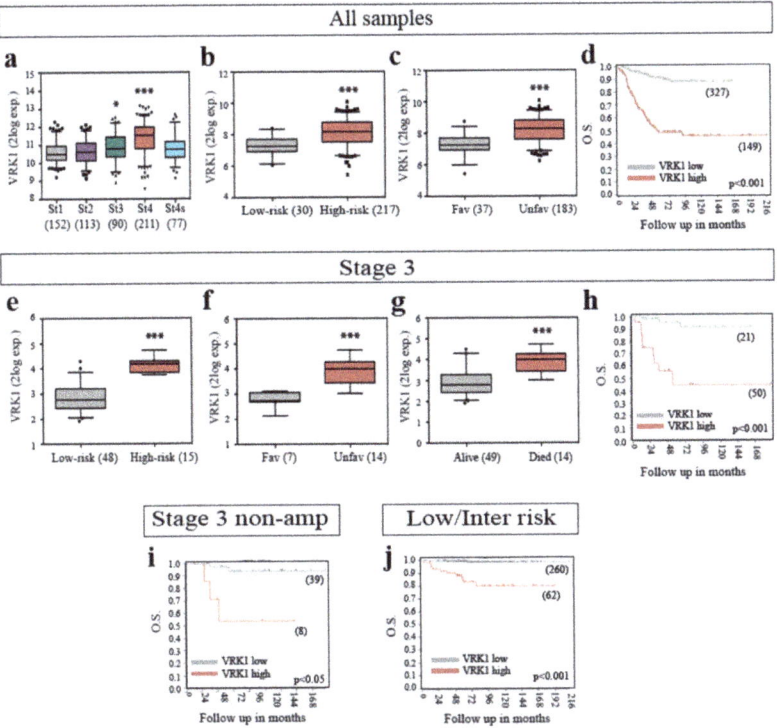

Figure 1. VRK1 mRNA expression correlates with neuroblastoma (NB) progression in patient tumor samples. (**a–c**) VRK1 expression in patient tumor samples of all stages separated by the International Neuroblastoma Staging System (INSS) stage a, the International Neuroblastoma Risk Group Staging System (INRGSS) risk b or histology c. GSE62564 and GSE3446 datasets used; (**d**) Kaplan curve showing overall survival probability from patients stratified according to VRK1 expression (GSE62564); (**e–g**) stage 3 patient tumor samples separated by risk (**e**) histology (**f**) or outcome (**g**). GSE62564 and GSE3446 datasets used; (**h–j**) Kaplan curve showing overall survival probability from stage 3 patients (**h**) stage 3 MYCN nonamplified patients (**i**) or low/intermediate risk patients (**j**) stratified according to VRK1 expression (GSE62564). Number of samples shown in brackets. *: $p < 0.05$; ***: $p < 0.001$.

High VRK1 expression levels were also able to significantly stratify patients with high-risk, unfavorable histology, poor survival and worse outcome (Figure 1b–d and Figure S1b), indicating a strong correlation between VRK1 expression and NB unfavorable prognosis and aggressiveness. Same results were obtained with all patient datasets tested. A proportion of patients classified at diagnosis as INSS Stage 3 present progression of the disease later on. Strategies to stratify these patients early on would be beneficial to anticipate treatment. VRK1 expression alone could identify, among INSS stage 3 patients, those with high-risk, unfavorable histology, worse outcome and low survival probability, indicating the potential of VRK1 expression as a prognostic factor (Figure 1e–h). High VRK1 expression is also indicative of worse survival probability among the patients with stage 3 tumors without MYCN amplification and among low- and intermediate-risk patients (Figure 1i,j). VRK1 expression also identifies patients with worse survival when classified into age at diagnosis groups, including groups in which it would be important to find new prognostic markers to identify patients with tumor progression, such as the ones diagnosed before 12 months of age (Figure S1c).

In addition to mRNA expression, VRK1 protein detection by immunohistochemistry on our own collection of 36 human neuroblastoma tumor samples shows high VRK1 expression in M stage tumors and patient-derived xenografts (PDXs) derived from high-grade NB patients, compared to L1 tumors (Figure 2a). Interestingly, we observed a decrease in VRK1 expression in samples obtained after treatment, when compared to the ones obtained at diagnosis, but high VRK1 expression on samples from patients with relapses and worse outcome (Figure S1d).

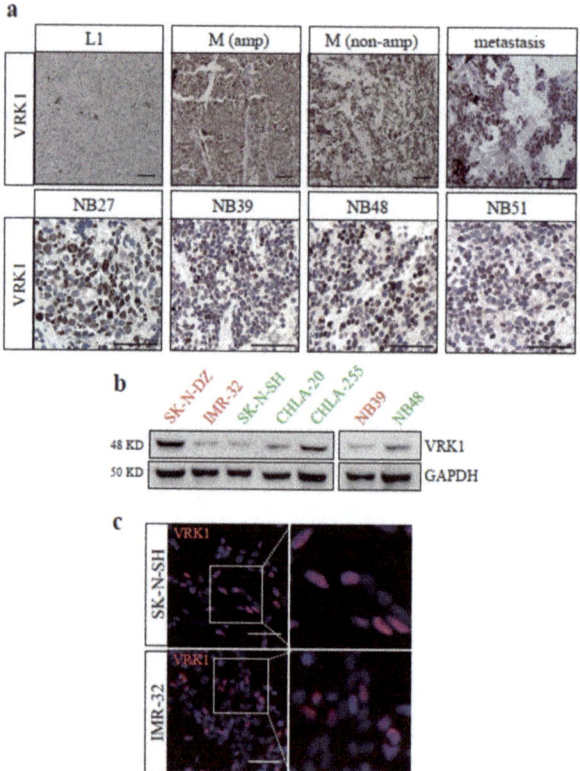

Figure 2. VRK1 protein expression in NB samples and cells. (**a**) Immunohistochemistry showing VRK1 expression in examples of NB tumor patient samples from the indicated International Neuroblastoma Risk Group Staging System (INRGSS) stages (top row) or patient-derived xenografts (PDXs) samples (bottom row), from our in-house collection. Scale bars: 60 µM. (**b**) Western blot showing VRK1 expression in cell lysates from different NB cell lines or PDX-derived cells. In red, MYCN-amplified cell lines. In green, nonamplified cell lines. (**c**) Immunofluorescence showing VRK1 expression (red) in NB cell lines. Nuclear staining is shown in blue. Scale bar: 60 µM.

We finally analyzed VRK1 protein levels in a panel of commonly used neuroblastoma cell lines and primary PDX-derived cells. VRK1 expression was variable among the cell lines and does not seem to correlate with MYCN amplification, but the kinase was expressed in all neuroblastoma cell lines and PDX samples tested (Figure 2b,c). We decided to perform functional studies in SK-N-SH and IMR-32 cell lines, with similar levels of VRK1, a moderate expression and different MYCN-amplification status.

2.2. VRK1 is Associated with NB Tumor Cell Proliferation

A role for VRK1 in the control of cell division has been proposed in cells from diverse origin [12]. To analyze the specific implication of VRK1 in neuroblastoma tumors, we first took an indirect approach in which, using different human neuroblastoma expression datasets, we analyzed the function of genes whose expression were significantly correlated to the one of *VRK1* across the samples, creating a *VRK1*-high-expression signature (Figure 3a and Table S4). A signaling pathway analysis performed with these genes showed a significant enrichment in pathways related to cell cycle, DNA replication, DNA repair and differentiation. There was a strong positive correlation in NB tumors and PDX-derived cells between *VRK1* expression and the expression of the proliferation marker *Ki67*, as well as the mitotic index in the tumors, observed both by mRNA and immunohistochemistry (Figure 3b–d).

VRK1 is an essential gene in many cellular contexts, and a total abrogation of VRK1 expression has been shown to be detrimental for cells [15,26]. Therefore, we used transient siRNA transfection to partially reduce the expression of VRK1 in neuroblastoma cells and study the functional consequences. VRK1 downregulation in NB cells by specific siRNA diminishes cell division, observed as a significant reduction in cell culture confluency, cell viability and cycling Ki67-positive cells (Figure 3e,f). Competition assays performed with SK-N-SH cells labeled either with Green Fluorescent Protein (GFP) or Red fluorescent Protein (RFP), and depleting VRK1 with siRNA only in one of the two populations, showed an enrichment in cells transfected with control siRNA after 96 h in culture (Figure S2a). Single-cell clonogenic proliferation assays also showed an NB cell proliferation dependence on VRK1 (Figure S2b). Cell cycle and apoptosis analysis by FACS showed that cells depleted of VRK1 do not experience an increase in apoptosis (Figure S3).

All together, these functional assays demonstrate an important role for VRK1 in NB cell proliferation. Concordant with this, transient and moderate VRK1 knockdown induces a downregulation of cell cycle progression protein levels, such as cyclin D1 or mdm2, and an increase in cell cycle suppressors like *p*53 and its target *p*21 (Figure 3g). Interestingly, the downregulation of VRK1 also provokes a drop in MYCN protein expression.

2.3. VRK1 Downregulation Impairs Neuroblastoma Tumorigenesis in a Xenograft Model

Given the association of VRK1 with malignancy, we investigated whether VRK1 depletion on neuroblastoma cells would impact tumor progression. Neuroblastoma cells were treated with siRNA against VRK1 or with control siRNA before xenograft transplantation on recipient immunocompromised mice (Figure 4). Tumor onset was delayed on mice injected with VRK1-depleted cells, and resulting tumors in these mice were significantly smaller. A histological analysis showed that tumors grown from VRK1-RNAi-treated cells were less proliferative. Surprisingly, depletion of VRK1 with siRNA is transitory and tumors were collected after 8 weeks, indicating that VRK1 downregulation is somehow maintained in tumors and might have a profound and long-lasting influence on tumor establishment and growth.

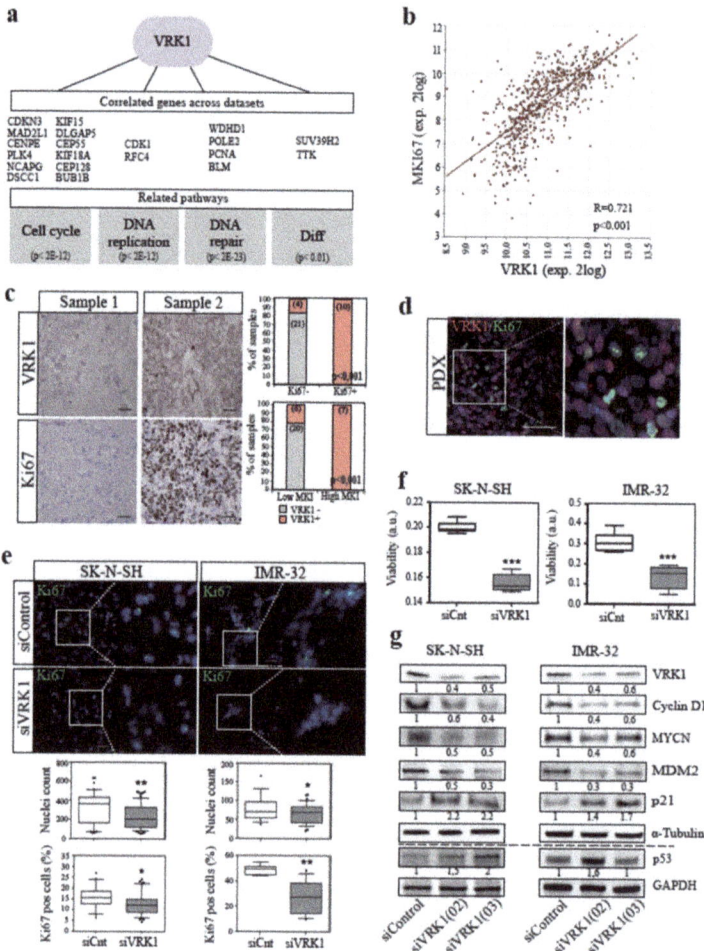

Figure 3. VRK1 associates with neuroblastoma tumor cell proliferation. (**a**) Representative genes correlated with VRK1 expression across NB sample datasets and their associated pathways. p values for signaling Gene Expression Omnibus (GEO) terms are shown; (**b**), mRNA expression correlation between VRK1 and Ki67 in human NB tumors (GSE45547); (**c**) immunohistochemical detection of the proliferation marker Ki67 and VRK1 in serial sections of NB patient samples. Representative negative (left) and positive (right) cases have been selected. Quantifications show correlation between VRK1 protein expression and Ki67 expression or mitotic-karyorrhexis index (MKI) per sample. Number of samples per group shown in brackets; (**d**) immunofluorescence staining showing a VRK1 and Ki67 cellular staining in a PDX tumor sample. Scale bar: 250 µM; (**e**) immunofluorescence staining and quantification of Ki67-positive cells in NB cell lines after 96 h transfection with either VRK1 or control siRNAs. Nuclei are counterstained with DAPI. Scale bar: 100 µM. ** $p < 0.01$; * $p < 0.05$; (**f**) Viability of NB cells after VRK1 downregulation by siRNA. *** $p < 0.001$; (**g**) Western blot analysis showing the levels of the indicated proteins after transient VRK1 downregulation. Quantification of representative blots shown. Note average 50% reduction in VRK1 expression.

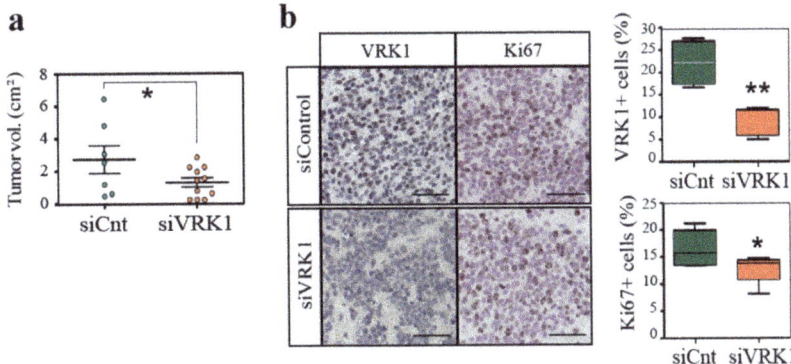

Figure 4. VRK1 downregulation impairs neuroblastoma tumorigenesis in a xenograft model. (**a**) Volume of tumors in mice collected after flank injection with SK-N-SH cells 24 h after transfection with either VRK1 or control siRNA; (**b**) Immunohistochemical staining showing VRK1 and Ki67 protein expression in representative tumors from each condition. Percentage of positive cells are shown. Scale bars: 60 μM.

2.4. VRK1 Associates with Neuroblastoma Progression Independently of MYCN Amplification

We have previously seen that *VRK1* expression strongly correlates with aggressiveness in neuroblastoma tumors. *VRK1* expression is also significantly higher in *MYCN*-amplified versus nonamplified neuroblastoma tumors (Figure 5a). However, the correlation of *VRK1* expression with malignant traits was still maintained when only the *MYCN* nonamplified tumors were analyzed (Figure 5b). This indicates that, despite the possible relationship between *VRK1* and *MYCN*, *VRK1* expression strongly correlates with neuroblastoma unfavorable prognosis and aggressiveness independently of the *MYCN* amplification status.

We decided to further explore the connection between *MYCN* transcription factor and VRK1 in neuroblastoma. Amplification of *MYCN* in neuroblastoma tumors correlates with high *VRK1* gene expression and aggressiveness, although the levels of *VRK1* do not correlate with the levels of *MYCN* expression in nonamplified tumors (Figure 5c). In neuroblastoma PDX tissues, all MYCN-positive cells showed expression of VRK1 (Figure 5d). These could be explained because *VRK1* has been identified as a MYCN transcriptional target with an E-box MYCN response element in the gene promoter [25]. Analysis of *VRK1* gene promoter methylation status in an NB tumor panel shows a region, downstream of the *VRK1* transcription start site, that is hypomethylated in high-risk tumors with *MYCN* amplification and is defined by a single CpG probe (cg26685539, mean methylation difference 0.2 (*b*), $q < 0.001$)) (Figure 6a, Table S5). According to MYCN ChIP-seq data from three neuroblastoma cell lines (Be(2)-C, Kelly and NGP), this region does not map to the uniformly hypomethylated *MYCN*-binding site, and possibly indicates the binding of additional transcription factors or coactivators. Significant negative correlation between cg26685539 methylation and VRK1 expression indicates the presence of a promoter downstream correlated region (pdCR) [27] with high potential for *VRK1* gene transcription regulation (Figure 6b). This opens the possibility to synergistic actions regulating cell proliferation in neuroblastoma cells. *MYCN*-amplified neuroblastoma cell lines are more sensitive to VRK1 inhibition than cells with no *MYCN* amplification, reinforcing this possibility (Figure 6c).

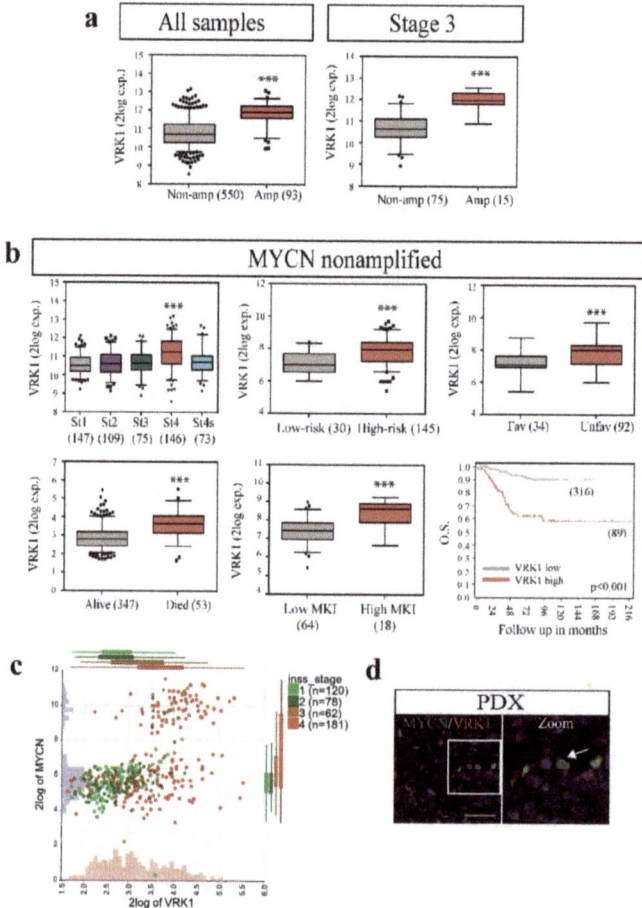

Figure 5. VRK1 associates with neuroblastoma progression independently of MYCN amplification. (**a**) Expression of VRK1 in MYCN-amplified or MYCN nonamplified NB tumors (GSE45547); (**b**) VRK1 expression on patient tumor samples without MYCN amplification separated by INSS stage (GSE45547), risk, histology, outcome (GSE62564) or mitotic-karyorrhexis index (MKI) (GSE3446). Kaplan curves show overall survival probability from patients stratified according to VRK1 expression (GSE45547). Number of samples shown in brackets. ***: $p < 0.001$; (**c**) two gene (VRK1 and MYCN) expression analyses in tumor samples (dataset GSE49710). Number of samples in each INSS stage are shown and separated by colors; (**d**) immunofluorescence showing MYCN and VRK1 staining in a representative PDX sample.

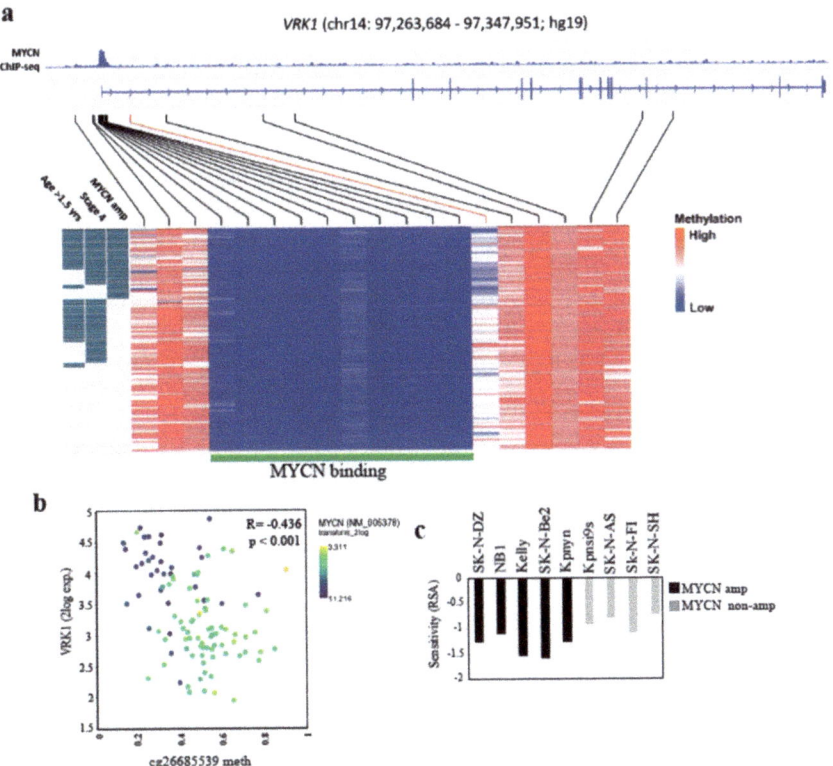

Figure 6. VRK1 promoter is hypomethylated in MYCN-amplified NB tumors. (**a**) Graphic representation of the VRK1 gene promoter region and colour-coded methylation levels on 16 regional CpG probes across 105 NB tumor samples. The MYCN binding site according to MYCN ChIP-seq in neuroblastoma cell lines Be(2)-C, Kelly and NGP is depicted in green with exemplary Be(2)-C MYCN ChIP-seq signal at the top. cg2668539 probe is shown in red; (**b**) Correlation between VRK1 expression and the methylation of the probe cg26685539 in NB tumors. Each dot represents a patient sample and is colored code according to MYCN gene expression; (**c**) MYCN status-dependent sensitivity (RSA) for VRK1 knockdown in 9 NB cell lines. Negative RSA values indicate viability reduction upon knockdown.

3. Discussion

Recurrent mutations or alterations in known oncogenes are not common in neuroblastoma. High *MYCN* expression occurs in about 20% of neuroblastoma and is a clear indication of bad prognosis. *MYCN* gene amplification confers a high probability of aggressive disease and metastasis [28]. However, there is still a proportion of NBs with poor survival but no clear molecular prognosis indicator at diagnosis or therapeutic target. We have shown that VRK1 kinase is highly expressed in NBs of high grade and poor survival, providing a potential new gene target with therapeutic value.

Our gene expression and ontology analysis predicts that *VRK1* expression is associated in neuroblastoma tumors with signaling pathways involved in cell cycle regulation, DNA replication or DNA repair. VRK1 has been described as a proliferation control protein in human fibroblasts and in some cancers like head and neck or myeloma [19,29,30]. We have identified that VRK1 is associated with cell proliferation in NB tumor cells and that it is an essential gene controlling cell division in these tumors. *VRK1* expression downregulation associates with cell cycle arrest, observed by a reduction of cyclin D1 and MDM2 and an increase of p 53 and p 21, while no increase in apoptosis was observed.

These indicate a possible cancer type-dependent action of VRK1, as higher apoptotic activity was detected in esophageal squamous cell carcinoma cells after VRK1 downregulation [22]. We found that VRK1 expression in NB also associates with genes belonging to signaling pathways related to differentiation. Given the importance of sympatoadrenal differentiation for the origin and development of NB, it would be interesting to study a possible role of VRK1 in this phenomenon.

A complete abrogation of VRK1 expression has been shown to be deleterious in cells and during development [15,18]. These have posed difficulties for the generation of knockout mice models or the use of CRISPR-Cas9 to study VRK1 biology. Surprisingly, a transient and partial reduction of VRK1 expression in NB cells was enough to significantly impaired tumor growth in a xenograft mouse model. Moreover, a sustained reduction in VRK1 expression in tumor cells in vivo could be observed long after transfection. It is possible that VRK1 downregulation elicits a long-lasting epigenetic effect on NB tumor cells or that a high VRK1 expression is needed for the successful establishment of the tumor in the initial steps. VRK1 is known to induce epigenetic changes in chromatin by histone phosphorylation and acetylation modulation [23,31]. We cannot rule out an influence of the tumor microenvironment on VRK1 expression and the proliferative potential of NB cells, not triggered in the case of tumor establishment with VRK1 knockdown cells. In any case, this could place VRK1 as an essential gene for NB progression, suggesting a possible use of transient inhibition of VRK1 for the treatment of NB. So far, we lack compounds to specifically inhibit the VRK family of proteins, but different efforts are underway to produce potent and specific inhibitors [11,32].

Interestingly, *VRK1* expression alone stratified patients originally diagnosed as intermediate risk or INSS stage 3, allowing the identification of patients with worse outcome. Although most stage 3 patients respond well to therapy and become disease free, about 10-15% of them do not respond adequately to current treatments, many of them but not all, corresponding to patients with *MYCN* amplified tumors. *VRK1* expression, together with known prognostic factors, might contribute to a better and more precise stratification of intermediate risk patients. Further studies with bigger cohorts, especially in the case of stage 3 *MYCN* non-amplified tumors, could finally help to determine the potential use of VRK1 expression in the clinic.

VRK1 expression significantly correlates with malignancy in NB patient tumors, even in tumors without MYCN amplification, suggesting that VRK1 might be an indicative of poor survival, independent of MYCN status. We have observed a significantly higher expression of VRK1 gene in MYCN amplified tumors, although the correlation with MYCN gene expression disappears in tumors without amplification. The VRK1 gene promoter contains an E-BOX MYCN response sequence, and ChipSeq data from NB cells confirms MYCN binding to the VRK1 gene. Interestingly, VRK1 downregulation seems to also affect MYCN expression, raising the possibility of a regulatory feedback loop, similar to the one occurring between VRK1 and other regulators, like p 53 [33]. Both VRK1 and MYCN proteins could be cooperating in NB progression, although VRK1 gene expression does not seem to be entirely dependent on MYCN transcriptional activation. Interestingly, high levels of MYCN in MYCN-amplified tumors are associated with a specific epigenetic landscape in the VRK1 gene, characterized by hypomethylation of a region downstream of the promoter, which correlates with high expression of the kinase. This opens up the possibility for the presence of a new unknown transcription factor collaborating with MYCN to further activate VRK1 in MYCN-amplified NB tumors. MYCN-amplified tumor cells seem to be dependent on VRK1 expression for its exacerbated proliferation, raising the possibility of using VRK1 inhibitors for NB treatment as an alternative to MYCN targeting. Furthermore, the use of VRK1 inhibitors in combination with BET bromodomain domain inhibitors, with action against MYCN transcriptional activity, might also be a promising option [34,35].

4. Materials and Methods

4.1. Human Tumor Gene Expression and Methylation Analysis

VRK1 gene expression analysis was performed with the use of the R2: Genomics Analysis and Visualization Platform (Available on: http://r2.amc.nl; Academic Medical Centre, Amsterdam) and GEO Datasets (Gene Expression Omnibus; NCBI: National Centre for Biotechnology Information, Bethesda, MD, USA). Patient cohort datasets used are summarized in Table S1. Tumors on these datasets are clinically classified following the International Neuroblastoma Staging System (INSS) [36], classifying tumors in growing degree of aggressiveness into stages 1, 2, 3 or 4. 4S is a special metastatic benign stage. Risk information on these patient samples according to the INRG stratification system is also used [37]. Gene ontology and pathway analysis were performed with the help of the Reactome Pathway Database (Available on: https://reactome.org).

VRK1 gene promoter region methylation analysis by Illumina HumanMethylation450 BeadChip was performed with data from [38]. Differential DNA methylation was performed applying the dmpFinder function of the minfi R package with limits q-val < 0.05 and mean methylation difference > 0.1 (beta value). MYCN ChIP-seq data from neuroblastoma cell lines was derived from GEO ID GSE80154 [39].

4.2. Cell Culture and siRNA Transfection

The human NB cell lines SK-N-SH, SK-N-DZ and IMR-32 were obtained from the EACC (Salisbury, UK) and grown at 37 °C in 5% CO_2 in Dulbecco's Modified Eagle Medium (GIBCO) + 10% fetal bovine serum (FBS). CHLA20 and CHLA-255 NB cell lines were obtained from the COG Cell Line and Xenograft Repository (Texas Tech University Health Sciences Center, Lubbock, TX, USA) and were grown in IMDM media (GIBCO) + 15%FBS and 1 × ITS (5 µg/mL insulin, 5 µg/mL transferrin y 5 ng/mL selenic acid). All media was supplemented with 2 mM glutamine (GIBCO BRL, Gaithersburg, MD, USA), 100 U/mL of penicillin and 100 µg/mL of streptomycin. Cell lines expressing fluorescent proteins were generated by transfection and selection with the corresponding vectors (pEGFPN1 and pERFPN1 from Clontech, Mountain View, CA, USA). NB39T and NB48T PDX primary cell lines were derived from freshly obtained tumors and have been described previously [5].

Two siRNAs targeting VRK1 (named siVRK1(02) and siVRK1(03), respectively) and a control siRNAs (named siControl) were obtained from Dharmacon (Thermo Scientific, Waltham, MA, USA). Transient transfections were performed using Lipofectamine 2000 (Invitrogen, Carlsbad, CA, USA) according to the manufacturer's instructions with final siRNAs concentration of 100 nM. Knock down of the protein was checked and assays performed 72 h post-transfection, unless indicated otherwise. The sequences of VRK1 siRNAs and control siRNAs were: siVRK1(02) (CAAGGAACCUGGUGUUGAA; UUCAACACCAGGUUCCUUG), siVRK1(03) (GGAAUGGAAAGUAGGAUUA; UAAUCCUACUUUCCAUUCC), siControl-ontarget plus#4 (UGGUUUACAUGUUUUCCUA; UAGGAAAACAUGUAAACCA).

For NB cell line sensitivity to VRK1 knockdown, data from the DRIVE data portal was collected [40].

4.3. Western Blot and Cellular Assays

Western blot analysis was performed from cell lysates using the following antibodies: mouse anti-VRK1 (1F6) (1:1000, #3307, Cell Signaling Technology, Danvers, MA, USA), mouse anti-Cyclin D1 (1:500, Santa Cruz Biotechnology, Santa Cruz, CA, USA), rabbit anti-MDM2 (1:500, R&D Systems), rabbit anti-p 21 (1:500, Abcam), mouse anti-Nestin (1:500, R&D Systems), mouse anti-MYCN (1:500, Millipore, Burlington, MA, USA), mouse anti-α-Tubulin (1:5000, Sigma) and rabbit anti-GAPDH (1:5000, Trevigen, Gaithersburg, MD, USA).

Cell viability was measured with the use of AlamarBlue reagent (Thermo Scientific, Waltham, MA, USA) 96 h post-transfection, following recommended instructions.

For clone formation assays, cells were transfected with siRNA as described and after 72 h 5×10^4 cells per well were seeded on a 6-well plate and grown for 7 days before pictures of the cell clones formed were taken under the microscope.

Apoptosis assay was performed with the Phycoerythrin (PE) AnnexinV Apoptosis Detection kit (BD Pharmigen, San Diego, CA, USA). The original Western blot figures can be found in the Supplementary Materials (Figure S4).

4.4. Tumor Xenografts

6–8 weeks-old CB-17 SCID mice were acquired from Harlan Laboratories. Each mouse was injected in the right flank with 4×10^5 SK-N-SH, 24 h after transfection with the corresponding siRNAs. Efficiency of knock-down was demonstrated in parallel. After 8 weeks, all mice were sacrificed humanely and tumors excised and measured. Tissue samples were included in paraffin for immunohistochemical analysis.

The generation and maintenance of PDXs was described previously [5]. Four different generated PDXs were used (Table S2). PDX tumor samples were obtained and treated similarly than xenograft.

4.5. Immunofluorescence and Immunohistochemistry

For immunofluorescence, cells or frozen sections were fixed with 4% paraformaldehyde, permeabilized with 0.2% Triton X-100 in PBS, blocked with 1% BSA in PBS and incubated with the corresponding antibodies. The following antibodies were used: rabbit anti-VRK1 (1:500, Sigma, San Luis, MO, USA), rabbit anti-Ki67 (1:500, Thermo Scientific, Waltham, MA, USA), mouse anti-MYCN (1:500, Millipore, Burlington, MA, USA). Nuclei were stained with DAPI (Life Technologies, Carlsbad, CA, USA; 1:1000). Secondary antibodies used were Alexa488-donkey-anti-mouse-IgG and Alexa568-goat-anti-rabbit-IgG (Life Technologies, Carlsbad, CA, USA; 1:1000). Images were obtained with an epifluorescence microscope (Olympus BX-61, IX-71 or Nikon TiE2000). Images were analyzed with ImageJ software (National Institutes of Health, Bethesda, WA, USA) and Cell Profiler [41].

Immunohistochemical detection in patient samples was performed using a cohort of 31 primary paraffin-embedded neuroblastoma cancer tissue sections, placed in duplicate on a tissue microarray (TMA) (Table S3) or PDXs. Tumors on the TMA were clinically classified into the more recent International Neuroblastoma Risk Groups staging system (INRGSS), dividing patients into L1, L2, M or MS stages [42]. For immunohistochemistry staining, paraffin-embedded sections were obtained from tissues, hydrated, treated for antigen retrieval with citrate buffer (pH 6) and incubated with the corresponding antibodies. Vectastain ABC kit and DAB peroxidase substrate kit (Vector Laboratories, Burlingame, CA, USA) were used following recommended procedures. Consecutive sections were used when appropriate. Antibodies used were rabbit anti VRK1 (Sigma, San Luis, MO, USA; 1:500) and rabbit anti Ki67 (Thermo Scientific, Waltham, MA, USA; 1:500). Secondary antibodies used were biotinylated-conjugated anti-mouse and biotinylated-conjugated anti-rabbit (Vector Laboratories Burlingame, CA, USA; 1:1000). Pathologists scored the samples using a scale that combines the percentage of positive cells and the intensity of the reaction product [43].

4.6. Statistical Analysis

Statistical analysis was performed on R2 genomics platform or Graphpad Prism software. One-way (two-way on grouped differentiation data) analysis of variance ANOVA or the unpaired *t*-test were used for statistical analysis. Results were assumed significant when $p < 0.05$. Fisher's exact test was used for the analysis of positive and negative tumor samples. In gene expression analysis plots, box and whiskers graphs show median, 10–90 percentiles and outliers as dots. Scan was used to identify Kaplan survival curves cutoff, and p-values are Bonferroni corrected. Bar graphs show average ± SEM in all cases. Number of measurements or samples (n) is indicated in each case.

4.7. Ethics Approval and Consent to Participate

All animal experiments were conducted according to procedures approved by the Ethics Committee from the University of Seville (CEEA_US2014-012) and complying with all animal use guidelines. Fresh neuroblastoma tumor samples were managed and obtained from the Andalusian tissue Biobank (Andalusian Public Health System Biobank and ISCIII-Red de Biobancos PT13/0010/0056, Seville, Spain) after informed consent was obtained from subjects' guardians following all established regulations. Clinical information on patient cohorts is available for research use and has been anonymized.

5. Conclusions

Overall, our findings identify VRK1 as an essential protein for NB cell proliferation, and establish a complex relationship and possible collaboration with the MYCN oncogene driving NB progression.

Supplementary Materials: The following are available online at http://www.mdpi.com/2072-6694/12/11/3465/s1, Figure S1: Expression of VRK1 in NB tumors. Figure S2: VRK1 downregulation abrogates proliferation. Figure S3: Apoptosis assay after VRK1 downregulation. Figure S4: Uncropped Western Blotting figures. Table S1: Data cohorts of NB patient samples used for VRK1 gene expression analysis. Table S2: Characteristics of the original tumor biopsies used for stablishing the PDX used in the study. Table S3: Anatomo-pathological characteristics of the human tumors included in the TMA. Table S4: Correlation of gene expression with VRK1 across different NB patient cohorts and gene ontology. Table S5: CpGs VRK1 promoter and association with VRK1 gene expression.

Author Contributions: F.M.V. and R.P. designed and supervised the study and wrote the manuscript. F.M.V. and A.C.-R. developed methodology. F.M.V., A.C.-R., M.A.G.-M. and I.R.-P. acquired data. D.P.-V. and E.R. contributed to the immunohistochemistry data and analysis. K.-O.H. and F.W. were involved in promoter analysis and expression data analysis. K.O. performed computational analysis. I.R.-P., M.A.G.-M. and A.A.-Á. provided technical support and F.M.V., A.C.-R. and R.P. analyzed and interpreted the data. All authors have read and agreed to the published version of the manuscript.

Funding: This research is supported by grants from the "Junta de Andalucía-Universidad de Sevilla-FEDER" (US-1262985) and the Spanish Ministry of Science and Innovation (SAF2016-80412-P and PID2019-110817R). A.C. is the recipient of a FPI fellowship from the Spanish Ministry of Science and Innovation. MAG is supported by a fellowship from the "Asociación de familiares y amigos de pacientes con Neuroblastoma (NEN)". A.A. is the recipient of a FPU fellowship from the Spanish Ministry of Education.

Acknowledgments: We thank Pedro A. Lazo from Centro de Investigación del Cáncer in Salamanca, for kindly providing reagents and helpful discussion. We are grateful to the Andalusian tissue Biobank at Virgen del Rocío University Hospital for their help with the human tumor samples and tissue histology. We thank Catalina Márquez, Gema Ramírez and Rosa Cabello, from the Virgen del Rocío University Hospital, for their insight and help obtaining NB samples.

Conflicts of Interest: The authors declare no conflict of interest. The funders had no role in the design of the study; in the collection, analyses, or interpretation of data; in the writing of the manuscript or in the decision to publish the results.

References

1. Johnsen, J.I.; Dyberg, C.; Wickström, M. Neuroblastoma-A neural crest derived embryonal malignancy. *Front. Mol. Neurosci.* **2019**, *12*, 9. [CrossRef] [PubMed]
2. Matthay, K.K.; Maris, J.M.; Schleiermacher, G.; Nakagawara, A.; Mackall, C.L.; Diller, L.; Weiss, W.A. Neuroblastoma. *Nat. Rev. Dis. Prim.* **2016**, *2*, 16079. [CrossRef] [PubMed]
3. Kamijo, T.; Nakagawara, A. Molecular and genetic bases of neuroblastoma. *Int. J. Clin. Oncol.* **2012**, *17*, 190–195. [CrossRef] [PubMed]
4. Van Groningen, T.; Koster, J.; Valentijn, L.J.; Zwijnenburg, D.A.; Akogul, N.; Hasselt, N.E.; Broekmans, M.; Haneveld, F.; Nowakowska, N.E.; Bras, J.; et al. Neuroblastoma is composed of two super-enhancer-associated differentiation states. *Nat. Genet.* **2017**, *49*, 1261–1266. [CrossRef]

5. Vega, F.M.; Colmenero-Repiso, A.; Gómez-Muñoz, M.A.; Rodríguez-Prieto, I.; Aguilar-Morante, D.; Ramírez, G.; Márquez, C.; Cabello, R.; Pardal, R. CD44-high neural crest stem-like cells are associated with tumour aggressiveness and poor survival in neuroblastoma tumours. *EBioMedicine* **2019**, *49*, 82–95. [CrossRef] [PubMed]
6. Gröbner, S.N.; Project, I.P.-S.; Worst, B.C.; Weischenfeldt, J.; Buchhalter, I.; Kleinheinz, K.; Rudneva, V.A.; Johann, P.D.; Balasubramanian, G.P.; Segura-Wang, M.; et al. The landscape of genomic alterations across childhood cancers. *Nat. Cell Biol.* **2018**, *555*, 321–327. [CrossRef]
7. Louis, C.U.; Shohet, J.M. Neuroblastoma: Molecular pathogenesis and therapy. *Annu. Rev. Med.* **2015**, *66*, 49–63. [CrossRef]
8. Tomolonis, J.A.; Agarwal, S.; Shohet, J.M. Neuroblastoma pathogenesis: Deregulation of embryonic neural crest development. *Cell Tissue Res.* **2018**, *372*, 245–262. [CrossRef]
9. Delloye-Bourgeois, C.; Castellani, V. Hijacking of embryonic programs by neural crest-derived neuroblastoma: From physiological migration to metastatic dissemination. *Front. Mol. Neurosci.* **2019**, *12*, 52. [CrossRef]
10. Klerkx, E.P.F.; Lazo, P.A.; Askjaer, P. Emerging biological functions of the vaccinia-related kinase (VRK) family. *Histol. Histopathol.* **2009**, *24*, 749–759. [CrossRef] [PubMed]
11. Campillo-Marcos, I.; Lazo, P.A. Implication of the VRK1 chromatin kinase in the signaling responses to DNA damage: A therapeutic target? *Cell. Mol. Life Sci.* **2018**, *75*, 2375–2388. [CrossRef] [PubMed]
12. Valbuena, A.; Sanz-García, M.; López-Sánchez, I.; Vega, F.M.; Lazo, P.A. Roles of VRK1 as a new player in the control of biological processes required for cell division. *Cell. Signal.* **2011**, *23*, 1267–1272. [CrossRef] [PubMed]
13. Aihara, H.; Nakagawa, T.; Mizusaki, H.; Yoneda, M.; Kato, M.; Doiguchi, M.; Imamura, Y.; Higashi, M.; Ikura, T.; Hayashi, T.; et al. Histone H2A T120 Phosphorylation promotes oncogenic transformation via upregulation of cyclin D1. *Mol. Cell* **2016**, *64*, 176–188. [CrossRef] [PubMed]
14. Dobrzynska, A.; Askjaer, P. Vaccinia-related kinase 1 is required for early uterine development in Caenorhabditis elegans. *Dev. Biol.* **2016**, *411*, 246–256. [CrossRef] [PubMed]
15. Vega, F.M.; Gonzalo, P.; Gaspar, M.L.; Lazo, P.A. Expression of the VRK (vaccinia-related kinase) gene family of p53 regulators in murine hematopoietic development. *FEBS Lett.* **2003**, *544*, 176–180. [CrossRef]
16. Choi, Y.H.; Park, C.-H.; Kim, W.; Ling, H.; Kang, A.; Chang, M.W.; Im, S.-K.; Jeong, H.-W.; Kong, Y.-Y.; Kim, K.-T. Vaccinia-related kinase 1 is required for the maintenance of undifferentiated spermatogonia in mouse male germ cells. *PLoS ONE* **2010**, *5*, e15254. [CrossRef]
17. Vinograd-Byk, H.; Sapir, T.; Cantarero, L.; Lazo, P.A.; Zeligson, S.; Lev, D.; Lerman-Sagie, T.; Renbaum, P.; Reiner, O.; Levy-Lahad, E. The spinal muscular atrophy with pontocerebellar hypoplasia gene VRK1 regulates neuronal migration through an amyloid-β precursor protein-dependent mechanism. *J. Neurosci.* **2015**, *35*, 936–942. [CrossRef]
18. Vinograd-Byk, H.; Renbaum, P.; Levy-Lahad, E. Vrk1 partial knockdown in mice results in reduced brain weight and mild motor dysfunction, and indicates neuronal VRK1 target pathways. *Sci. Rep.* **2018**, *8*, 11265. [CrossRef]
19. Santos, C.R.; Rodríguez-Pinilla, M.; Vega, F.M.; Rodríguez-Peralto, J.L.; Blanco, S.; Sevilla, A.; Valbuena, A.; Hernandez, A.S.; Van Wijnen, A.J.; Li, F.; et al. VRK1 Signaling pathway in the context of the proliferation phenotype in head and neck squamous cell carcinoma. *Mol. Cancer Res.* **2006**, *4*, 177–185. [CrossRef]
20. Valbuena, A.; López-Sánchez, I.; Vega, F.M.; Sevilla, A.; Sanz-García, M.; Blanco, S.; Lazo, P.A. Identification of a dominant epitope in human vaccinia-related kinase 1 (VRK1) and detection of different intracellular subpopulations. *Arch. Biochem. Biophys.* **2007**, *465*, 219–226. [CrossRef]
21. Lee, N.; Kwon, J.-H.; Kim, Y.B.; Kim, S.-H.; Park, S.J.; Xu, W.; Jung, H.-Y.; Kim, K.-T.; Wang, H.J.; Choi, K.Y. Vaccinia-related kinase 1 promotes hepatocellular carcinoma by controlling the levels of cell cycle regulators associated with G1/S transition. *Oncotarget* **2015**, *6*, 30130–30148. [CrossRef] [PubMed]
22. Liu, Z.-C.; Cao, K.; Xiao, Z.-H.; Qiao, L.; Wang, X.-Q.; Shang, B.; Jia, Y.; Wang, Z. VRK1 promotes cisplatin resistance by up-regulating c-MYC via c-Jun activation and serves as a therapeutic target in esophageal squamous cell carcinoma. *Oncotarget* **2017**, *8*, 65642–65658. [CrossRef] [PubMed]
23. Salzano, M.; Vázquez-Cedeira, M.; Sanz-García, M.; Valbuena, A.; Blanco, S.; Fernández, I.F.; Lazo, P.A. Vaccinia-related kinase 1 (VRK1) confers resistance to DNA-damaging agents in human breast cancer by affecting DNA damage response. *Oncotarget* **2014**, *5*, 1770–1778. [CrossRef]

24. Campillo-Marcos, I.; Lazo, P.A. Olaparib and ionizing radiation trigger a cooperative DNA-damage repair response that is impaired by depletion of the VRK1 chromatin kinase. *J. Exp. Clin. Cancer Res.* **2019**, *38*, 1–16. [CrossRef] [PubMed]
25. Wei, J.S.; Song, Y.K.; Durinck, S.; Chen, Q.-R.; Cheuk, A.T.C.; Tsang, P.; Zhang, Q.; Thiele, C.J.; Slack, A.; Shohet, J.; et al. The MYCN oncogene is a direct target of miR-34a. *Oncogene* **2008**, *27*, 5204–5213. [CrossRef]
26. Vega, F.M.; Sevilla, A.; Lazo, P.A. p53 Stabilization and accumulation induced by human vaccinia-related kinase 1. *Mol. Cell. Biol.* **2004**, *24*, 10366–10380. [CrossRef]
27. Hovestadt, V.; Jones, D.T.W.; Picelli, S.; Wang, W.; Kool, M.; Northcott, P.A.; Sultan, M.; Stachurski, K.; Ryzhova, M.; Warnatz, H.-J.; et al. Decoding the regulatory landscape of medulloblastoma using DNA methylation sequencing. *Nat. Cell Biol.* **2014**, *510*, 537–541. [CrossRef]
28. Lee, J.W.; Son, M.H.; Cho, H.W.; Ma, Y.E.; Yoo, K.H.; Sung, K.W.; Koo, H.H. Clinical significance of MYCN amplification in patients with high-risk neuroblastoma. *Pediatr. Blood Cancer* **2018**, *65*, e27257. [CrossRef]
29. Valbuena, A.; López-Sánchez, I.; Lazo, P.A. Human VRK1 is an early response gene and its loss causes a block in cell cycle progression. *PLoS ONE* **2008**, *3*, e1642. [CrossRef]
30. Liu, J.; Wang, Y.; He, S.; Xu, X.; Huang, Y.; Tang, J.; Wu, Y.; Miao, X.; He, Y.; Wang, Q.; et al. Expression of vaccinia-related kinase 1 (VRK1) accelerates cell proliferation but overcomes cell adhesion mediated drug resistance (CAM-DR) in multiple myeloma. *Hematology* **2016**, *21*, 603–612. [CrossRef]
31. Kim, W.; Chakraborty, G.; Kim, S.; Shin, J.; Park, C.-H.; Jeong, M.-W.; Bharatham, N.; Yoon, H.S.; Kim, K.-T. Macro histone H2A1.2 (MacroH2A1) protein suppresses mitotic kinase VRK1 during interphase. *J. Biol. Chem.* **2011**, *287*, 5278–5289. [CrossRef] [PubMed]
32. Couñago, R.M.; Allerston, C.K.; Savitsky, P.; Azevedo, H.; Godoi, P.H.; Wells, C.I.; Mascarello, A.; Gama, F.H.D.S.; Massirer, K.B.; Zuercher, W.J.; et al. Structural characterization of human Vaccinia-Related Kinases (VRK) bound to small-molecule inhibitors identifies different P-loop conformations. *Sci. Rep.* **2017**, *7*, 1–12. [CrossRef] [PubMed]
33. Valbuena, A.; Vega, F.M.; Blanco, S.; Lazo, P.A. p53 Downregulates its activating vaccinia-related kinase 1, forming a new autoregulatory loop. *Mol. Cell. Biol.* **2006**, *26*, 4782–4793. [CrossRef] [PubMed]
34. Henssen, A.G.; Althoff, K.; Odersky, A.; Beckers, A.; Koche, R.; Speleman, F.; Schäfers, S.; Bell, E.; Nortmeyer, M.; Westermann, F.; et al. Targeting MYCN-driven transcription by BET-bromodomain inhibition. *Clin. Cancer Res.* **2015**, *22*, 2470–2481. [CrossRef] [PubMed]
35. Puissant, A.; Frumm, S.M.; Alexe, G.; Bassil, C.F.; Qi, J.; Chantery, Y.H.; Nekritz, E.A.; Zeid, R.; Gustafson, W.C.; Greninger, P.; et al. Targeting MYCN in neuroblastoma by BET bromodomain inhibition. *Cancer Discov.* **2013**, *3*, 308–323. [CrossRef] [PubMed]
36. Brodeur, G.M.; Pritchard, J.; Berthold, F.; Carlsen, N.L.; Castel, V.; Castelberry, R.P.; De Bernardi, B.; Evans, A.E.; Favrot, M.; Hedborg, F. Revisions of the international criteria for neuroblastoma diagnosis, staging, and response to treatment. *J. Clin. Oncol.* **1993**, *11*, 1466–1477. [CrossRef]
37. Cohn, S.L.; Pearson, A.D.J.; London, W.B.; Monclair, T.; Ambros, P.F.; Brodeur, G.M.; Faldum, A.; Hero, B.; Iehara, T.; Machin, D.; et al. The International Neuroblastoma Risk Group (INRG) classification system: An INRG task force report. *J. Clin. Oncol.* **2009**, *27*, 289–297. [CrossRef]
38. Henrich, K.-O.; Bender, S.; Saadati, M.; Dreidax, D.; Gartlgruber, M.; Shao, C.; Herrmann, C.; Wiesenfarth, M.; Parzonka, M.; Wehrmann, L.; et al. Integrative genome-scale analysis identifies epigenetic mechanisms of transcriptional deregulation in unfavorable neuroblastomas. *Cancer Res.* **2016**, *76*, 5523–5537. [CrossRef]
39. Zeid, R.; Lawlor, M.A.; Poon, E.; Reyes, J.M.; Fulciniti, M.; Lopez, M.A.; Scott, T.G.; Nabet, B.; Erb, M.A.; Winter, G.E.; et al. Enhancer invasion shapes MYCN-dependent transcriptional amplification in neuroblastoma. *Nat. Genet.* **2018**, *50*, 515–523. [CrossRef]
40. Iii, E.R.M.; De Weck, A.; Schlabach, M.R.; Billy, E.; Mavrakis, K.J.; Hoffman, G.; Belur, D.; Castelletti, D.; Frias, E.; Gampa, K.; et al. Project DRIVE: A compendium of cancer dependencies and synthetic lethal relationships uncovered by large-scale, deep RNAi screening. *Cell* **2017**, *170*, 577–592. [CrossRef]
41. Carpenter, A.E.; Jones, T.R.; Lamprecht, M.R.; Clarke, C.; Kang, I.H.; Friman, O.; Guertin, D.A.; Chang, J.H.; Lindquist, R.A.; Moffat, J.; et al. CellProfiler: Image analysis software for identifying and quantifying cell phenotypes. *Genome Biol.* **2006**, *7*, R100. [CrossRef] [PubMed]

42. Monclair, T.; Brodeur, G.M.; Ambros, P.F.; Brisse, H.J.; Cecchetto, G.; Holmes, K.; Kaneko, M.; London, W.B.; Matthay, K.K.; Nuchtern, J.G.; et al. The International Neuroblastoma Risk Group (INRG) staging system: An INRG task force report. *J. Clin. Oncol.* **2009**, *27*, 298–303. [CrossRef] [PubMed]
43. Allred, D.C.; Harvey, J.M.; Berardo, M.; Clark, G.M. Prognostic and predictive factors in breast cancer by immunohistochemical analysis. *Mod. Pathol.* **1998**, *11*, 155–168. [PubMed]

Publisher's Note: MDPI stays neutral with regard to jurisdictional claims in published maps and institutional affiliations.

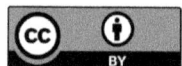

© 2020 by the authors. Licensee MDPI, Basel, Switzerland. This article is an open access article distributed under the terms and conditions of the Creative Commons Attribution (CC BY) license (http://creativecommons.org/licenses/by/4.0/).

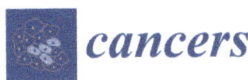

Article

Sunitinib-Containing Carborane Pharmacophore with the Ability to Inhibit Tyrosine Kinases Receptors FLT3, KIT and PDGFR-β, Exhibits Powerful In Vivo Anti-Glioblastoma Activity

Catalina Alamón [1,†], Belén Dávila [1,†], María Fernanda García [2], Carina Sánchez [1], Mariángeles Kovacs [3], Emiliano Trias [3], Luis Barbeito [3], Martín Gabay [4], Nidal Zeineh [4], Moshe Gavish [4], Francesc Teixidor [5], Clara Viñas [5,*], Marcos Couto [1,5,*] and Hugo Cerecetto [1,2,*]

1. Grupo de Química Orgánica Medicinal, Instituto de Química Biológica, Facultad de Ciencias, Universidad de la República, Montevideo 11400, Uruguay; calamon@pasteur.edu.uy (C.A.); bdavila@fcien.edu.uy (B.D.); Csanchez@fcien.edu.uy (C.S.)
2. Área de Radiofarmacia, Centro de Investigaciones Nucleares, Facultad de Ciencias, Universidad de la República, Montevideo 11400, Uruguay; mfgarcia@fcien.edu.uy
3. Laboratorio de Neurodegeneración, Institut Pasteur de Montevideo, Montevideo 11400, Uruguay; mkovacs@pasteur.edu.uy (M.K.); etrias@pasteur.edu.uy (E.T.); barbeito@pasteur.edu.uy (L.B.)
4. Molecular Pharmacology, Faculty of Medicine, Technion Institute of Technology, Haifa 3200003, Israel; mgabay@campus.technion.ac.il (M.G.); nidalz@campus.technion.ac.il (N.Z.); mgavish@technion.ac.il (M.G.)
5. Institut de Ciència de Materials de Barcelona, ICMAB-CSIC, Campus UAB, 08193 Bellaterra, Spain; teixidor@icmab.es
* Correspondence: clara@icmab.es (C.V.); mcouto@fcien.edu.uy (M.C.); hcerecetto@cin.edu.uy (H.C.)
† Equivalent contribution.

Received: 21 October 2020; Accepted: 13 November 2020; Published: 18 November 2020

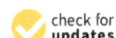

Simple Summary: Glioblastoma is one of the most aggressive central nervous system tumors. Combinations of therapies, such as tyrosine kinase receptor inhibition and boron neutron capture therapy (BNCT), could offer greater patients benefits over single-therapies. The aim of our study was to assess the potential of sunitinib-carborane hybrid compound **1** as an anti-glioblastoma agent. We confirmed for **1** the ability to inhibit tyrosine kinase receptors, which could promote canonical and non-canonical effects, absence of mutagenicity, ability to cross the blood–brain barrier, and powerful in vivo anti-glioblastoma activity. The overall attractive profile of **1** makes it an interesting compound for a bimodal therapeutic strategy against high grade gliomas.

Abstract: Malignant gliomas are the most common malignant and aggressive primary brain tumors in adults, the prognosis being—especially for glioblastomas—extremely poor. There are no effective treatments yet. However, tyrosine kinase receptor (TKR) inhibitors and boron neutron capture therapy (BNCT), together, have been proposed as future therapeutic strategies. In this sense in our ongoing project of developing new anti-glioblastoma drugs, we identified a sunitinib-carborane hybrid agent, **1**, with both in vitro selective cytotoxicity and excellent BNCT-behavior. Consequently, we studied the ability of compound **1** to inhibit TKRs, its promotion of cellular death processes, and its effects on the cell cycle. Moreover, we analyzed some relevant drug-like properties of **1**, i.e., mutagenicity and ability to cross the blood–brain barrier. These results encouraged us to perform an in vivo anti-glioblastoma proof of concept assay. It turned out to be a selective FLT3, KIT, and PDGFR-β inhibitor and increased the apoptotic glioma-cell numbers and arrested sub-G1-phase cell cycle. Its in vivo activity in immunosuppressed mice bearing U87 MG human glioblastoma evidenced excellent anti-tumor behavior.

Keywords: carborane; FLT3; sub-G1 arrest; anti-tumor activity

1. Introduction

Even though glioblastoma is one of the most frequent and aggressive adult primary central nervous system tumors, with no more than two years of survival in a low percentage (3–5%) group of patients [1], there are still no adequate therapeutic strategies. Some studied therapeutic tools include surgery, chemotherapy, boron neutron capture therapy (BNCT), radiotherapy, tumor treating fields therapy, photodynamic therapy, and combined strategies. Regarding chemotherapy, the first-line drug is the alkylating agent temozolomide (**Tmz**, Figure 1) which shows clear disadvantages, drug resistance in patients [2] being the most relevant. As second-line chemotherapeutics, tyrosine kinase receptors (TKRs) inhibitors have been used [3–5], i.e., vascular endothelial growth factor (VEGF) receptor (VEGFR1 and 2) inhibitors. In this sense, the anti-tumor and anti-angiogenic agent sunitinib (**Sun**, Figure 1) inhibits VEGFR1, 2, and 3, PDGFR-α and β, KIT, FLT3, RET, and CSF1R [6]. It was studied on a preclinical neuroendocrine tumor model, thereby displaying a reduction in the glioma cells' invasive capacity [6–8]. Nevertheless, it has not been active in newly diagnosed glioblastoma patients [9] and in a single-arm phase II trial **Sun** displayed minimal anti-glioblastoma activity with high toxicity [10].

On the other hand, as an alternative therapeutic approach, BNCT emerges as an opportunity to treat high-grade gliomas [11]. The BNCT therapy occurs when cells accumulating ^{10}B are irradiated with thermal neutrons to produce ^{4}He and ^{7}Li. [11,12] The resulting energy is about 100 million times more than was put in. The generated radiation destroys malignant cells containing the boron compound (approximately 10^9 atoms of ^{10}B/cell) and results in a therapeutic effect. Thus, highly boron-enriched molecules with an adequate vector might allow the selective delivery of a consistent amount of boron to the tumor without loading healthy cells. The fact that new irradiation facilities are becoming accessible at hospitals due to the recent advances in particles technology [13,14] and in medical imaging and in computing [15–17], makes radiotherapies such as BNCT a feasible choice for cancer medical therapy that may work especially well for tumors, which are resistant to chemotherapy and conventional radiotherapy. All these indications foresee BNCT as an accessible leading-edge technology.

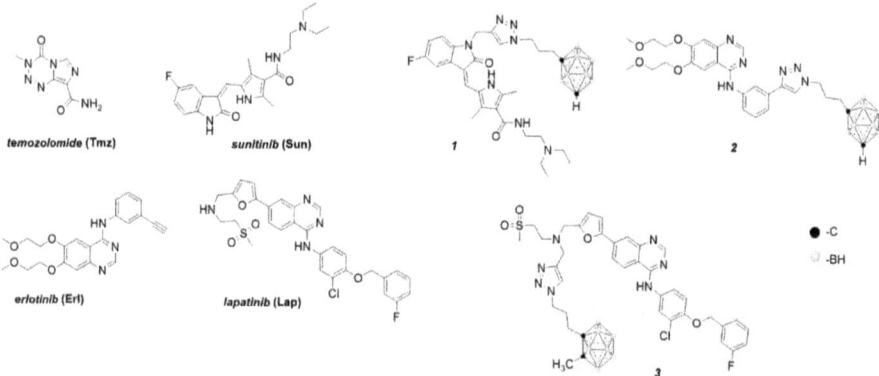

Figure 1. Chemical structures of glioblastoma drug temozolomide (**Tmz**); some relevant tyrosine kinase receptor inhibitors, sunitinib (**Sun**), erlotinib (**Erl**), and lapatinib (**Lap**); and a previous hybrid TKI–boron cluster [18–22].

For an efficient BNCT, a ^{10}B containing drug that accumulates selectively into target cells is necessary. Regarding this subject, we have previously investigated and developed hybrid agents that provide dual therapeutic actions (chemotherapy plus BNCT), i.e., tyrosine kinase receptor inhibitors such as chemotherapeutics and boron clusters, as BNCT agents. The substructures derived of the TKRs inhibitors, which were combined with icosahedral boron clusters for potential use in BNCT, are sunitinib (**Sun**, Figure 1), erlotinib (**Erl**, Figure 1), and lapatinib (**Lap**, Figure 1) [18–22].

Moving to the workflow of our investigation, herein we describe some studies on compound **1** that allow us to think that it could be used as an anti-glioblastoma drug using combined therapies. We first examined its in vitro ability to inhibit 468 human protein kinases, the kind of cellular death triggered in glioblastoma cells and in a simulated tumor microenvironment, i.e., glioma cells-astrocytes, and the effects on the cell cycle for both kinds of cells. Secondly, we analyzed some relevant drug-like properties of **1**, such as mutagenicity and the ability to cross the blood–brain barrier. Based on the good results obtained in the previous experiments, thirdly we performed an in vivo proof of concept of compound **1** as an anti-glioblastoma agent, using an immunosuppressed mouse bearing U87 MG human glioblastoma.

2. Results

Recently, we designed a series of hybrid compounds (Figure 2), which combine substructures derived from **Sun** and icosahedral boron clusters [22], to be tested as bifunctional-boron-cluster-based compounds with relevant activities in cells expressing tyrosine kinase proteins. The substituent at the C-3-indol system and the indolin-2-one motive are important for effective kinase inhibition by Sun. Both structural characteristics play relevant roles in protein-binding processes [9,23–25]. Moreover, the substituent at the C-3-indol system influences the compound solubility too [23,24]. The icosahedral boron-cluster $C_2B_{10}H_{12}$ isomers (*ortho*, *meta*, and *para*) are white solids that rank among the most chemically and biologically stable molecular compounds known. Icosahedral carboranes are hydrophobic [26] and have an icosahedral shape with a depth of about 0.5 nm and a volume similar to the one of benzene in rotation with twice the number of atoms [27]. Carboranes display 3D aromaticity [28,29]. Furthermore, the inorganic 3D neutral $C_2B_{10}H_{12}$ clusters and their derivatives can produce hydrogen and dihydrogen bonds C-H···X and B-H···H-X (X = N, C, O, and S [30,31]) and B-H···π and C-H···π hydrogen bonds [32]. The unique rigid and spherical form of the carborane cluster plus the possibility it offers to produce these weak intramolecular interactions could provide extra beneficial interactions with target receptors. Consequently, in the new hybrid compounds (**Sun** + boron-cluster), the carborane cage could be located in the target-pocket exploring unique regions of chemical space, i.e., in the **Sun** indolin-2-one region, establishing extra-interactions with kinases that cannot be achieved with purely organic compounds [22]. Two types of substructures—(i) flexible and polar backbones (methyl-1,2,3-triazolylalkyl moieties), and (ii) a rigid and hydrophobic system (2-propynylphenylmethyl linker)—have been selected as connectors between indolin-2-one system and carborane clusters. Moreover, three different icosahedral boron clusters were selected to introduce chemical diversity into the target: the neutral *o* and *m*-carboranes, and the anionic cobaltabis(dicarbollide). The designed hybrid compounds, **1** and **4–11**, carrying the tyrosine kinase receptor inhibitors plus the boron cluster moiety, were synthesized as shown in the Supplementary Material (Figure S1). Figure 2 displays the formulae of the synthesized **Sun**-icosahedral boron cluster hybrids.

Further, the in vitro activity of the bifunctional-boron-cluster-based compounds (**1, 4–11**) against different tyrosine kinase-overexpressing tumor cells HT-29, C6, and U98 MG, was evaluated (see Table S1) [22]. Hybrid **1** was the most active against U87 MG glioblastoma cells of the full **Sun**-boron-cluster-based compound (**1, 4–11**) series and was at least four times more active than the parent **Sun**. Table 1 summarizes the in vitro activity of the parent **Sun**, **Erl**, and **Lap** tyrosine kinase receptor inhibitors and the most active compounds of each family of hybrids compounds derived from these TKRs inhibitors. The incorporation of boron cluster resulted in hybrid compounds, such as carboranes **1–3** (Figure 1), with enhanced in vitro activity against TKR-overexpressing cells with respect to the corresponding parents [18–22]. In these studies, compound **1** stood out, especially against glioma cells, compared to **Erl** and **Lap** derivatives, i.e., **2** and **3**, and compared to the rest of the **Sun** derivatives (Table 1, Table S1).

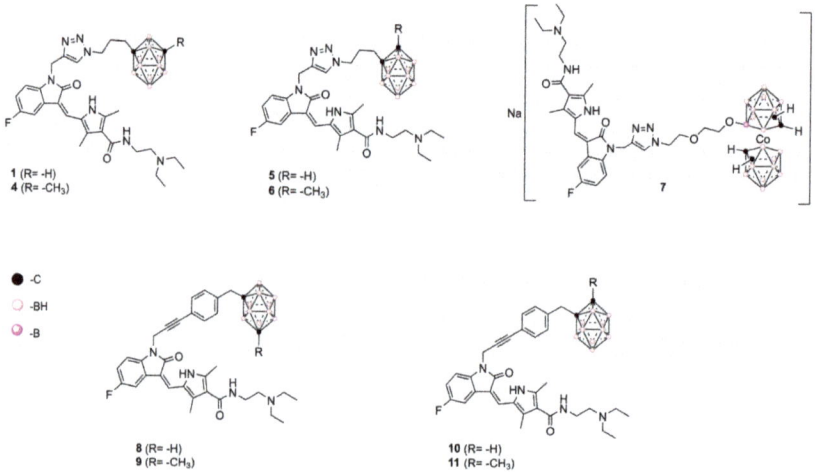

Figure 2. Representation of **Sun**-icosahedral boron cluster hybrids [22].

Table 1. In vitro activity of the most relevant hybrid TKI–boron clusters and the corresponding parent compounds against different TKR-overexpressing tumor cells, U87 MG, C6, and HT-29.

Compound	IC$_{50,\text{U87 MG}}$ (µM) [1,2]	IC$_{50,\text{C6}}$ (µM) [1,2]	IC$_{50,\text{HT-29}}$ (µM) [1,2]	References
1	8.0 ± 0.3	6.9 ± 0.5	<6.25 (0.45 ± 0.04%)	[22]
Sun	32 ± 4	36 ± 10	6.25 ± 0.04	[18,20]
2	70 ± 5	30 ± 5	25.0 ± 5.0	[18,20]
Erl	63 ± 5	>100	>100 [3]	[18,20]
3	10.0 ± 0.2	11.8 ± 0.4	>100 (73 ± 6)	[21]
Lap	54 ± 14	>100 (89 ± 5)	6.25 ± 0.05	[21]

[1] Concentrations, in µM, required to inhibit the cellular growth by 50%. They were determined from dose–response curves, and represent the mean ± SD. All experiments were repeated at least three times. [2] Values in parentheses are the percentages of cell survival at 100 µM. [3] Higher doses than 100 µM could not be evaluated due to solubility problems. The colors in the cells show the level of activity in each studied cell (green: highest activity; yellow: intermediate activity; pink: lowest activity).

Later, the potential use as a BNCT agent was checked using compound **1** as the model compound (Table S2). When compound **1** was incubated on F98-glioma cells the boron accumulation increased with time, reaching its maximum (6 µg of B/mg protein) after 4 h of incubation, while the amount of boron on astrocytes decreased, the ratio of glioma/astrocyte being 2.12 at that time.

2.1. Kinases' Binding Affinity for Compound 1

The previously evidenced relationship between the lipophilicity and cellular-toxicity of the studied carboranes [22] made us think that, beyond the aspect related to the process of crossing the cell membrane, mechanistically the interaction with a bio-receptor could be involved in the activity. Consequently, in order to inquire the tyrosine kinase inhibition ability of compound **1**, it was extensively profiled in a high-throughput competition-binding assay against a panel of 468 kinases (KINOMEscan®) at 10 µM. It demonstrated high inhibitory activity against 33 out of the 468 analyzed bio-targets (Figure 3, Table 2, Table S3), with a final selectivity score, or "S," of 0.04. This result is highly relevant as most tumors can circumvent the inhibition of a specific kinase either by de novo resistance, which refers to the failure of drugs to produce any detectable response after initial treatment, or by acquired resistance [33].

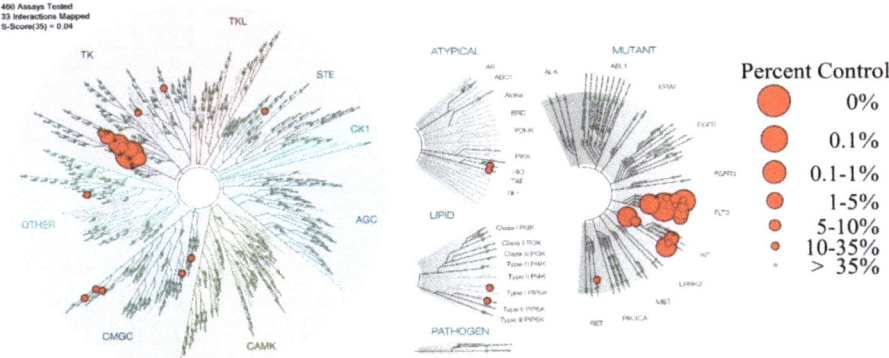

Figure 3. Selectivity profile of compound **1** against 468 protein kinases. Relative binding affinities are indicated by red circles in a phylogenetic kinome tree for wild-type enzymes (**left**) and atypical/mutant/lipo/pathogen variants (**right**). The sizes of the red circles are proportional to the strength of the binding; the larger circles indicate higher affinity. A total of 33 of the best interactions with binding levels 35% greater than the control (red circles) at a fixed 10 µM concentration of test compound were mapped. Selectivity factor (S), S35 = 0.04. Image generated using TREEspot™ Software Tool and reprinted with permission from KINOMEscan®, a division of DiscoveRx Corporation, © DiscoveRx Corporation 2010.

Table 2. Primary screening results [1] of KINOMEScan assay for compound **1**, at 10 µM, for the most inhibited TKRs.

DiscoveRx Gene Symbol	Entrez Gene Symbol	Percent of Remaining Enzymatic Activity [2]
PDGFR-α	PDGFRA	2.6
PDGFR-β	PDGFRB	0.05
FLT1 [3]	FLT1	14
FLT3	FLT3	2.1
FLT3(D835V)	FLT3	0.1
FLT3(ITD)	FLT3	2.3
FLT3(ITD,D835V)	FLT3	0.55
FLT3(ITD,F691L)	FLT3	0
KIT	KIT	0.25
KIT(V559D)	KIT	0.45
KIT(V559D,T670I)	KIT	1.4

[1] Assay performed by DiscoveRx. [2] With respect to untreated tyrosine kinase receptor. [3] Included in order to compare with other FLTs.

Like **Sun** [6], compound **1** displays inhibition capacity against FLT3, PDGFR-α and β, KIT, CSF1R (classified as type III receptor tyrosine kinase), and VEGFR2 (Table 2). Specifically, the best inhibition ability of **1** was against the FMS-like tyrosine kinase 3 (FLT3) internal tandem duplication mutation of the gatekeeper residue F691 (FLT3-ITD, F691L) involved in acute myeloid leukemia, among others [34]. Secondly, **1** inhibited in a good manner PDGFRs (especially PDGFR-β) and the mutations that occur in the exon 11 of the KIT gene, which encodes the juxta-membrane domain (V559D and L576P) (Table S3) involved, for example, in gastrointestinal stromal tumors [35].

Compound **1** is a multi-tyrosine-kinase inhibitor, but unlike **Sun**, with a "S" score of 0.57 (Figure S2) [36], it is selective against the aforementioned bio-systems. Additionally, **1** displays lower inhibition of AMP-activated protein kinase (AMPK) and ribosomal S6 kinase RSK1 than **Sun** at the assayed dose (near to 15% and lower than 17%, respectively, of inhibition at 10 µM; Table S3). **Sun** cardiotoxicity could be the result of the AMPK and RSK1 inhibitions ($IC_{50,Sun,AMPK}$ = 0.32 µM, $IC_{50,Sun,RSK1}$ = 0.36 µM) [37,38]; consequently, we would expect that compound **1** does not display this off-target secondary effect of tyrosine kinase inhibitors.

To confirm it, compound **1** was challenged directly against the isolated FLT3 and PDGFR-β receptors; using the ADP-Glo kinase assay system, we observed IC_{50} values of 3.1 and 2.1 µM, respectively. These results are consistent with the dose used for the KINOMEscan®assay (Figure S3).

2.2. Effect of Compound 1 on Co-Cultures of Tumor Cells and Normal Astrocytes

U87 MG cells, stained with PKH26 dye, were co-cultured with neonatal murine astrocytes to resemble the cellular environment of a developing brain tumor. This system was incubated with compound **1** or **Sun** or dimethylsulfoxide (DMSO) as a control (vehicle-treated cells) at the corresponding IC_{50} doses against U87 MG for 24 h [22]. Very different behavior was observed by confocal microscopy among the studied **1** and **Sun** and the control (DMSO) (Figure 4). As expected, PKH26 dye revealed a decrease of U87 MG population upon **1** or **Sun** treatment when compared to the control. Additionally, GFAP staining, which highlights astrocyte activation [39,40], indicated that the population of these tumor-associated astrocytes was observed mainly in the cells incubated with **Sun**, and in a lower level, in the control, but astrocyte activation was not observed in the co-culture' cells treated with compound **1**. Accordingly, it was concluded that astrocytes become reactive by the action of **Sun** but not by sunitinib-carborane hybrid **1**. These results highlighted the particular biological behavior of compound **1** against the astrocytes–glioma cells system. Finally, DAPI nuclei staining showed for both **Sun** and **1** treatments, chromatin condensation, which could be associated with the onset of apoptosis.

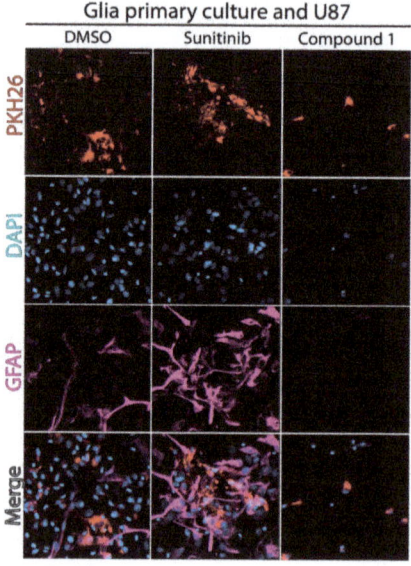

Figure 4. Effect of compound **1** on co-cultures of astrocytes with U87 MG tumor cells. Confocal images showing the co-culture of U87 MG cells (PKH26) and mouse neonatal reactive astrocytes (GFAP). The nucleuses were stained with DAPI. Co-cultured cells were treated at $IC_{50,U87\,MG}$ doses of **Sun** or compound **1** or with DMSO as a control, for 24 h. Scale bar: 20 µm.

2.3. Study of Cellular Death Mechanism Triggered by Compound 1

To confirm the kind of cell death promoted by compound **1** in U87 MG cells and in U87 MG co-cultured with astrocytes, mitochondrial membrane potential change studies and phosphatidylserine exposure analysis, respectively, were performed. The results showed that compound **1** produced cell death of U87 MG tumor cells via apoptotic mechanism given the 4 h of contact at IC$_{50}$ dose (Figure 5a). Additionally, it was observed that in co-cultured experiments (mixed of U87 MG and astrocytes) compound **1**, at IC$_{50}$ dose (8.0 µM), significantly increased the percentage of U87 MG cells undergoing early apoptosis from 17% to 63% and the percentage of cells undergoing late apoptosis from 4% to 34% with respect to control samples (Figure 5b,c). Consequently, approximately 97% of the total U87 MG cell population became apoptotic after treatment with compound **1**. Similar results were observed after treatment with **Sun** at the IC$_{50}$ dose (32.0 µM), the main phenomenon being early apoptosis. Both compound **1** and **Sun** have the same kind of effect on glial cells regarding death (Figure 5b,c).

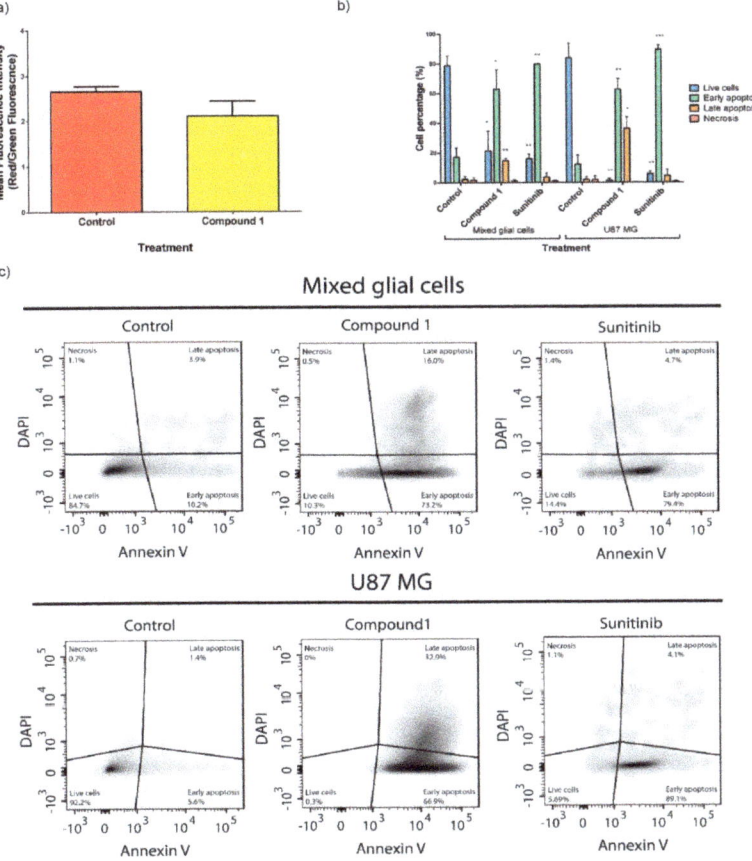

Figure 5. (**a**) Collapse of the mitochondrial membrane potential results for untreated and compound **1**-treated U87 MG cells. Compound **1** was evaluated at IC$_{50}$ doses (8.0 ìM) incubated for 4 h. (**b**) Quantitative analysis of flow cytometry results (three independent experiments). (*) $p < 0.05$; (**) $p < 0.01$; (***) $p < 0.001$ when compared to the negative control by two-way analysis of variance (ANOVA). (**c**) Phosphatidylserine exposure results for mixed glial cells (top) and U87 MG (bottom). Compound **1** and **Sun** were evaluated at their IC$_{50}$ doses (8.0 ìM and 32.0 ìM, respectively) after incubation for 24 h.

2.4. Compound 1's Effect on the Cell Cycle

To determine the effect of compound **1** on the cell cycle, we investigated the cell cycle distribution of compound **1** against astrocytes and U87 MG cells by using flow cytometry analysis. Both cell lines showed a sub-G1 phase arrest after treatment with **1**. Astrocytes showed a significant increase in the percentage of cells in sub-G1 and G1 phases after 24 h incubation with compound **1** at IC_{50} doses (8.0 µM) (Figure 6a,b). Similarly, as it can be seen in Figure 6c,d, the percentage of U87 MG cells in sub-G1 phase upon treatment with compound **1** was higher than the corresponding percentage for untreated cells, which were mainly in a G2/M phase. **Sun** provoked an increase in the percentage of both astrocytes and U87 MG cells in the sub-G1 phase after 24 h of incubation at IC_{50} (32 µM).

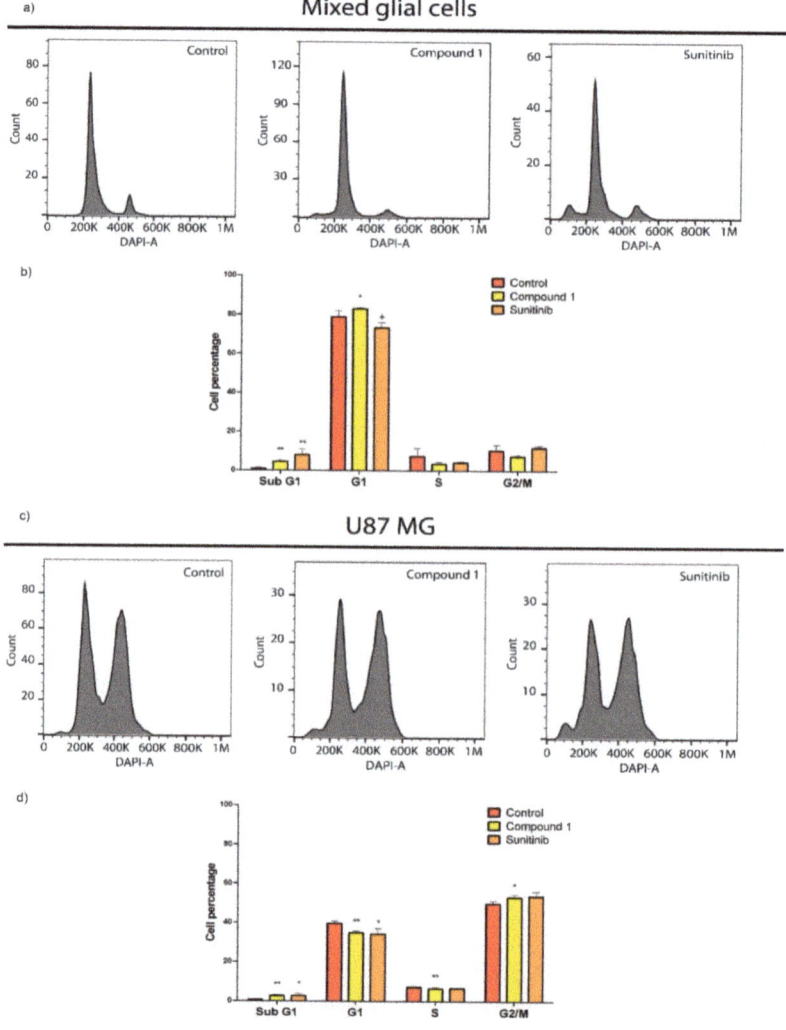

Figure 6. Effects on cell cycle in mixed glial cells (**a**,**b**) and U87 MG cells (**c**,**d**) treated with compounds **1** or **Sun**. Values correspond to the averages ± SEMs of three independent experiments. Cell debris was omitted from analyses; 10,000 events were analyzed per sample. ** $p < 0.05$, * $p < 0.1$, + $p = 0.1245$, when compared to the negative control group by multiple T-test.

These results could be indicating the FLT-inhibition non-canonical effects. Hedgehog signaling cascade is able, via the FLT3/PI3k pathway, to non-canonically upregulate glioma zinc finger (GLI) transcription factors [41]. GLIs, and especially GLI1 in human brain gliomas, play important roles in cell-cycle and apoptosis regulation [42,43]. GLI1-upregulating agents lead to G1 and sub-G1 phase arrest and apoptosis in different kinds of cancers [43–45].

2.5. Drug-Like Properties of Compound 1

The special in vitro biological-behavior of compound **1**, significantly different from its parent compound **Sun** (i.e., different tyrosine kinases inhibition profile, better cellular cytotoxicity, and ability to be used as BNCT agent [22]), led us to study deeper into its use as a drug. Consequently, some drug-like properties of **1** were theoretically and experimentally analyzed.

On the one hand, theoretical predictions of drug-like properties [46] showed that compound **1** shared drug-like properties with **Sun**, mainly the absence of toxicities and adequate water solubility (Table 3). Secondly, as displayed at Table 4, compound **1** has proven not to be mutagenic, using an Ames test with two different *S. typhimurium* strains, another desirable characteristic that would act in favor of this compound as a drug [47]. Finally, and thinking in the potential use of **1** as anti-glioblastoma agent, we studied its ability to cross the brain blood barrier (BBB) using a reported artificial endothelial-cell model [48–51]. According to the results, compound **1** has the ability to cross the BBB, as ≈3-times more compound translocates across the artificial BBB after hybrid **1** exposure in the feeding side of the membrane for 24 h at room temperature in the dark and without stirring (Table 4). These results encouraged us to study compound **1** in an animal model of glioblastoma.

Table 3. Predicted drug-like properties of compound **1**, **Sun**, and **Tmz**.

Cpd	HIA [1]	Subcellular Localization	CYP-Subs [2]	hERG [3]	Carc [4]	LD$_{50}$ [5]	LogS [6]	Viol, Rule 5 [7]
1	(+)	Mit [8]	3A4	w	(−)	2.69	−3.48	1 [9]
Sun	(+)	Mit	3A4	w	(−)	2.66	−3.24	0
Tmz	(+)	Mit	-	w	(−)	2.53	−1.63	0

[1] Human intestinal absorption: If the compound has an HIA% less than 30%, it is labeled as (−); otherwise it is labeled as (+) [52]. [2] Ability to be a substrate of cytochrome P450 isoenzymes (CYP450 2C9, CYP450 2D6, and CYP450 3A4) [53]. Shown is the predicted isoform of CYP for which the compound potentially acts as substrate. [3] Human ether-a-go-go-related gene (hERG) inhibition [54,55]. Weak-inhibition is labeled as "w." [4] Potential as carcinogens [56]. Non-carcinogen is labeled as (−) [5] Rat acute toxicity by oral exposure [57], expressed as mol/kg. [6] Aqueous solubility [58]. [7] Number of violations of Lipinski's "rule of five." [8] Mit: mitochondria. [9] MW higher than 500 Da.

Table 4. Summary of Ames and BBB permeability tests for compound **1**.

	Ames Test		BBB [1]	
	TA98	TA100		
Dose (μg/plate)	Number of revertants		before BBB	[1] = 15 ± 5 μM
Positive control [2]	295 ± 11	704 ± 6	after BBB	[1] = 48 ± 4 μM
0.45	12 ± 1	67 ± 3		
0.15	9 ± 1	56 ± 3		
0.05	7.5 ± 1.5	46.5 ± 1.5		
0.016	6 ± 1	37 ± 6		
0.005	8 ± 1	29.5 ± 0.5		
0 [3]	12 ± 2	95.6 ± 5.7		
Mutagenic	(−)	(−)		

[1] The concentration of compound **1** in the assay milieu before and after the BBB translocation was measured by HPLC. [2] 4-Nitro-o-phenylendiamine (NPD). [3] Negative control: phosphate buffer and DMSO (10% v/v) (no effect on cell growth was observed by this mixture of solvents).

2.6. Study of the In Vivo Anti-Glioblastoma Activity of Compound 1

In vivo anti-glioblastoma activity of compound **1** was evaluated in immunosuppressed mice bearing human U87 MG tumors [59]. The antitumor activity was evaluated using both the evolution of the tumor volumes and the animal survival.

Compound **1** was intraperitoneallt administered at 1 mg/kg/day three times a week for as long as the mice lived (in the best cases eight weeks). In this assay, **Tmz** was used as a positive therapy reference and administered in the same conditions but at 4 mg/kg/day (Figure 7a). The volumes were determined by bioluminescence imaging weekly. We found that treatment with **1** significantly reduced glioblastoma growth when compared to untreated animals (Figure 7b,c). The tumor volumes were significantly different three weeks after cell injection.

Additionally, compound **1**, at a dose four times lower than the dose of **Tmz** and in the same administration conditions, significantly prolonged the survival of unhealthy mice by between 2 to 1.8 times, with an average survival time of 45 days (Figure 7d). In comparison, **Tmz**-treated and untreated control groups showed median survivals of 23 and 25 days, respectively (Figure 7d). Furthermore, **1** provoked increases of 70% and 89% of mouse survival time, from 30 and 27 to 51 days, and increases of 32% and 43% for the time to mouse deaths, from 25 and 23 to 33 days, respectively. These results strongly suggest an anti-glioblastoma activity of compound **1**. Furthermore, we aimed to proving that compound **1** did not induce apparent toxicity effects such as death, seizures, convulsions decreased/increased motor activity, or dehydratation, which was monitored based on body weight before and after treatment, on mice during the trail. This fact may indicate that it is well tolerated (Figure S4). Importantly, all mice treated with compound **1** survived the study period.

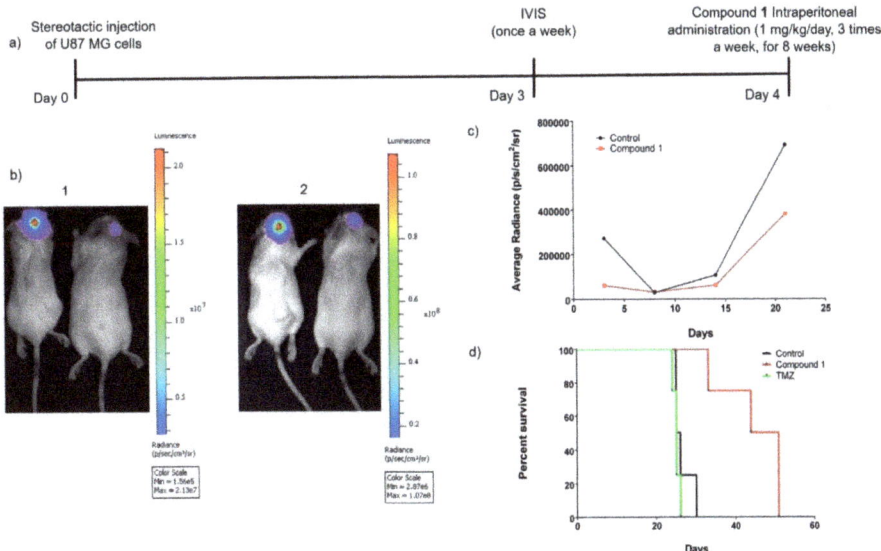

Figure 7. (**a**) Dosification schedule. (**b**) Selected images of the evolution of glioblastoma correspond to 14 days (**1**) and to 21 days (**2**) after cell injection; in each case the left mouse was an untreated control and the right one was treated with compound **1**. (**c**) Weekly evolution of glioblastoma sizes; in black untreated control and in red treated with **1**. In the third week (day 21st) the study was ended because all the untreated animals died. (**d**) Kaplan–Meier survival curves of mice bearing glioblastoma receiving different treatments. Black: untreated animals; green: **Tmz** (4 mg/kg/day)-treated animals; red: compound **1** (1 mg/kg/day)-treated animals. The study showed a significant difference either between compound **1** and control (untreated animals) or **1** and **Tmz** ($p < 0.01$). Data were analyzed by log-rank test.

3. Discussion

A series of hybrid compounds with potential anti-glioblastoma activity has been developed [22]. Among them emerged the novel compound **1**, which is a multi-tyrosine-kinase inhibitor, especially inhibiting FLT3, KIT, and PDGFR-β. In the U87 MG/astrocyte co-cultured experiments, resembling the tumor cellular environment, reactive astrocytes were inhibited by compound **1**, contrary **Sun**'s behavior, this being a very important fact due to reactive astrocytes being associated with enhanced proliferation and cells with abnormal mitoses [60]. Additionally, compound **1** promoted U87 MG early apoptosis and late apoptosis with both different death profiles in associated astrocytes, a lower level of late apoptosis and some grade of necrosis. For **Sun**, almost exclusively early apoptosis in both cellular systems. The effects on the cell cycle on U87 MG and astrocytes, showed that compound **1** increased the number of cells in sub-G1 phase. According to the U87 MG cellular death mechanism and the effect on the cell cycle promoted by compound **1**, the non-canonical effect by the inhibition of FLT3, via GLI1 upregulation, could be an operative extra-effect of compound **1** besides the classical FLT3-canonical. Future research to investigate the Hedgehog-GLI1 signaling status, by RT-PCR or Western blot analysis, should be done. Additionally, to fully characterize the mechanisms of action of compound **1**, and on-target and off-target effects, proteomics-based assays will be carried out.

The in vivo behavior of compound **1** showed that, beyond further use in combination with BNCT, it possesses anti-glioblastoma activity per se. This result opens the use of **1** as a new therapeutic agent via TKRs inhibitions, which in the case of combination with BNCT could further improve the therapeutic efficacy against one of the most lethal cancers. Ongoing studies will focus on the preparation of compound **1** ^{10}B-enriched and assessment of BNCT's in vivo efficacy that may result in significant clinical benefits.

4. Materials and Methods

4.1. Chemistry

Compound **1** was synthesized according to literature [22].

4.2. Biology

In vitro cytotoxicity assays on EGFR-expressing cells [22]. Cells (C6, U87 MG, or HT-29) were seeded in 96-well plates (7000–10,000 cells/well depending on the cell line) in 100 µL final volume of growing milieu and were allowed to grow for 24 h. After that, 125 µL of fresh culture milieu was added and the cells were allowed to grow for additional 24 h. Then, 25 µL of a solution 10× of desired final concentration of the tested compounds in culture milieu was added to the culture. Cells were further incubated for 24 h. Afterwards, culture milieu was removed and cells were washed twice with 200 µL of PBS. Cells were then fixed with 50 µL of ice-cold trichloroacetic acid for 1 h at 4 °C; the plates were washed five times in distilled water and allowed to dry at room temperature. Sulphorhodamine B (SRB) solution (50 µL, 0.4 *w/v* in aqueous solution of acetic acid (1 %, *v/v*)) was added to each well of the dried 96-well plates. Staining was performed at room temperature for 30 min. The SRB solution and unbound dye were removed by washing the plates quickly with an aqueous solution of acetic acid (1 %, *v/v*) at least five times (until excess dye was fully removed). The washed plates were allowed to dry in the air for at least 24 h. Finally, the bound SRB was solubilized by adding Tris base buffer (pH 10, 10 mM, 100 µL) to each well and the resulting solution was shaken for 5 min on a shaker platform. The optical density (OD) of each well solution was read in a 96-well plate reader at λ = 540 nm. The OD of SRB solution in each well was directly proportional to the cell number. Cell viability percentage was calculated according to the following equation: C.V.% = ($A_{540\,nm}$ −B/C−B), where C.V.% stands for cell viability percentage, $A_{540\,nm}$ corresponds to OD of a particular well, B is the OD of untreated wells with no cells seeded onto them, and C is the OD of control wells treated only with 1% of DMSO. C.V.% values were plotted against compound concentration and the IC_{50} values were determined.

Cell line and culture conditions. Human malignant glioblastoma cell line (U87 MG, ATCC® HTB-14™) was cultured in Dulbecco's modified Eagle's milieu high glucose (4.5 g/L), with stable glutamine, with sodium pyruvate milieu supplemented with 10% inactivated fetal bovine serum (FBS) and penicillin/streptomycin (1%). The cells were kept at 37 °C under a 5% CO_2 humidified environment, changing the milieu every 2–3 days. Cells were sub cultured once they reached 90–95% confluence.

Astrocytes were isolated from newborn mice. The mice were terminally anesthetized, the cerebral cortexes were dissected with the meninges previously removed. Cerebral cortexes were mechanically chopped then enzymatically dissociated using 0.25% trypsin for 10 minutes at 37 °C. To halt trypsin digestion a mix of DMEM with FSB 10% was added. After repetitive pipetting to disaggregate the tissue, it was strained through an 80 µm mesh and centrifuged. The pellet was resuspended in complete DMEM milieu.

4.2.1. Kinases Assays

For most assays, kinase-tagged T7 phage strains were grown in parallel in 24-well blocks in an *E. coli* host derived from the BL21 strain. *E. coli* were grown to log-phase and infected with T7 phage from a frozen stock (multiplicity of infection = 0.4) and incubated with shaking at 32 °C until lysis (90–150 min). The lysates were centrifuged (6000× *g*) and filtered (0.2 µm) to remove cell debris. The remaining kinases were produced in HEK-293 cells and subsequently tagged with DNA for qPCR detection. Streptavidin-coated magnetic beads were treated with biotinylated small molecule ligands for 30 min at room temperature to generate affinity resins for kinase assays. The liganded beads were blocked with excess biotin and washed with blocking buffer (SeaBlock (Pierce, MA, USA), 1% BSA, 0.05% Tween 20, 1 mM DTT) to remove unbound ligand and to reduce non-specific phage binding. Binding reactions were assembled by combining kinases, liganded affinity beads, and test compound in 1× binding buffer (20% SeaBlock, 0.17× PBS, 0.05% Tween 20, 6 mM DTT). Test compound was prepared as 40× stocks in 100% DMSO and directly diluted into the assay. All reactions were performed in polypropylene 384-well plates in a final volume of 0.02 mL. The assay plates were incubated at room temperature with shaking for 1 h and the affinity beads were washed with wash buffer (1× PBS, 0.05% Tween 20). The beads were then re-suspended in elution buffer (1× PBS, 0.05% Tween 20, 0.5 µM non-biotinylated affinity ligand) and incubated at room temperature with shaking for 30 min. The kinase concentration in the eluates was measured by qPCR. Compound **1** was screened at 10 µM, and results for primary screen binding interactions were reported as percentages of control (PoC). PoC = (test compound signal-positive control signal)/(DMSO signal-positive control signal). PoC values at 10 µM for all kinases were visualized using TREEspot (DiscoveRx, San Diego, CA, USA).

4.2.2. PDGFR-β and FLT3 Enzymatic Assays

The wild-type PDGFR-β kinase enzyme system (Catalog. V3731) and FLT3 kinase enzyme system (Catalog. V4064) were purchased from Promega Corporation (Fitchburg, WI, USA). The experiments were performed according to the manufacturer's instructions. For more detailed and complete protocols, see the ADP-Glo™ kinase Assay Technical Manual and the active kinase datasheet available at: http://www.promega.com/KESProtocol. Briefly, for the kinase reaction step serial dilutions of the compound **1**—1000, 100, 10, 1, 0.1, and 0.01 µM for FLT3, and 100, 10, 1, 0.1, and 0.01 for PDGFR-β—were prepared. A 5 µL enzyme reaction mixture was performed containing 1 mL of the compound dilution (5% DMSO), 2 µL of the enzyme dilution, and 2 µL of the ATP/substrate solution to get a final concentration of 50 µM ATP, 0.2 g/mL of Poly(Glu, Tyr) substrate, and 5 mg/mL of enzyme. Each reaction was performed by triplicate on a 384-well plate and incubated during 1 h at room temperature. The kinase reaction was stopped with 5 µL of ADP-Glo™ during 40 min, followed by the addition of 10 µL of Kinase Detection Reagent. **Sun** was used as a positive control. Luminescence was measured after 40 min on a BioTek®FLx800 Multi-Detection Microplate Reader (Integration time 0.5–1 s). Curve fitting and data presentations were performed using GraphPad Prism version 5.0 (GraphPad Software, Inc., San Diego, CA, USA).

4.2.3. Confocal Microscopy of Treated Co-Cultures of U87 MG and Astrocytes

Astrocytes (3×10^4 cells) were seeded into p35 dishes and were allowed to grow until 80% confluence. Next, 5×10^4 U87 MG stained cells with PKH26 dye were seeded onto a p35 dish containing a growing primary cell culture of astrocytes. After a 48 h-incubation in fresh growing milieu, the p60 dishes were treated with the IC$_{50}$ doses of compound **1** or **Sun**. A p60 dish treated with 1% DMSO served as a negative control. Treated cells were incubated for further 24 h. After that, treated co-cultures were fixed for 20 min at 4 °C with PFA and washed 2 times with PBS. Then, samples were permeabilized for 10 min at room temperature with 0.1% Triton X-100 in PBS, passed through washing PBS, blocked with 5% BSA:PBS for 1 h at room temperature, and incubated overnight in a solution of 1% BSA:PBS containing the primary antibody and DAPI at 4 °C. After washing, treated cells were incubated in 1:500-diluted secondary antibody during 2 h at room temperature. The following antibodies were used for immunofluorescence staining: primary antibody 1:400 mouse monoclonal anti-GFAP (Sigma-Aldrich, Darmstadt, Germany) and secondary antibody conjugated to AlexaFluor 633 (Invitrogen, Carlsbad, CA, USA). DAPI was used at a 1:1000 dilution. Antibodies were detected by confocal microscopy using a confocal Olympus FV300 microscope.

4.2.4. Cellular Death Mechanisms

Cell death mechanism triggered by either compound **1** or **Sun** were evaluated by collapse of the mitochondrial membrane potential ($\Delta\Psi$m) assay and phosphatidylserine exposure analysis.

Collapse of the ΔΨm

As a measure of the initiation of the mitochondrial apoptosis cascade, the cationic lipophilic 5,5′,6,6′-tetrachloro-1,1′,3,3′-tetraethylbenzimidazolylcarbo cyanine chloride (JC-1) dye was utilized as an indicator of changes in ΔΨm, as previously described [61]. In intact cells with high ΔΨm, JC-1 can enter the mitochondria and reversibly form aggregates with intense red fluorescence (emission at 590 nm; orange-red fluorescence). In case of mitochondrial membrane potential collapse, JC-1 remains in the cytosol as a monomer and emits at 527 nm (green fluorescence). To access the possible effect of compound **1** on mitochondrial membrane potential a growing culture of U87 MG cells (2×10^6 cells) were treated at IC_{50} dose. After a 4 h-incubation with compound **1**, cells were trypsinized, centrifuged ($660 \times g$, 5 min, 4 °C), and collected. Cells were resuspended and incubated with 400 µL of JC-1 dye (1/500 dilution) for 30 min. Then, the cells were centrifuged, resuspended in 500 µL of PBS, and transferred into FACS tubes. The mean fluorescence intensity of JC-1 labeling was measured by FACS. The results were analyzed using FlowJo software (FlowJo LLC, Ashland, OR, USA).

Phosphatidylserine Exposure Assay

Astrocytes (6×10^4 cells) were seeded into p60 dishes and were allowed to grow until 80% confluence. Next, 1×10^5 U87 MG stained cells with PKH26 dye were seeded onto a p60 dish containing a growing primary cell culture of astrocytes. After a 48 h incubation in fresh growing milieu, the p60 dishes were treated with the IC_{50} doses of compound **1** or **Sun**. A p60 dish treated with 1% DMSO served as a negative control. Treated cells were incubated for further 24 h. Then, cells were harvested with trypsin (0.05%, supplemented with EDTA, 0.38 mg/mL), and centrifuged at 250 g speed. The resulting pellet was resuspended in an appropriate volume of Annexin binding buffer (0.01 M Hepes pH 7.4, 0.14 M NaCl, and 2.5 mM $CaCl_2$) as to get a cell suspension of 1×10^6 cells per mL. After cell counts, samples were divided and cells alone and isotype-matched control samples were generated to control for nonspecific binding of antibodies and for autofluorescence. An Annexin V-FITC antibody solution (catalog number: A13199) was used at a 1:20 concentration. After 30 min of incubation with the aforementioned antibody at 4 °C, samples were incubated with DAPI at a 1:5000 concentration and immediately after were submitted to flow cytometry analysis. To perform the analysis, cells were first gated for PKH26 in order to tell apart U87 MG cells from astrocytes. In each type of cells, the following markers were used to define four different populations: for living cells DAPI low, Annexin V low; for necrotic cells DAPI high, Annexin V low; for early apoptotic cells DAPI low, Annexin V high; and finally, for late apoptotic cells, DAPI high, Annexin V high. Samples were acquired using FACSAria Fusion flow cytometer and BD FACSDiva ™ software.

4.2.5. Measurement of Cell Cycle/DNA Content

In order to investigate how compound **1** affects cell cycle, a co-culture of astrocytes and U87 MG was performed to simulate tumor microenvironment. The DNA content in G1/G0, S, and G2/M phases was analyzed using flow cytometry.

U87 MG cells were stained with CFSE using CellTrace™ CFSE Cell Proliferation Kit (Thermo Fisher Scientific, Waltham, MA, USA) and seeded into p60 dishes (3×10^5 cells) containing a growing culture of glia. Co-cultured cells were incubated for 48 h and then treated with compound **1** or **Sun** at $IC_{50,U87\,MG}$ doses for 24 h. The harvested cells were washed with PBS, fixed with 2% PFA solution at 4 °C for 20 min. Subsequently, the cells were resuspended in fresh staining buffer (1 µg/mL DAPI and 0.1% Triton X prepared in PBS) and incubated in the dark for 30 min at room temperature. Cell cycle distribution analysis was performed with an Attune NxT flow cytometer using Attune NxT Software for data acquisition. For each sample, cellular aggregates were gated out and 10,000 cells were counted and plotted on a single parameter histogram. The percentages of cells in the G1/G0, S, and G2/M phases and the sub-G1 peak were then calculated using FlowJo 7.6.

4.3. Drug-Like Properties

4.3.1. Prediction

Drug-like properties were predicted using admetQSAR tool kit (http://lmmd.ecust.edu.cn/admetsar1/predict/) from the molecule SMILE code generated with ChemDraw Standard 14.0 software.

4.3.2. Ames Test

Salmonella *typhimurium* TA98 and TA100 strains were incubated in agar minimum glucose milieu solution (Difco Bacto® agar) and aqueous glucose solution (40%). First of all, the direct toxicity of the compound **1** against S. *typhimurium* TA 98 strain was studied. From these data, the mutagenic assay was performed. Briefly, **1** in phosphate buffer (0.1 M, pH 7.4) and DMSO (10%, *v/v*) at five doses, 0.450, 0.150, 0.050, 0.016, and 0.005 µg/plate, starting at the highest doses without toxic effects (0.450 µg/plate), were studied in triplicate. Controls: positive control in the assay: NPD (20.0 mg/plate for TA98 strain and 2.0 mg/plate for TA100 strain); negative control: phosphate buffer and DMSO (10% *v/v*) (no effect on cells growth was observed by this mixture of solvents). The revertants were counted and the studied system was considered mutagenic if the colonies number was at least doubled the natural revertants (negative control) for two or more consecutive doses.

4.3.3. BBB In Vitro Passage Assay

BBB Artificial Model

Isolation and culture of glial cells from newborn rats. Cerebral cortex of ten 1-day-old Wistar newborn rats were taken with aseptic operation and then were cut to pieces. After stripped the pia mater, cerebral cortex were digested by 1 mL of 0.25% trypsin at 37 °C for 10 min. Next, dispersed cell suspension was made by mechanical method. Cell suspensions were seeded into 12-well plates coated with L-polylysine, at a cell density of 1×10^5 cell per well.

Isolation and Culture of Porcine Brain Micro Vessel Endothelial Cells

Pig brains were obtained fresh from the abattoir, washed in ethanol 70% and transported on ice in PBS (with Ca^{2+}/Mg^{2+}). The hemispheres of three brains were washed, the cerebellum removed, and meninges peeled off and discarded. White matter was carefully removed. The grey matter was collected in milieu M-199 Earle's salts (Biological industries, Beit Ha'emek, Israel) with added penicillin (100 U/mL) and streptomycin (100 µg/mL) and forced through a 20 mL syringe. The homogenized, was centrifuged and filtered successively through 160 and 80 µm nylon meshes. The resulting micro vessels were seeded in T75 culture flasks, previously coated over night with calf skin collagen (Sigma cat. C-8919), in M-199 milieu with 10% newborn calf serum, penicillin (100 U/mL), streptomycin (100 mg/mL), glutamine (2 mM) and puromycin (2 mg/mL) and cultured until 80% confluence. Endothelial cells were detached by brief trypsinisation and seeded into rat tail collagen coated Transwell filter inserts 2.5×10^5 cells/filter (0.5 mL). Trans-endothelial electrical resistance (TEER) was measured as indication of membrane stability with EVOM2 epithelial voltohmmeter (World precision instruments, Inc., Sarasota, FL, USA).

Assembling of the Artificial BBB Model

After 3 days, filters with endothelial cells were transferred to 12-well plates containing primary glial cells, and the milieu was changed to serum-free milieu DMEM:F12 supplemented with penicillin (100 U/mL), streptomycin (100 mg/mL), glutamine (2 mM) and hydrocortisone (550 nM). After 3 days of co-culture, TEER was measured and treated given to the cells (epithelial side) for 24 h. When ending the experiment, TEER was measured again in order to check the stability of membrane after treatment, and media from both sides of membrane were collected.

BBB-Passage Protocol

Compound **1** (400 µM) was incubated in the upper layer for 24 h at room temperature in the dark and without stirring. After that, aliquots from the upper and lower layers were analyzed and quantified by reverse phase-high performance liquid chromatography (RP-HPLC). RP-HPLC was done on an Agilent 1200 Series Infinity Star equipped with GABI detector, a UV detector and a ThermoScientific Hypersil ODS reverse phase C18 column (300 mm × 4.6 × 10 microns). A gradient mode (flow rate 1 mL/min), beginning with a mobile phase consisting of an aqueous solution of TFA 0.1% (A) that gradually was converted to acetonitrile (B) (0 to 100% in 20 min) was used. The injection volume was 50 µL and the detection was performed at a wavelength of 220 nm. Calibration curve was made with compound **1** prior performing the BBB quantification.

4.4. In Vivo Anti-Glioblastoma Studies

Animals. All protocols for animal experimentation were carried out in accordance with experimentation procedures approved by Technion Institute of Technology Ethical Commission in the Use of Animal, Israel (Protocol number IL-143-10-17 Technion). All animal experimental protocols followed the principles outlined in the Declaration of Helsinki. Animals were housed in wire mesh cages at 20 ± 2 °C with 12 h artificial light-dark cycles. The animals were fed ad libitum to standard pellet diet and water and were used after a minimum of 5 days acclimation to the housing conditions.

In Vitro glioblastoma U87 MG cell growing. Glioblastoma U87 MG cells are grown in full milieu, MEM-eagle with fetal cow serum (9%), glutamine (2%), and gentamycin (0.05%) (Biological Industries, Beit Ha'emek, Israel). The cells were thawed and grown. After three days, the cells were split and grown for additional 4 more days until the injection. The culture milieu was changed every two days. To prepare the cells for injection into the mouse brain, they were counted and suspended in PBS.

Stereotactic surgery—cell injection in brain. The mice were anesthetized either by inhalation of isoflurane or injection of ketamine-xylazine mixture in physiological saline (ketamine 1 mg/mL: xylazine 20 mg/mL). Eye ointment was applied to maintain adequate moisture during the procedure. Using a sterile scalpel, a sagittal incision was preformed over the parieto-occipital bone, approximately 1 cm long. The exposed skull surface was then cleaned. With stereotactic surgery, coordinates where the cells were injected were marked (1.5 mm right and 1.5 mm backward bregma). A volume of 3 mL containing 2.5–3.0 × 10^5 U87 MG cells was injected into a depth of 2.5 mm skull. After the cell injection we waited 4 minutes until taking the syringe out.

4.4.1. Treatments

The experiments were carried out on 7–8 weak-old BALB/c female mice (17.6–18.0 g of body weight, bw) bred under specific pathogen-free conditions. At the end of experiments, they were anaesthetized with isoflurane and sacrificed by cervical dislocation. When tumors begin to develop, according to bioluminescence imaging (3rd day after cell inoculation), six mice per group were located in one cage and the treatments began the next day. Three groups of treatment were defined: (i) compound **1**, dissolved in sterile physiological saline:Tween 80 (4:1, *v/v*), administered at 1 mg/kg bw ip; (ii) **Tmz**, dissolved in sterile physiological saline:Tween 80 (4:1, *v/v*), administered at 4 mg/kg bw ip; (iii) negative control (vehicle, sterile physiological saline:Tween 80 (4:1, *v/v*)). The animals were dosed three days a week every two days, with resting-days, for as long as the mice lived. Days of treatments after cells inoculation: 4th, 6th, 8th, 11th, 13th, 15th, 18th, 20th, 22th, 25th, etc.

4.4.2. Anti-Tumor Evaluation

The antitumor activity was evaluated using both the evolution of the tumor volumes and the animal survival. Tumor volumes were determined by bioluminescence imaging weekly. The bioluminescence imaging was based on the oxidation of luciferin [d-(-)-2-(6-hydroxy-2-benzothiazolyl)-thiazole-4-carboxylic acid] in the presence of oxygen and adenosine triphosphate. This reaction is catalyzed by the enzyme luciferase, which converts chemical energy into photons with resultant emission of light. Luciferase is present only in the injected cancer cells (that were pre transfected with plasmid encoding for the enzyme). Bioluminescence monitoring was done once a week beginning two days after cell injection until mouse death. After the administration of luciferin (d-luciferin potassium salt, 150 mg/kg) via intraperitoneal injection, mice were anesthetized with isoflurane. Measurements are taken every minute until 24 min after luciferin injection. Regions of interest encompassing the intracranial area of signal were defined using Living Image software, and the total photons/s/sr/cm2 (photons per second per radian per square cm) was recorded.

4.5. Statistical Analysis

All results are expressed as the averages of independent experiments ± SEM. Differences between populations were calculated with two-tailed Student's *t*-test. Kaplan–Meier survival curve and comparisons were performed by log-rank test. GraphPad Prism 6 was used for data analysis.

5. Conclusions

Many divesting tumors in humans, such as high-grade gliomas, are not yet treated satisfactorily by conventional therapeutic approaches. In our ongoing project of R+D of drugs with dual action (chemotherapy + radiotherapy combination), a new anti-glioblastoma agent was identified. This agent inhibiting TKRs, which produces canonical and non-canonical effects, is able to overcome the in vivo behavior of the first-line drug temozolomide.

This **Sun**-carborane cluster bifunctional hybrid compound, which exploits the TKR-interaction/inhibition ability plus the previously reported selective boron accumulation for the BNCT process, would act as an anticancer bimodal agent (chemo + radiotherapy) to result in significant clinical benefits by reducing the drug doses to get the same therapeutic effect while diminishing the side effects to the patient.

Supplementary Materials: The following are available online at http://www.mdpi.com/2072-6694/12/11/3423/s1. Figure S1: Synthetic procedures for preparation of compounds **1** and **4–11**, Figure S2: Profile of **Sun** against 468 protein kinases, Figure S3: Inhibition studies of FLT3 and PDGFR-β kinases, Figure S4: Animals' body weight evolutions during the in vivo anti-glioblastoma assays, Table S1: In vitro activity of studied compounds against different TKR-overexpressing HT-29, C6, and U87 MG tumor cells, Table S2: Effect on F98-cell survival after post-neutron irradiation (2 Gy) in different conditions, Table S3: Complete list of kinases and primary screening results of KINOMEScan assay performed by DiscoveRx in 468 selected kinases for compound **1**.

Author Contributions: Conceptualization, E.T., L.B., M.G. (Moshe Gavish), F.T., C.V., M.C., and H.C.; methodology, C.A., B.D., M.F.G., C.S., M.K., M.G. (Martín Gabay), and N.Z.; formal analysis, C.A., B.D., M.F.G., C.S., M.K., E.T., L.B., M.G. (Martín Gabay), N.Z., M.G. (Moshe Gavish), F.T., C.V., M.C., and H.C.; writing—original draft preparation, C.V., M.C., and H.C.; writing—review and editing, C.A., B.D., M.F.G., M.K., E.T., L.B., M.G. (Martín Gabay), F.T., C.V., M.C., and H.C. All authors have read and agreed to the published version of the manuscript.

Funding: This research was funded by Agencia Nacional de Investigación e Innovación (ANII, Uruguay), grant numbers FCE_3_2018_1_148288 and POS_NAC_2015_1_110068, Institut Pasteur de Montevideo—FOCEM, and Comisión Sectorail de Investigación Científica-Universidad de la República (Uruguay). M.C., M.F.G., E.T., L.B., and H.C. are Sistema Nacional de Investigadores-ANII researchers.

Conflicts of Interest: The authors declare no conflict of interest.

References

1. Fitzmaurice, C.; Dicker, D.; Pain, A.; Hamavid, H.; Moradi-Lakeh, M.; MacIntyre, M.F.; Allen, C.; Hansen, G.M.; Woodbrook, R.; Wolfe, C.; et al. The global burden of cancer 2013. *JAMA Oncol.* **2015**, *1*, 505–527. [CrossRef]
2. Stupp, R.; Mason, W.P.; van den Bent, M.J.; Weller, M.; Fisher, B.; Taphoorn, M.J.B.; Belanger, K.; Brandes, A.A.; Marosi, C.; Curschmann, J.; et al. Radiotherapy plus concomitant and adjuvant Temozolomide for glioblastoma. *N. Engl. J. Med.* **2005**, *352*, 987–996. [CrossRef]

3. Batchelor, T.T.; Mulholland, P.; Neyns, B.; Nabors, L.B.; Campone, M.; Wick, A.; Mason, W.; Mikkelsen, T.; Phuphanich, S.; Ashby, L.S.; et al. Phase III randomized trial comparing the efficacy of Cediranib as monotherapy, and in combination with Lomustine, versus Lomustine alone in patients with recurrent glioblastoma. *J. Clin. Oncol.* **2013**, *31*, 3212–3218. [CrossRef]
4. Lombardi, G.; Pambuku, A.; Bellu, L.; Farina, M.; Della Puppa, A.; Denaro, L.; Zagonel, V. Effectiveness of antiangiogenic drugs in glioblastoma patients: A systematic review and meta-analysis of randomized clinical trials. *Crit. Rev. Oncol./Hematol.* **2017**, *111*, 94–102. [CrossRef]
5. Goodwin, C.R.; Rath, P.; Oyinlade, O.; Lopez, H.; Mughal, S.; Xia, S.; Li, Y.; Kaur, H.; Zhou, X.; Ahmed, A.K.; et al. Crizotinib and Erlotinib inhibits growth of c-Met + /EGFRvIII + primary human glioblastoma xenografts. *Clin. Neurol. Neurosurg.* **2018**, *171*, 26–33. [CrossRef]
6. Papaetis, G.S.; Syrigos, K.N. Sunitinib: A multitargeted receptor tyrosine kinase inhibitor in the era of molecular cancer therapies. *BioDrugs* **2009**, *23*, 377–389. [CrossRef]
7. Giannopoulou, E.; Dimitropoulos, K.; Argyriou, A.A.; Koutras, A.K.; Dimitrakopoulos, F.; Kalofonos, H.P. An in vitro study, evaluating the effect of sunitinib and/or lapatinib on two glioma cell lines. *Investig. New Drugs* **2010**, *28*, 554–560. [CrossRef] [PubMed]
8. de Bouard, S.; Herlin, P.; Christensen, J.G.; Lemoisson, E.; Gauduchon, P.; Raymond, E.; Guillamo, J.-S. Antiangiogenic and anti-invasive effects of sunitinib on experimental human glioblastoma. *Neuro-Oncol.* **2007**, *9*, 412–423. [CrossRef] [PubMed]
9. Balaña, C.; Gil, M.J.; Perez, P.; Reynes, G.; Gallego, O.; Ribalta, T.; Capellades, J.; Gonzalez, S.; Verger, E. Sunitinib administered prior to radiotherapy in patients with non-resectable glioblastoma: Results of a phase II study. *Target Oncol.* **2014**, *9*, 321–329. [CrossRef] [PubMed]
10. Hutterer, M.; Nowosielski, M.; Haybaeck, J.; Embacher, S.; Stockhammer, F.; Gotwald, T.; Holzner, B.; Capper, D.; Preusser, M.; Marosi, C.; et al. A single-arm phase II Austrian/German multicenter trial on continuous daily sunitinib in primary glioblastoma at first recurrence (SURGE 01-07). *Neuro-Oncol.* **2014**, *16*, 92–102. [CrossRef] [PubMed]
11. Cerecetto, H.; Couto, M. Medicinal chemistry of boron-bearing compounds for BNCT-glioma treatment: Current challenges and perspectives. In *Glioma: Contemporary Diagnostic and Therapeutic Approaches*; Omerhodzic, I., Arnautovic, K., Eds.; IntechOpen: London, UK, 2018. [CrossRef]
12. Barth, R.F.; Vicente, M.H.; Harling, O.K.; Kiger, W.S.; Riley, K.J.; Binns, P.J.; Wagner, F.M.; Suzuki, M.; Aihara, T.; Kato, I.; et al. Current status of boron neutron capture therapy of high grade gliomas and recurrent head and neck cancer. *Radiat. Oncol.* **2012**, *7*, 1–21. [CrossRef]
13. Capoulat, M.E.; Sauzet, N.; Valda, A.A.; Gagetti, L.; Guillaudin, O.; Lebreton, L.; Maire, D.; Mastinu, P.; Praena, J.; Riffard, Q.; et al. Neutron spectrometry of the ^{9}Be(d (1.45 MeV), n)^{10}B reaction for accelerator-based BNCT. *Nucl. Instrum. Methods Phys. Res. B Beam Interact. Mater. At.* **2019**, *445*, 57–62. [CrossRef]
14. Kumada, H.; Naito, F.; Hasegawa, K.; Kobayashi, H.; Kurihara, T.; Takada, K.; Onishi, T.; Sakurai, K.; Matsumura, A.; Sakae, T. Development of LINAC-based neutron source for boron neutron capture therapy in University of Tsukuba. *Plasma Fusion Res.* **2018**, *13*, 2406006. [CrossRef]
15. Gordillo, N.; Montseny, E.; Sobrevilla, P. State of the art survey on MRI brain tumor segmentation. *Magn. Reson. Imaging* **2013**, *31*, 1426–1438. [CrossRef] [PubMed]
16. Maas, A.I.R.; Stocchetti, N.; Bullock, R. Moderate and severe traumatic brain injury in adults. *Lancet Neurol.* **2008**, *7*, 728–741. [CrossRef]
17. Price, E.W.; Orvig, C. Matching chelators to radiometals for radiopharmaceuticals. *Chem. Soc. Rev.* **2014**, *43*, 260–290. [CrossRef] [PubMed]
18. Couto, M.; Mastandrea, I.; Cabrera, M.; Cabral, P.; Teixidor, F.; Cerecetto, H.; Vinas, C. Small-molecule kinase-inhibitors-loaded boron cluster as hybrid agents for glioma-cell-targeting therapy. *Chem. Eur. J.* **2017**, *23*, 9233–9238. [CrossRef] [PubMed]
19. Couto, M.; García, M.F.; Alamón, C.; Cabrera, M.; Cabral, P.; Merlino, A.; Teixidor, F.; Cerecetto, H.; Vinas, C. Discovery of potent EGFR inhibitors through the incorporation of a 3D-aromatic-boron-rich-cluster into the 4-anilinoquinazoline scaffold: Potential drugs for glioma treatment. *Chem. Eur. J.* **2018**, *24*, 3122–3126. [CrossRef]
20. Couto, M.; Alamón, C.; Sánchez, C.; Dávila, B.; Fernández, M.; Lecot, N.; Cabral, P.; Teixidor, F.; Viñas, C.; Cerecetto, H. Carboranylanilinoquinazoline EGFR-inhibitors: Toward "lead-to-candidate" stage in the drug-development pipeline. *Future Med. Chem.* **2019**, *11*, 2273–2285. [CrossRef]

21. Couto, M.; Alamón, C.; García, M.F.; Kovacs, M.; Trias, E.; Nievas, S.; Pozzi, E.C.; Curotto, P.; Thorp, S.I.; Dagrosa, M.A.; et al. Closo-carboranyl- and metallacarboranyl (1,2,3)triazolyl-decorated Lapatinib-scaffold for cancer therapy combining tyrosine kinase inhibition and boron neutron capture therapy. *Cells* **2020**, *9*, 1408. [CrossRef]
22. Couto, M.; Alamón, C.; Nievas, S.; Perona, M.; Dagrosa, M.A.; Teixidor, F.; Cabral, P.; Vinas, C.; Cerecetto, H. Bimodal therapeutic agents against glioblastoma, one of the most lethal forms of cancer. *Chem. Eur. J.* **2020**. [CrossRef] [PubMed]
23. Laird, A.D.; Vajkoczy, P.; Shawver, L.K.; Thurnher, A.; Liang, C.; Mohammadi, M.; Schlessinger, J.; Ullrich, A.; Hubbard, S.R.; Blake, R.A.; et al. SU6668 is a potent antiangiogenic and antitumor agent that induces regression of established tumors. *Cancer Res.* **2000**, *60*, 4152–4160. [PubMed]
24. Sun, L.; Liang, C.; Shirazian, S.; Zhou, Y.; Miller, T.; Cui, J.; Fukuda, J.Y.; Chu, J.-Y.; Nematalla, A.; Wang, X.; et al. Discovery of 5-[5-Fluoro-2-oxo-1,2-dihydroindol-(3Z)-ylidenemethyl]-2,4-dimethyl-1*H*-pyrrole-3-carboxylic acid (2-diethylaminoethyl)amide, a novel tyrosine kinase inhibitor targeting vascular endothelial and platelet-derived growth factor receptor tyrosine kinase. *J. Med. Chem.* **2003**, *46*, 1116–1119. [CrossRef] [PubMed]
25. Drevs, J.; Medinger, M.; Schmidt-Gersbach, C.; Weber, R.; Unger, C. Receptor tyrosine kinases: The main targets for new anticancer therapy. *Curr. Drug Targets.* **2003**, *4*, 113–121. [CrossRef] [PubMed]
26. Issa, F.; Kassiou, M.; Rendina, L.M. Boron in drug discovery: Carboranes as unique pharmacophores in biologically active compounds. *Chem. Rev.* **2011**, *111*, 5701–5722. [CrossRef]
27. Scholz, M.; Hey-Hawkins, E. Carbaboranes as pharmacophores: Properties, synthesis, and application strategies. *Chem. Rev.* **2011**, *111*, 7035–7062. [CrossRef]
28. Poater, J.; Solà, M.; Viñas, C.; Teixidor, F. Hückel's rule of aromaticity categorizes aromatic *closo* boron hydride clusters. *Chem. Eur. J.* **2016**, *22*, 7437–7443. [CrossRef]
29. Poater, J.; Viñas, C.; Bennour, I.; Escayola, S.; Solà, M.; Teixidor, F. Too persistent to give up: Aromaticity in boron clusters survives radical structural changes. *J. Am. Chem. Soc.* **2020**, *142*, 9396–9407. [CrossRef]
30. Fox, M.A.; Hughes, A.K. Cage C–H$\cdots$X interactions in solid-state structures of icosahedral carboranes. *Coord. Chem. Rev.* **2004**, *248*, 457–476. [CrossRef]
31. Donati, A.; Ristori, S.; Bonechi, C.; Panza, L.; Martini, G.; Rossi, C. Evidences of strong C–H$\cdots$O bond in an *o*-carboranyl β-lactoside in solution. *J. Am. Chem. Soc.* **2002**, *124*, 8778. [CrossRef]
32. Zhang, X.; Dai, H.; Yan, H.; Zou, W.; Cremer, D. B–H$\cdots\pi$ interaction: A new type of nonclassical hydrogen bonding. *J. Am. Chem. Soc.* **2016**, *138*, 4334–4337. [CrossRef]
33. Knight, Z.A.; Lin, H.; Shokat, K.M. Targeting the cancer kinome through polypharmacology. *Nat. Rev. Cancer.* **2010**, *10*, 130–137. [CrossRef] [PubMed]
34. Gilliland, D.G.; Griffin, J.D. The roles of FLT3 in hematopoiesis and leukemia. *Blood* **2002**, *100*, 1532–1542. [CrossRef] [PubMed]
35. Heinrich, M.C.; Corless, C.L.; Demetri, G.D.; Blanke, C.D.; von Mehren, M.; Joensuu, H.; McGreevey, L.S.; Chen, C.-J.; Abbeele, A.D.V.D.; Druker, B.; et al. Kinase mutations and imatinib response in patients with metastatic gastrointestinal stromal tumor. *J. Clin. Oncol.* **2003**, *21*, 4342–4349. [CrossRef] [PubMed]
36. Karaman, M.W.; Herrgard, S.; Treiber, D.K.; Gallant, P.; Atteridge, C.E.; Campbell, B.T.; Chan, K.W.; Ciceri, P.; Davis, M.I.; Edeen, P.; et al. A quantitative analysis of kinase inhibitor selectivity. *Nat. Biotechnol.* **2008**, *26*, 127–132. [CrossRef] [PubMed]
37. Kerkela, R.; Woulfe, K.C.; Durand, J.-B.; Vagnozzi, R.; Kramer, D.; Chu, T.F.; Beahm, C.; Chen, M.H.; Force, T. Sunitinib-induced cardiotoxicity is mediated by off-target inhibition of AMP-activated protein kinase. *Clin. Transl. Sci.* **2009**, *2*, 15–25. [CrossRef] [PubMed]
38. Hasinoff, B.B.; Patel, D.; O'Hara, K.A. Mechanisms of myocyte cytotoxicity induced by the multiple receptor tyrosine kinase inhibitor Sunitinib. *Mol. Pharmacol.* **2008**, *74*, 1722–1728. [CrossRef]
39. Chen, Z.; Zhong, D.; Li, G. The role of microglia in viral encephalitis: A review. *J. Neuroinflamm.* **2019**, *16*, 76. [CrossRef]
40. Brandao, M.; Simon, T.; Critchley, G.; Giamas, G. Astrocytes, the rising stars of the glioblastoma microenvironment. *Glia* **2019**, *67*, 779–790. [CrossRef]

41. Latuske, E.-M.; Stamm, H.; Klokow, M.; Vohwinkel, G.; Muschhammer, J.; Bokemeyer, C.; Jucker, M.; Kebenko, M.; Fiedler, W.; Wellbrock, J. Combined inhibition of GLI and FLT3 signaling leads to effective anti-leukemic effects in human acute myeloid leukemia. *Oncotarget* **2017**, *8*, 29187–29201. [CrossRef]
42. Nagao, H.; Ijiri, K.; Hirotsu, M.; Ishidou, Y.; Yamamoto, T.; Nagano, S.; Takizawa, T.; Nakashima, K.; Komiya, S.; Setoguchi, T. Role of GLI2 in the growth of human osteosarcoma. *J. Pathol.* **2011**, *224*, 169–179. [CrossRef] [PubMed]
43. Wang, K.; Pan, L.; Che, X.; Cui, D.; Li, C. Gli1 inhibition induces cell-cycle arrest and enhanced apoptosis in brain glioma cell lines. *J. Neuro-oncol.* **2010**, *98*, 319–327. [CrossRef] [PubMed]
44. Lim, C.B.; Prêle, C.M.; Baltic, S.; Arthur, P.G.; Creaney, J.; Watkins, D.N.; Thompson, P.J.; Mutsaers, S.E. Mitochondria-derived reactive oxygen species drive GANT61-induced mesothelioma cell apoptosis. *Oncotarget* **2015**, *6*, 1519–1530. [CrossRef] [PubMed]
45. Zhou, X.; Zhou, L.-F.; Yang, B.; Zhao, H.-J.; Wang, Y.-Q.; Li, X.-Y.; Ye, Y.-P.; Chen, F.-Y. The loss of a sugar chain at C(3) position enhances Stemucronatoside K-induced apoptosis, cell cycle arrest and hedgehog pathway inhibition in HT-29 cells. *Chem. Biodivers.* **2016**, *13*, 1484–1492. [CrossRef] [PubMed]
46. Cheng, F.; Li, W.; Zhou, Y.; Shen, J.; Wu, Z.; Liu, G.; Lee, P.W.; Tang, Y. AdmetSAR: A comprehensive source and free tool for assessment of chemical ADMET properties. *J. Chem. Inf. Model.* **2012**, *52*, 3099–3105. [CrossRef]
47. Organisation for Economic Co-Operation and Development (OECD). OECD Guidelines for Testing of Chemicals: Acute Oral Toxicity—Acute Toxic Class Method. OECD 423, 2001. Available online: https://ntp.niehs.nih.gov/iccvam/suppdocs/feddocs/oecd/oecd_gl423.pdf (accessed on 1 January 2020).
48. Malina, K.C.K.; Cooper, I.; Teichberg, V.I. Closing the gap between the in-vivo and in-vitro blood-brain barrier tightness. *Brain Res.* **2009**, *1284*, 12–21. [CrossRef]
49. Aparicio-Blanco, J.; Romero, I.A.; Male, D.K.; Slowing, K.; García-García, L.; Torres-Suárez, A. Cannabidiol enhances the passage of lipid nanocapsules across the blood-brain barrier both in vitro and in vivo. *Mol. Pharm.* **2019**, *16*, 1999–2010. [CrossRef]
50. Le Joncour, V.; Karaman, S.; Laakkonen, P.M. Predicting in vivo payloads delivery using a blood-brain tumor-barrier in a dish. *J. Vis. Exp.* **2019**, *146*, e59384. [CrossRef]
51. Bhupathiraju, N.V.S.D.K.; Hu, X.; Zhou, Z.; Fronczek, F.R.; Couraud, P.-O.; Romero, I.A.; Weksler, B.; Vicente, M.G.H. Synthesis and in vitro evaluation of BBB permeability, tumor cell uptake, and cytotoxicity of a series of carboranylporphyrin conjugates. *J. Med. Chem.* **2014**, *57*, 6718–6728. [CrossRef]
52. Shen, J.; Cheng, F.; Xu, Y.; Li, W.; Tang, Y. Estimation of ADME properties with substructure pattern recognition. *J. Chem. Inf. Model.* **2010**, *50*, 1034–1041. [CrossRef]
53. Carbon-Mangels, M.; Hutter, M.C. Selecting relevant descriptors for classification by Bayesian estimates: A comparison with decision trees and support vector machines approaches for disparate data sets. *Mol. Inform.* **2011**, *30*, 885–895. [CrossRef] [PubMed]
54. Robinson, R.L.M.; Glen, R.C.; Mitchell, J.B.O. Development and comparison of hERG blocker classifiers: Assessment on different datasets yields markedly different results. *Mol. Inform.* **2011**, *30*, 443–458. [CrossRef] [PubMed]
55. Wang, S.; Li, Y.; Wang, J.; Chen, L.; Zhang, L.; Yu, H.; Hou, T. ADMET evaluation in drug discovery. 12. Development of binary classification models for prediction of hERG potassium channel blockage. *Mol. Pharm.* **2012**, *9*, 996–1010. [CrossRef] [PubMed]
56. Lagunin, A.; Filimonov, D.; Zakharov, A.; Xie, W.; Huang, Y.; Zhu, F.; Shen, T.; Yalo, J.; Poroikov, V.V. Computer-aided prediction of rodent carcinogenicity by PASS and CISOC-PSCT. *QSAR Comb. Sci.* **2009**, *28*, 806–810. [CrossRef]
57. Zhu, H.; Martin, T.M.; Ye, L.; Sedykh, A.; Young, D.M.; Tropsha, A. Quantitative structure-activity relationship modeling of rat acute toxicity by oral exposure. *Chem. Res. Toxicol.* **2009**, *22*, 1913–1921. [CrossRef]
58. Wang, J.; Krudy, G.; Hou, T.; Zhang, W.; Holland, G.; Xu, X. Development of reliable aqueous solubility models and their application in druglike analysis. *J. Chem. Inf. Model.* **2007**, *47*, 1395–1404. [CrossRef]
59. Vainshtein, A.; Veenman, L.; Shterenberg, A.; Singh, S.; Masarwa, A.; Dutta, B.; Island, B.; Tsoglin, E.; Levin, E.; Leschiner, S.; et al. Quinazoline-based tricyclic compounds that regulate programmed cell death, induce neuronal differentiation, and are curative in animal models for excitotoxicity and hereditary brain disease. *Cell Death Discov.* **2015**, *1*, 15027. [CrossRef]

60. Sosunov, A.; Wu, X.; McGovern, R.; Mikell, C.; McKhann, G.M.; Goldman, J.E. Abnormal mitosis in reactive astrocytes. *Acta Neuropathol. Commun.* **2020**, *8*, 47. [CrossRef]
61. Zeno, S.; Zaaroor, M.; Leschiner, S.; Veenman, L.; Gavish, M. $CoCl_2$ induces apoptosis via the 18 kDa translocator protein in U118MG human glioblastoma cells. *Biochemistry* **2009**, *48*, 4652–4661. [CrossRef]

Publisher's Note: MDPI stays neutral with regard to jurisdictional claims in published maps and institutional affiliations.

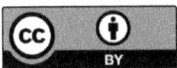

© 2020 by the authors. Licensee MDPI, Basel, Switzerland. This article is an open access article distributed under the terms and conditions of the Creative Commons Attribution (CC BY) license (http://creativecommons.org/licenses/by/4.0/).

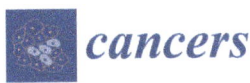

Article

VRK1 Phosphorylates Tip60/KAT5 and Is Required for H4K16 Acetylation in Response to DNA Damage

Raúl García-González [1,2], Patricia Morejón-García [1,2], Ignacio Campillo-Marcos [1,2], Marcella Salzano [3] and Pedro A. Lazo [1,2,*]

1. Molecular Mechanisms of Cancer Program, Instituto de Biología Molecular y Celular del Cáncer, CSIC-Universidad de Salamanca, Campus Miguel de Unamuno, 37007 Salamanca, Spain; garciaraul@usal.es (R.G.-G.); pmoreg@usal.es (P.M.-G.); ignacio_cm@usal.es (I.C.-M.)
2. Área de Cancer, Instituto de Investigación Biomédica de Salamanca-IBSAL, Hospital Universitario de Salamanca, 37007 Salamanca, Spain
3. Enfermedades Digestivas y Hepáticas, Vall d'Hebron Institut de Recerca, Hospital Universitari Vall d'Hebron, Universidad Autónoma de Barcelona, 08035 Barcelona, Spain; marcella.salzano@vhir.org
* Correspondence: pedro.lazo@csic.es; Tel.: +34-923-294-804

Received: 17 August 2020; Accepted: 13 October 2020; Published: 15 October 2020

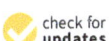

Simple Summary: Dynamic remodeling of chromatin requires epigenetic modifications of histones. DNA damage induced by doxorubicin causes an increase in histone H4K16ac, a marker of local chromatin relaxation. We studied the role that VRK1, a chromatin kinase activated by DNA damage, plays in this early step. VRK1 depletion or MG149, a Tip60/KAT5 inhibitor, cause a loss of H4K16ac. DNA damage induces the phosphorylation of Tip60 mediated by VRK1 in the chromatin fraction. VRK1 directly interacts and phosphorylates Tip60. This phosphorylation of Tip60 is lost by depletion of VRK1 in both *ATM +/+* and *ATM−/−* cells. Kinase-active VRK1, but not kinase-dead VRK1, rescues Tip60 phosphorylation induced by DNA damage independently of ATM. The VRK1 chromatin kinase is an upstream regulator of the initial acetylation of histones, and an early step in DNA damage responses.

Abstract: Dynamic remodeling of chromatin requires acetylation and methylation of histones, frequently affecting the same lysine residue. These alternative epigenetic modifications require the coordination of enzymes, writers and erasers, mediating them such as acetylases and deacetylases. In cells in G0/G1, DNA damage induced by doxorubicin causes an increase in histone H4K16ac, a marker of chromatin relaxation. In this context, we studied the role that VRK1, a chromatin kinase activated by DNA damage, plays in this early step. VRK1 depletion or MG149, a Tip60/KAT5 inhibitor, cause a loss of H4K16ac. DNA damage induces the phosphorylation of Tip60 mediated by VRK1 in the chromatin fraction. VRK1 directly interacts with and phosphorylates Tip60. Furthermore, the phosphorylation of Tip60 induced by doxorubicin is lost by depletion of VRK1 in both *ATM +/+* and *ATM−/−* cells. Kinase-active VRK1, but not kinase-dead VRK1, rescues Tip60 phosphorylation induced by DNA damage independently of ATM. The Tip60 phosphorylation by VRK1 is necessary for the activating acetylation of ATM, and subsequent ATM autophosphorylation, and both are lost by VRK1 depletion. These results support that the VRK1 chromatin kinase is an upstream regulator of the initial acetylation of histones, and an early step in DNA damage responses (DDR).

Keywords: phosphorylation; histone H4; acetylation; DNA-damage response; nucleosomal histone kinase-1

1. Introduction

Chromatin remodeling underlines all biological processes of the genome. The dynamic reorganization of chromatin requires several different, or alternative, epigenetic modifications of histones, which include acetylation, methylation, ubiquitination, and phosphorylation. Different combinations of these epigenetic marks are associated to the compaction or relaxation of chromatin and its biological functions including transcription, replication, differentiation, telomere protection, genome stability and DNA damage repair (DDR) [1–4]. Each individual cell has to remodel its chromatin to adjust to its particular functional situation. The pattern of histone modifications determines the tumor epigenome in tumor cells [5,6], which is also reflected in the tumor cell heterogeneity [7]. Some of these alternative epigenetic modifications frequently affect the same lysine residue in the targeted histone [8–10], such as acetylations and methylations, and there is crosstalk among these different histone modifications [2,4].

This dynamic chromatin remodeling involves at least four different enzyme families with several members, which includes writers such as lysine acetyl transferases (KAT) and methyl transferases (KMT), as well as erasers such as lysine deacetylases (HDAC) and demethylases (KDM) [2,4,11]. All of them are active target for pharmacological development in cancer [3,12]. The transition from one epigenetic histone modification to another requires the coordination of two, or four, of these enzymes, depending on the types of modifications in a specific lysine residue. However, the coordinators of these alternative enzymes and their functional and temporal organization are unknown.

Kinases are likely candidates to regulate, or coordinate, the balance of alternative histone epigenetic modifications, depending on the individual cell functional needs, by phosphorylation in Ser or Thr residues in nucleosomal histones [3], as well as by the regulation of the enzymes implicated in these modifications. Among them, human VRK1 (Q99986) [13], also known as nucleosomal-histone kinase 1 (NHK1) in *Drosophila melanogaster* [14], a very abundant nuclear/chromatin kinase [15], is well situated to participate in these processes. Human VRK1 is involved in the regulation of cell proliferation [16–18], and DNA damage responses [19–22]. VRK1 also specifically phosphorylates and regulates several transcription factors such as p53 [23–25], c-Jun [26], ATF2 [27], CREB [28], and Sox2 [18]. Furthermore, VRK1 also phosphorylates BAF, which is involved in regulation of the nuclear envelope assembly and chromosome attachment, and their disruption cause DNA chromosomal alterations [29–31]. The kinase activity of VRK1 is induced by different types of DNA damage able to cause single or double strand breaks or alkylating lesions [19]. In response to DNA damage, VRK1 directly phosphorylates histones H3 [21,32–34], H2AX [14,35], NBS1 [20], and 53BP1 [19,36]. VRK1 also phosphorylates hnRNPA1 in telomerase activation [37]. The VRK1 kinase activity is regulated by interactions of its C-terminal regulatory region with different proteins [38], such as the macroH2A histone variant [18,39], or with nuclear Ran [40].

When DNA damage occurs, each individual cell has to respond independently of its particular situation regarding resting or dividing, differentiation stage and the heterogeneity of its cellular or protein interactions. The initial response to DNA damage implicates a local chromatin relaxation that is associated to histone H4 acetylation in K16 [41–43]. Therefore, H4K16 hypo-acetylation is associated with defective DNA repair [36,44]. The importance of H4K16ac in order to trigger a proper DNA-damage response in a locally altered chromatin indicates that this modification is tightly regulated. However, the regulation of histone H4 acetylation has to be indirect and mediated by regulation of the Tip60/KAT5 (Q92993) acetylase, as a potential candidate. The acetylation in K5 of H2AX by Tip60 is necessary for the recruitment of NBS1 to damaged chromatin [45]. Tip60 also regulates chromatin recognition by 53BP1 [46]. Impairment of H4K16ac interferes with the docking site of NBS1, which is required for recruitment of 53BP1 in DNA damage responses [47]. VRK1 depletion impairs both NBS1 [20] and 53BP1 [19] specific phosphorylation and activation in response to DNA damage. Moreover, Tip60 is necessary for the acetylation and activation by autophosphorylation of ATM in response to DNA damage [48], whereas VRK1 is also essential for ATM activation [19,20,36]. Overexpression of Tip60 is associated to a poorer prognosis [49] and to cisplatin resistance in tumor cells [50]. High levels of VRK1 are also associated to poor prognosis [51] and confer resistance to

DNA-damage based treatments [52]. All these data place VRK1 as a candidate to regulate Tip60 activity and H4K16ac.

In this work, we have studied the role that the VRK1 chromatin kinase played in the regulation of Tip60/KAT5, and its association to both very early upstream events in DNA-damage response, such as H4K16 acetylation (responsible for a local chromatin relaxation), and sequential steps in the context of the ATM pathway during DNA damage response.

2. Results

2.1. DNA Damage Induces Phosphorylation of Tip60 and Acetylation of H4K16

To address the role of human VRK1 in the chromatin relaxation associated to histone acetylation, it was determined whether the activation of Tip60 by doxorubicin, leading to the acetylation of H4K16, might be associated to Tip60 phosphorylation by a not yet identified kinase. To eliminate mitogenic signals that activate VRK1 [17], cells were serum-deprived for 48 h. In these conditions, cells accumulated in G0/G1, there is no expression of cyclinD1, and retinoblastoma is not phosphorylated [17]. The induction of DNA damage by doxorubicin was confirmed by determination of free DNA ends in TUNEL assays (Figure S1A), and the DDR was confirmed by determining the formation of 53BP1 foci induced by double–strand breaks caused by doxorubicin, a response that is prevented by VRK1 knockdown (Figure S1B). These cells were treated with doxorubicin and they responded with an increase in the phosphorylation of endogenous Tip60 (Figure 1A), as well as an increase in H4K16ac (Figure 1A). To confirm the role of Tip60, we tested the effect of two HAT inhibitors that target HATs associated to two different roles of VRK1, DDR, and transcription. The inhibitor MG149 that targets Tip60 [53] prevented H4K16 acetylation in response to DNA damage induced by doxorubicin, but this acetylation was not affected by C646 that inhibits p300 [54], in serum-deprived A549 cells (Figure 1B) and U2OS cells (Figure S2).

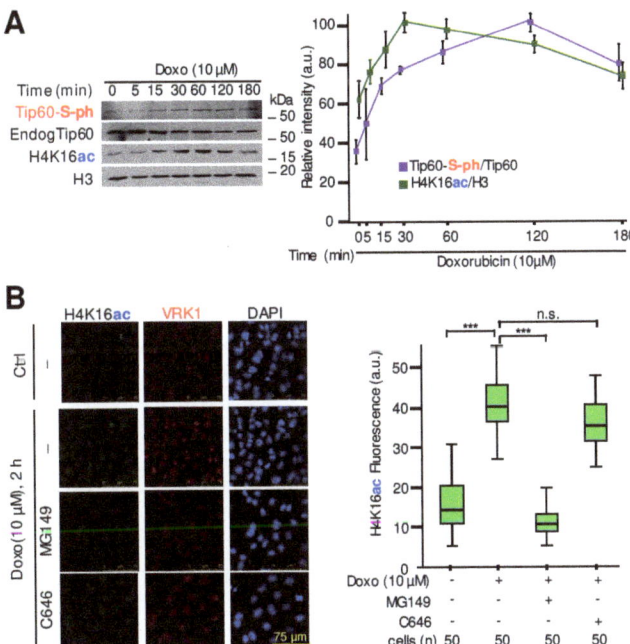

Figure 1. Effect of KAT (Lysine acetyl transferase) inhibitors on the acetylation of histone H4 induced by doxorubicin. (**A**). Time course of the effect of doxorubicin on the phosphorylation of endogenous Tip60

in serine detected with anti-phosphoserine antibody, and the acetylation of histone H4 in K16 in cells deprived of serum (0.5%) for 48 h and arrested in G0/G1 before treatment with doxorubicin (Doxo). Histones were prepared by acidic extraction. The reference value corresponds to the starting time point (0 min). (**B**). Induction of H4K16ac by treatment with doxorubicin (10 µM) and the effect of MG149 (Tip60 inhibitor, 2 µM) and C646 (p300 inhibitor, 10 µM) added ten hours before doxorubicin addition. The box plots show the quantification of the fluorescence using the Image J program. ns: Not significant. *** $p < 0.001$.

2.2. Kinase-Active VRK1 Rescues H4K16 Acetylation Induced by DNA Damage

Depletion of VRK1 caused a loss of H4K16ac in cells that were serum-deprived to prevent mitogenic activation of VRK1 [21,34]. Therefore, we hypothesized that VRK1 chromatin kinase might be a candidate kinase to regulate the acetylation of histone H4. The regulation of Tip60/KAT5 by a VRK1-mediated phosphorylation is a likely mechanism that regulates this acetylation. Therefore, to determine whether VRK1 can be a candidate kinase regulating Tip60 phosphorylation, its depletion should have a similar effect to that of Tip60 inhibitors on H4K16 acetylation. For this aim, it was determined whether H4K16ac induced by DNA damage and caused by doxorubicin [21], was sensitive to VRK1 depletion, and to MG149, an inhibitor of the histone acetylase Tip60. Depletion of VRK1 by two different siRNA caused a loss of H4K16ac induced by doxorubicin, and this effect mimicked that caused by MG149 and detected by immunofluorescence (Figure 2A). The effect of VRK1 depletion on the loss of H4K16ac level induced by doxorubicin was also confirmed using two different siRNA in Western blots (Figure 2B). This effect was confirmed using a different cell line, U2OS cells, which have a higher basal level of histone acetylation in the absence of doxorubicin treatment. In U2OS cells, depletion of VRK1, and the MG149 Tip60 inhibitor, had a similar effect and resulted in a significant reduction of H4K16ac (Figure S2).

To confirm that the H4K16ac induced by doxorubicin was dependent on the kinase activity of VRK1, we performed a rescue experiment. For this aim, endogenous human VRK1 was depleted in stable A549 cells expressing either murine VRK1 (mVRK1) wild-type or kinase-dead (K179E) [19,55]. Following depletion of the endogenous human VRK1, only wild-type mVRK1, but not kinase-dead mVRK1-K179E, was able to rescue H4K16ac induced by doxorubicin (Figure 2C).

2.3. VRK1 Directly Interacts with and Phosphorylates Tip60

To test whether VRK1 and Tip60 are directly related, we performed two types of assays with VRK1 and Tip60 human proteins. First, we performed an interaction assay from proteins expressed in bacteria and purified. In this experiment, a fixed amount of GST-VRK1 was incubated with increasing amounts of His-Tip60. The GST-VRK1 pulldown detected an increase in its interaction with His-Tip60 as the concentration of the latter was higher, and reaching a plateau as their concentrations became equimolar (Figure 3A). This indicated that both proteins are able to form a direct stable complex by themselves. To confirm the interaction in vivo, A549 cells were transfected with Tip60-V5 and VRK1-HA tagged human proteins, and a reciprocal immunoprecipitation was performed. The Tip60-VRK1 complex was detected in both reciprocal precipitations indicating it is stable by itself (Figure 3B). To confirm this interaction, the endogenous Tip60 was immunoprecipitated and the endogenous VRK1 detected in the immunoprecipitate (Figure 3C). In addition, we determined that the interaction between endogenous VRK1 and endogenous or transfected Tip60 was not affected by DNA damage (Figure 3D).

To demonstrate that the phosphorylation of Tip60 by VRK1 is also direct, we performed an in vitro kinase assay, with bacterially expressed and purified proteins. The assay was done with either active VRK1, or kinase-dead VRK1 (K179E) as negative control [19,40,55], and His-Tip60 as substrate. The phosphorylation of Tip60 was determined by immunoblot. Tip60 was phosphorylated by kinase-active VRK1, but not by kinase-dead VRK1 (K179E) (Figure 3E). Therefore, we concluded that VRK1 directly phosphorylates Tip60.

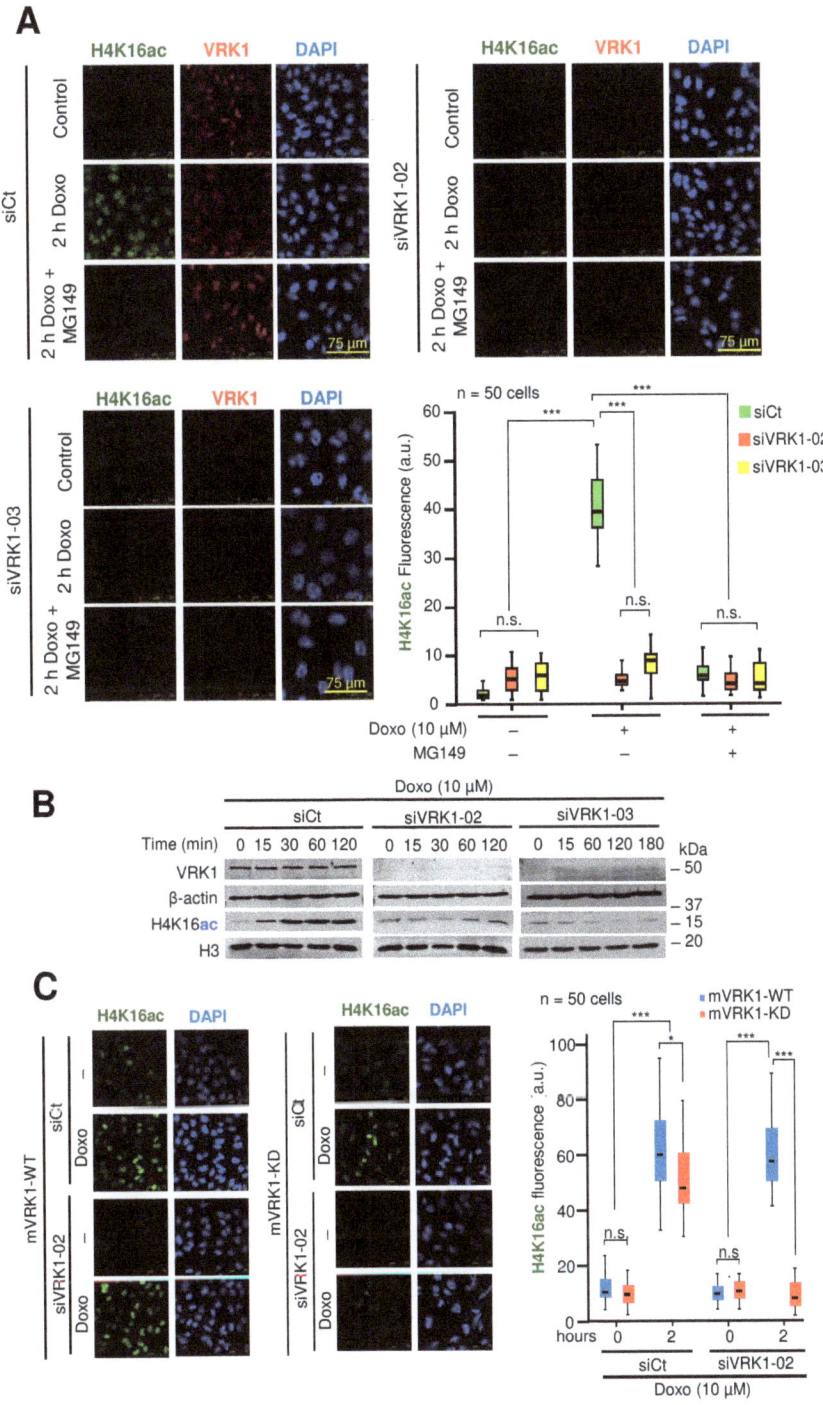

Figure 2. Effect of VRK1 depletion on H4K16 acetylation. (**A**). VRK1 was knockdown in A549 cells using siVRK1-02 (siV-02) and siVRK1-03 (siV-03). Serum-deprived (0.5% FBS for 48 h) cells were treated

with 10 µM doxorubicin (Doxo) for 3 h to induce DNA damage. MG149 (2 µM) was added to the cell culture at 12 h before doxorubicin. ns: Not significant, *** $p < 0.001$. (**B**). Effect of VRK1 depletion with two different siRNA on endogenous H4K16 acetylation induced by doxorubicin (Doxo) and detected by immunoblot. (**C**). Rescue of H4K16ac induced by doxorubicin in siVRK1-02 depleted cells and their rescue with either murine VRK1 or kinase-dead VRK1-KD (K179E) in stable A549 cell lines. All experiments were repeated three times. siCt: siControl. *** $p < 0.001$, * $p < 0.1$.

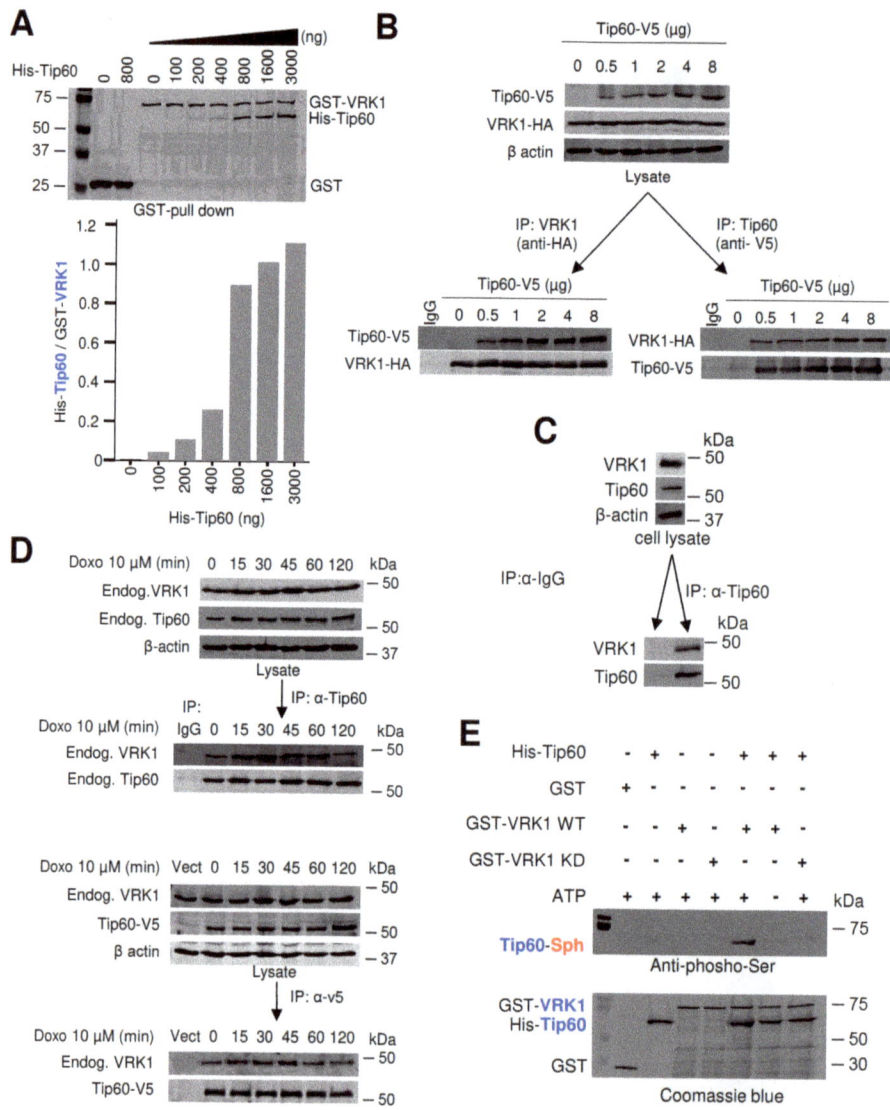

Figure 3. VRK1 direct interaction and phosphorylation of Tip60. (**A**). Binding of Tip60 to human VRK1. Increasing amounts of His-Tip60 were incubated with a fixed amount (1000 ng) of GST-VRK1, followed by a pulldown of GST-VRK1 and determination of Tip60. In the gel was included an assay with GST to rule out a non-specific interaction with His-Tip60. Proteins were detected by immunoblot with specific monoclonal antibodies for the GST and His epitopes. (**B**). Direct interaction between VRK1 and Tip60.

Cells were transfected with tagged plasmids expressing human VRK1-HA and Tip60-V5. The complex between these two proteins within cells was detected by reciprocal immunoprecipitations. (**C**). Immunoprecipitation of endogenous Tip60 with an anti-Tip60 antibody (ab137518) and detection of endogenous VRK1 in the immunoprecipitate. (**D**). Doxorubicin treatment does not alter the interaction between endogenous VRK1 and Tip60 (top) or between endogenous VRK1 and transfected Tip60-V5 (bottom). (**E**). Direct in vitro phosphorylation of Tip60 by VRK1 using bacterially expressed and purified proteins. Phosphorylated Tip60 was determined with an anti-phosphoserine antibody.

2.4. Kinase-Active VRK1 Mediates the Phosphorylation of Tip60 Induced by DNA-Damage

It is known that the kinase activity of VRK1 is induced by DNA damage independently of its type, including damage caused by doxorubicin [19]. Therefore, we tested whether incubation of A549 cells with doxorubicin was able to cause the phosphorylation of Tip60 in cells treated with doxorubicin. The treatment with doxorubicin did not alter the intracellular complex formed between the endogenous VRK1 and the transfected Tip60 determined by immunoprecipitation (Figure 4A). However, doxorubicin treatment induced an increase in the level of phosphorylated-Tip60 that is complexed with VRK1 (Figure 4A). Next, it was determined whether this Tip60 phosphorylation induced by doxorubicin was dependent on VRK1. For this aim, endogenous human VRK1 was depleted using two different siRNAs and the level of Tip60 phosphorylation induced by doxorubicin was determined in the immunoprecipitate. The increase of Tip60 phosphorylation induced by doxorubicin was lost in VRK1-depleted cells by using two different siRNA (Figure 4B).

Next, we performed a rescue experiment to confirm the effect of VRK1 on the phosphorylation of Tip60 in response to doxorubicin treatment. For this purpose, stable A549 cell lines were made, one expressing wild-type murine VRK1 (mVRK1), and the other by expressing kinase-dead murine VRK1-(K179E) [55]. In these cells, the effect of the murine VRK1 proteins was determined after depletion of the endogenous human VRK1. Wild-type murine VRK1 was able to rescue the phosphorylation of Tip60 induced by doxorubicin, but the kinase-dead mVRK1-(K179E) did not rescue Tip60 phosphorylation (Figure 4C).

2.5. VRK1 Depletion Prevents the Accumulation in Chromatin of Phospho-Tip60 Induced by DNA Damage

VRK1 is a nuclear kinase present in nucleoplasm and chromatin [21,32]. Therefore, it was determined whether the effect of VRK1 depletion on the nuclear localization of endogenous Tip60/KAT5 protein was dependent on its localization within nuclei. VRK1 was depleted with siRNA, and cells were treated with doxorubicin. In control cells, doxorubicin induced a significant accumulation of endogenous Tip60 in nuclei in response to DNA damage (Figure 5A). In VRK1 depleted cells, there was a loss of nuclear fluorescence associated to endogenous Tip60 (Figure 5A).

Next, it was determined whether the phosphorylated endogenous Tip60 was associated to the chromatin fraction of the nuclear protein. For this aim, the localization of phosphorylated Tip60 in response to doxorubicin was determined by fractionation of nuclei into chromatin and nucleoplasm fractions. The presence of phosphorylated endogenous Tip60 induced by doxorubicin was only detected in the chromatin fraction (Figure 5B right), but not in the nucleoplasm (Figure 5B left). Furthermore, this chromatin localization of endogenous Tip60 was lost by depletion of VRK1 (Figure 5B right). These data indicated that the phosphorylation of Tip60 occurred on chromatin where VRK1 is also present, but not in the nucleoplasm fraction.

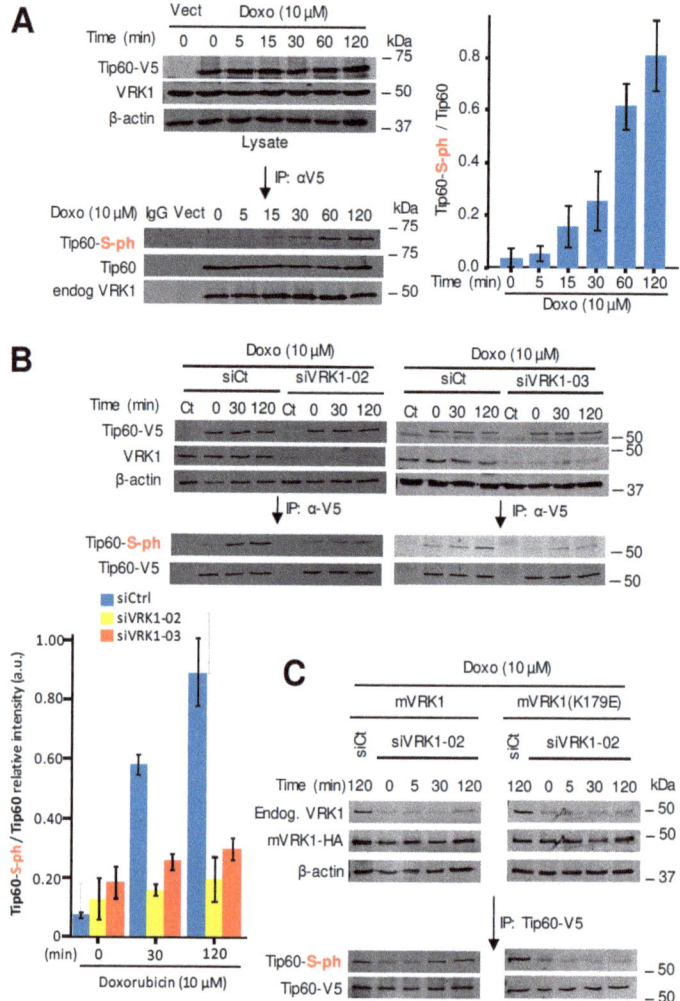

Figure 4. VRK1 mediates the phosphorylation of Tip60 induced by doxorubicin. (**A**). Time dependent phosphorylation of Tip60 in cells treated with doxorubicin. A549 cells were transfected with plasmid Tip60-V5 or empty vector (Ct); and to eliminate mitogenic signaling, cells were maintained in 0.5% serum for 48 h before the addition of doxorubicin to the culture. Cells were lysed at different time points and Tip60 was immunoprecipitated and determined its stable interaction with endogenous VRK1. The phosphorylation of the Tip60 after doxorubicin treatment and present in the immunoprecipitated Tip60-VRK1 complex was detected in Western blots. To the right it is shown the quantification from three independent experiments. Vect: Transfected with empty vector. Vect: Transfection control with empty vector. (**B**). Effect of VRK1 depletion on the phosphorylation of Tip60. A549 cells were treated with si-control (left), siVRK1-02 (center) or siVRK1-03 (right) followed by transfection with plasmid Tip60-V5, and cells were treated with doxorubicin at the indicated times. Transfected Tip60-V5 was immunoprecipitated and the phosphorylation of Tip60 determined in Western blots. The graph to the bottom-left shows the quantification of phosphorylated Tip60 from three different experiments. Vect: Transfected with empty vector. (**C**). Rescue of Tip60 phosphorylation induced by doxorubicin in two A549 stable cell lines expressing either murine kinase-active (left) or kinase-dead murine VRK1 (K179E) (right) in which endogenous human VRK1 was depleted. Experiments were repeated three times.

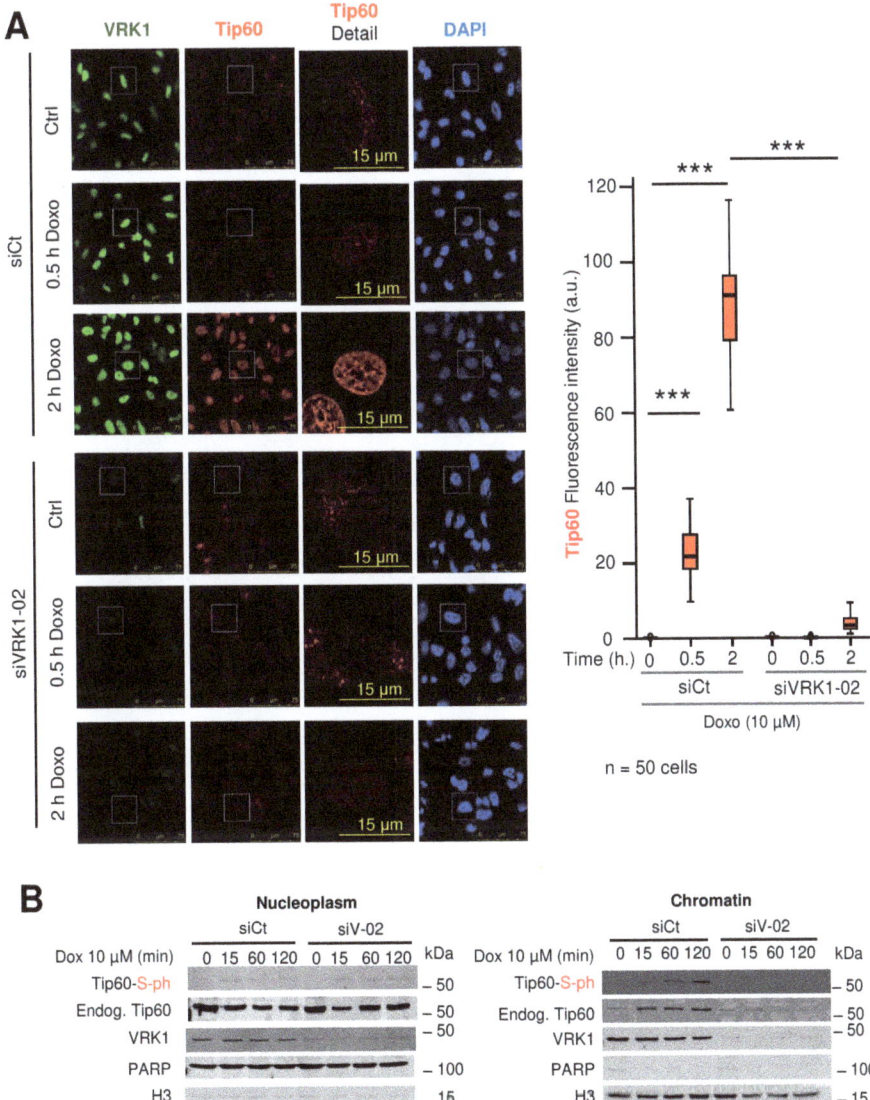

Figure 5. VRK1 knockdown prevents chromatin accumulation of endogenous Tip60 induced by doxorubicin. (**A**). Effect of doxorubicin on the Tip60 nuclear protein detected by immunofluorescence. siCt: si-control; si-V1-02: si-VRK1-02. The fluorescence was quantified in fifty cells using the Image J program. *** $p < 0.001$. (**B**). Effect of doxorubicin on the endogenous Tip60 and its phosphorylation in the nucleoplasm and chromatin fractions determined in control or VRK1-depleted A549 cells. In all time course experiments, the reference value is the one corresponding to the starting time point (0 min). All experiments were repeated four times.

2.6. The Phosphorylation of Tip60 by VRK1 is Induced by Doxorubicin in ATM Null Cells

The activation of ATM in DDR requires its previous acetylation in K3016 by Tip60 that induces its autophosphorylation in Ser1981 required for its kinase activity [56,57]. Moreover, the knockdown of VRK1 prevented the autophosphorylation of ATM in Ser1981 in DDR [19,20]. To rule out the possibility that the effect of VRK1 on Tip60 might be indirect and due to ATM, the induction of Tip60 phosphorylation in response to doxorubicin treatment was determined in the HT144 (*ATM−/−*) cell line. In these *ATM* deficient cells, doxorubicin induced the phosphorylation of Tip60 (Figure 6A), which indicated that ATM is not necessary for Tip60 phosphorylation. Next, we determined whether the Tip60 phosphorylation induced by doxorubicin in HT144 (*ATM−/−*) cells was also dependent on endogenous VRK1. The knockdown of VRK1 with two different siRNAs in HT144 (*ATM−/−*) cells resulted in the loss of Tip60 phosphorylation induced by doxorubicin (Figure 6B). This led to the conclusion that ATM does not mediate the phosphorylation of Tip60, and VRK1 is an upstream component in the pathway.

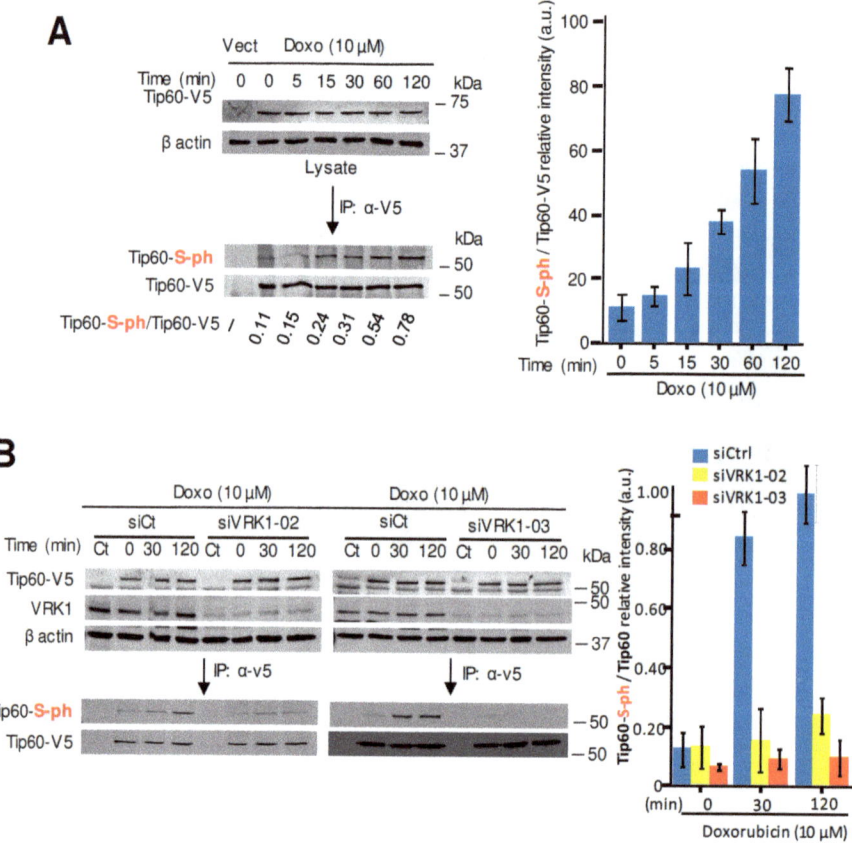

Figure 6. The phosphorylation of Tip60 is independent of ATM and lost by VRK1 depletion. (**A**). Time course of the phosphorylation of Tip60 by DNA damage induced by doxorubicin in HT144 cells (*ATM−/−*) deprived of serum (0.5% FBS) for 48 h before treatment. Tip60 was immunoprecipitated and its phosphorylation determined in Western blots. In the graph to the right is shown the relative increase in Tip60 phosphorylation from three independent experiments. Ct is a negative control of the transfection with an empty vector. (**B**). Depletion of VRK1 with two different siRNA causes a loss of Tip60 phosphorylation induced by doxorubicin in HT144 cells (*ATM−/−*). To the right is shown the quantification of the relative phosphorylation in siControl and siVRK1 in HT144 cells (*ATM−/−*). The graph to the right shows the relative increase in Tip60 phosphorylation from three independent experiments. Ct: Cells transfected with empty vector.

2.7. ATM Acetylation by Tip60 Is Insensitive to ATM Kinase Inhibitors but Is Lost by VRK1 Depletion or Tip60 Inhibition

Next, we used a different approach to demonstrate that the phosphorylation of Tip60 is independent of ATM kinase activity. Serum deprived A549 (*ATM +/+*) cells were treated with KU55933, an inhibitor of ATM [58,59], or caffeine that inhibits ATM/ATR activity [60,61]. In the absence of these inhibitors, and in response to doxorubicin treatment, there was acetylation of ATM in K3016 [56], and phosphorylation of Ser1981 in ATM (Figure 7A, left), as positive control, as well as the predicted phosphorylation of Tip60. ATM forms an inactive dimer and its acetylation in K3016 by Tip60 leads to ATM autophosphorylation in Ser1981 [57]. However, the addition of KU55933 or caffeine inhibited the activating autophosphorylation of ATM in Ser1981 without affecting ATM acetylation in K3016 or the phosphorylation of Tip60 (Figure 7A, center and right). To demonstrate that ATM modifications, acetylation and phosphorylation, required VRK1, a different approach was used. Following depletion of endogenous VRK1 with two different siRNA, their effect on ATM-K3016 acetylation and ATM-S1981 phosphorylation induced by doxorubicin was determined in the immunoprecipitated endogenous ATM. Depletion of VRK1 resulted in the loss of both ATM acetylation and autophosphorylation (Figure 7B). Additionally, determining the phosphorylation of CHK2 in T68, a downstream target of ATM, which was also lost by VRK1 depletion, confirmed this observation (Figure 7C).

Next, to confirm this observation at individual cell level, the phosphorylation of ATM induced by doxorubicin and its inhibition, by either VRK1 depletion or the Tip60 inhibitor MG149, were determined by immunofluorescence. VRK1 depletion (Figure 8A) or treatment with MG149 (Figure 8B) resulted in the loss of ATM-S1981 phosphorylation. The KU55933 ATM inhibitor does not affect H4K16 acetylation but prevents ATM-S1981 phosphorylation in the response to doxorubicin (Figure 8C). However, the MG149 Tip60 inhibitor (Figure 8C) prevents both H4K16 acetylation, and ATM-S1981 phosphorylation, which further supports that ATM acetylation precedes its phosphorylation as expected since acetylation of ATM is required for activation of this kinase [56].

2.8. The Kinase Activity of VRK1 Is Necessary to Rescue ATM Acetylation and Phosphorylation

To demonstrate that VRK1 is necessary for ATM acetylation and phosphorylation, a different experimental approach was used by performing a rescue experiment. Two A549-derived stable cell lines expressing murine VRK1 kinase active (mVRK1) and kinase-dead (mVRK1-K179E) were used. In these two stable cell lines, the endogenous human VRK1 was depleted and the effect of doxorubicin treatment on endogenous ATM acetylation and phosphorylation were studied, using Tip60 phosphorylation as an internal control. The kinase-active mVRK1 was able to rescue both the specific ATM–K3016 acetylation and ATM-S1981 phosphorylation in immunoblots (Figure 9A), and ATM-S1981 phosphorylation by immunofluorescence (Figure 9B). Neither of these two ATM modifications were rescued by the kinase-dead mVRK1-K179E (Figure 9A,B).

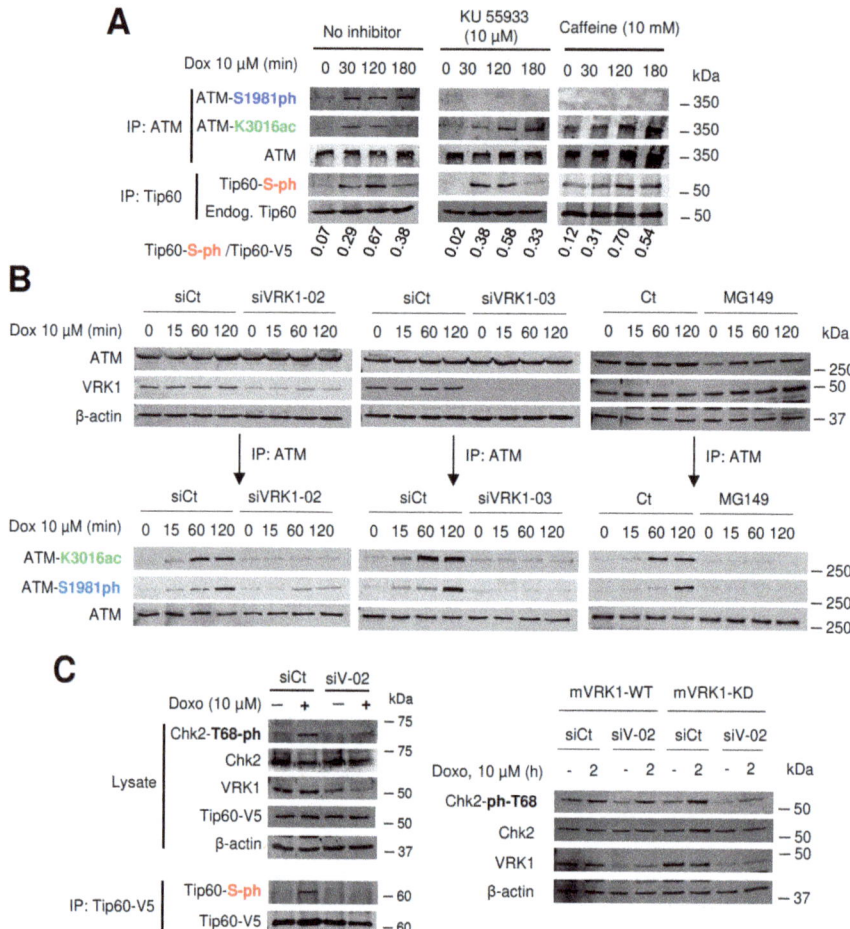

Figure 7. VRK1 is required for the acetylation of ATM by Tip60 in response to DNA damage induced by doxorubicin. (**A**). The phosphorylation and acetylation of ATM, and the phosphorylation of endogenous Tip60 were determined in A549 cells (ATM+/+) deprived of serum (0.5% FBS) for 48 h and treated with doxorubicin in combination with KU55933 or caffeine that inhibit ATM. The covalent modifications were detected in the immunoprecipitated endogenous proteins with specific antibodies. (**B**). Effect of VRK1 depletion with two different siRNA, and Tip60 inhibition with MG149, on the phosphorylation and acetylation of ATM in response to doxorubicin treatment in A549 cells. Treatment with the MG149 inhibitor was performed by its addition to cultures 12 h before cell lysis. (**C**). Effect of VRK1 depletion on the phosphorylation of CHK2 in T68, a downstream phosphorylation target of ATM in response to doxorubicin.

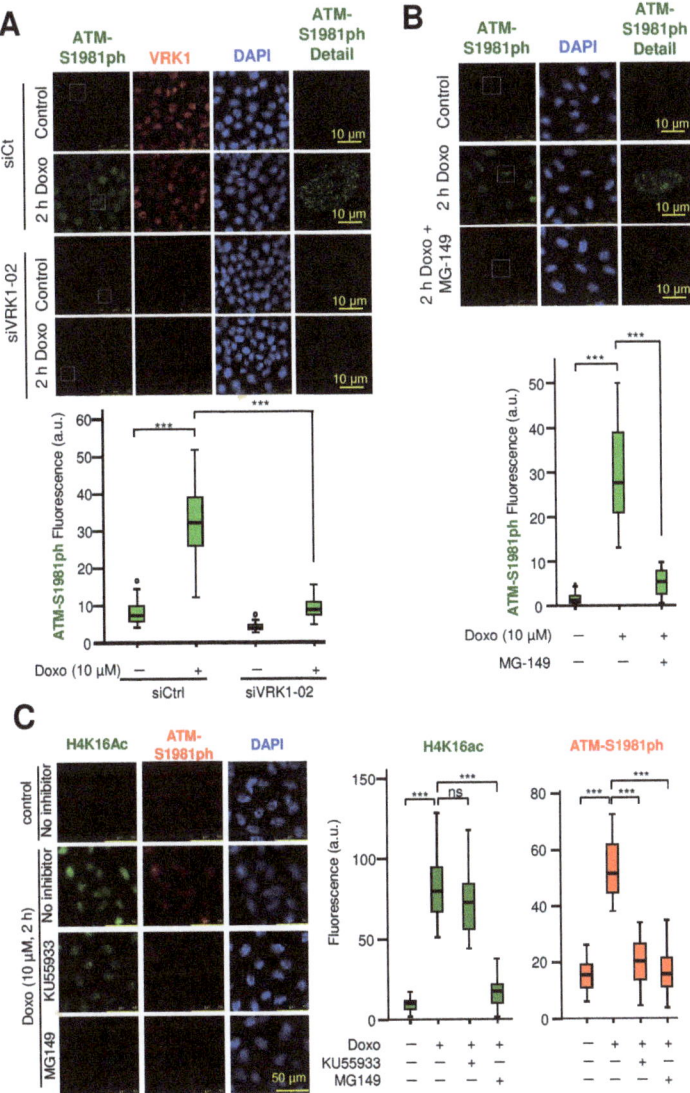

Figure 8. Phosphorylation of ATM is lost by depletion of VRK1 or inhibition of Tip60 in A549 (ATM+/+) cells. (**A**). Effect of VRK1 depletion or Tip60 inhibition on the phosphorylation of ATM in Ser1981. A549 cells deprived of serum (0.5% FBS) for 48 h were treated with doxorubicin and the effect of VRK1 depletion on the phosphorylation of ATM was determined by immunofluorescence. Field images and the selected individual cell are shown in Figure S3A. (**B**). Effect of the inhibition of Tip60 with MG149 on the phosphorylation of ATM in Ser1981 induced by doxorubicin and detected by immunofluorescence. Field images and the indicated individual cell are shown in Figure S3B. (**C**). Differential effect of KU55933 (ATM inhibitor) and MG149 (Tip60 inhibitor) on the acetylation of H4K6 and ATM phosphorylation in A549 cells treated with doxorubicin. The graphs show the quantification of 50 cells. ns: Not significant. *** $p < 0.001$. All experiments were repeated three times.

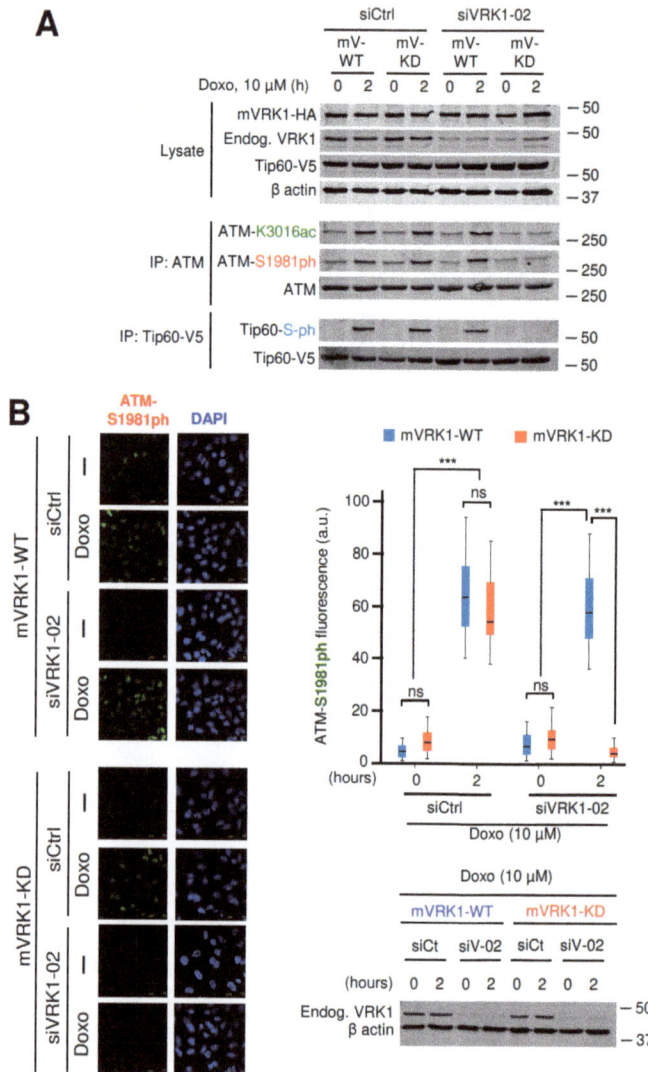

Figure 9. The acetylation and phosphorylation of ATM induced by doxorubicin are rescued by kinase-active VRK1. (**A**). Rescue of ATM acetylation and phosphorylation induced by doxorubicin in A549 stable cell lines expressing kinase-active (mV-WT) (left) or kinase-dead murine VRK1 (K179E) (mV-KD) (right) in which the endogenous human VRK1 was depleted. (**B**). Rescue of ATM phosphorylation induced by doxorubicin in A549 stable cell lines, which express either murine kinase-active (mVRK1) (top) or kinase dead murine VRK1 (K179E) (mVRK1-KD) (bottom), and in which endogenous human VRK1 was depleted. The graph to the right shows the quantification of fifty cells ns: Not significant. *** $p < 0.001$.

3. Discussion

Chromatin remodeling is a highly organized and regulated process. When DNA damage occurs, the cell has to respond to an aberrant alteration by a locally altered chromatin, which triggers a response aiming to its repair and that requires several sequential steps. The many different alternative covalent modifications of histones in chromatin underlie its dynamic changes associated to specific functions. These modifications require several different enzymatic activities that need to be coordinated and linked to specific cellular functions, ranging from transcription, replication, or chromatin compaction to DNA damage responses. There is a large group of lysine acetyl transferases (KAT) [62] and their regulation and coordination are unknown, but in both processes, phosphorylation is likely to play an important role that remains to be studied and understood. Kinases are well suited to orchestrate these roles and associate them to specific signaling pathways. The identification of the chromatin kinase VRK1, which participates in transcription, cell division and DNA repair, as a regulator of KAT5/Tip60 is a significant step in this context. Tip60 phosphorylation occurs in other biological processes. In apoptosis, GSK3 phosphorylates Tip60 and leads to the expression of PUMA (P53 Up-Regulated Modulator of Apoptosis) [63]. Tip60 is also phosphorylated by CDK9 and associated to gene transcription [64], and by cyclinB/cdc2 complexes in G2/M in cell cycle progression [65]. However, the regulation of Tip60 in DNA damage responses is initiated in a locally altered chromatin [48,66], as it occurs with VRK1 that is activated independently of the type of DNA damage [19].

Chromatin kinases are likely candidates to participate in early responses to DNA damage. The location of VRK1 as a kinase resident on chromatin places it in a very suitable situation to trigger, coordinate and organize the signals involved in sequential DDR steps. The colocalization of VRK1 [34] and Tip60 [42,67] on the chromatin fraction and its stable direct interaction indicate that Tip60 phosphorylation can contribute to its retention on this fraction, since VRK1 depletion results in the loss of Tip60 in the chromatin fraction. The complex between VRK1-Tip60 is activated by the structural change caused by the interaction of VRK1 with histones in nucleosomes located where DNA is altered by damage [21,39]. The kinase activity of VRK1 can be regulated by the interaction of its flexible C-terminus with histones [32,39]. These results indicated that the phosphorylation of Tip60 occurred on chromatin where VRK1 is also present and both form a basal complex, but an additional contribution of their nucleoplasm fraction cannot be rule out.

The chromatin kinase VRK1, which indirectly regulates histone acetylation in response to DNA damage in G0/G1, is a likely candidate to regulate Tip60. This KAT also regulates histone acetylation in DDR [45], and VRK1 depletion prevents H4K16 acetylation. The acetylation of H4K16, mediated by Tip60, is a marker of locally relaxed chromatin, facilitates the next steps, after deacetylation, for recruitment of 53BP1 to damaged DNA sites, and DNA repair by the NHEJ pathway [68,69]. Moreover, during progression of DDR, the deacetylation of H4K16 permits the dimethylation of H4K20 (me2) that facilitates later steps in the specific repair pathway [47,69]. Consistent with this role for H4K16ac, depletion of VRK1 impairs later steps in the specific pathway, such as the formation of 53BP1 foci in response to DNA damage by either ionizing radiation or doxorubicin [19–21,52], which is not rescued by kinase-dead VRK1 [55]. Thus, the interplay of histone acetylation and methylation can be associated to different functions in DDR, and is consistent with the role of VRK1 in NHEJ in cells in G0/G1. In this context, it will be important to study the role that VRK1 plays in the regulation of the methylase and demethylase that regulate K4H20me2.

The sequential order of Tip60 and ATM roles in the early response to DNA damage involving VRK1 is outlined in Figure 10. The interaction of VRK1 with histones regulates its kinase activity and permits the phosphorylation of Tip60, which by acetylation of H4 permits a local chromatin relaxation at the site of DNA damage. This locally relaxed chromatin permits the access to different components that participate in the sequential steps of DNA repair, from the initial DNA-end protection, damage identification and finally repair by facilitating the ATM acetylation and its subsequent autophosphorylation. In the case of DNA damage by doxorubicin that causes double-strand breaks, VRK1 depletion also alters the specific phosphorylation and formation of γH2AX [21], NBS1 [20] and 53BP1 foci [19,52], which represents sequential steps in the process downstream of H4K16ac. Inhibition of ATM, prevents its phosphorylation, but does not alter its acetylation by Tip60, which is lost by VRK1 depletion. Furthermore, there is a parallel cellular response mediated by VRK1 in response to DNA damage involving the specific phosphorylation of p53 in Thr18 [24], which prevents its interaction with mdm2, and facilitates subsequent phosphorylation by ATM/ATR to select specific transcriptional cofactors [70]. The initial phosphorylation of p53 in Thr18 by VRK1 [23,24,71] disrupting the interaction between p53 and the mdm2 ubiquitin ligase [72]. Additional phosphorylation of p53 in other N-terminus residues, such as Ser15 by ATR and Ser20 by ATM [73], determine the selection and affinity of p53 for specific transcriptional cofactors [70]. A similar order is likely to occur in the coordination of sequential steps in DDR. The sequential order of activation of kinases in DDR is consistent with their consecutive roles in the phosphorylation of p53 in response to DNA damage. This p53 activation by VRK1 contributes to induction of cell cycle arrest or apoptosis, depending on the magnitude of the DNA damage, and the ability of the cell to cope with it.

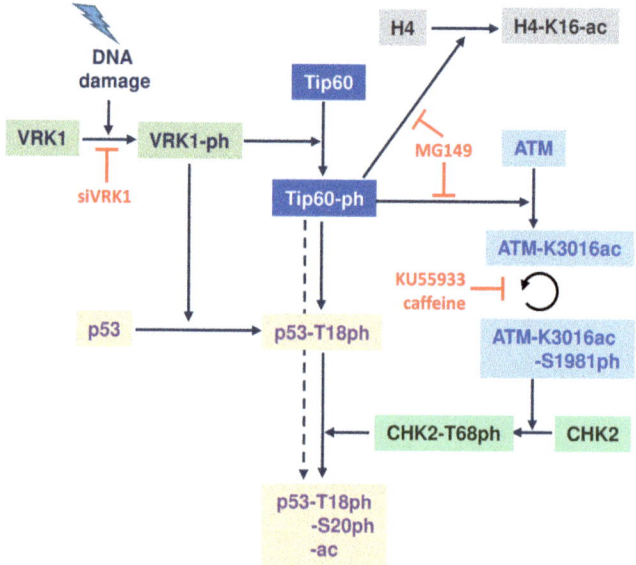

Figure 10. Sequential order of covalent modifications in response to DNA damage involving VRK1, Tip60, H4, ATM and p53. The site of action of siVRK1 and of specific acetylase and kinase inhibitors are indicated.

In this study, we have identified that VRK1 regulates the phosphorylation of Tip60 in the absence of ATM and in the presence of ATM inhibitors, indicating that VRK1 is an upstream component needed for the H4K16ac associated to the aberrant relaxation of damaged DNA and required for initiation of the specific sequential steps in DDR. This finding, the activation of Tip60/KAT5, a writer epigenetic enzyme, is a step in the coordination and regulation of alternative modifications in specific histone lysine residues. In those lysine residues with alternative epigenetic modifications, the coordination of four enzymes involved is still poorly known, but that is essential to understand how chromatin perform its transition from one configuration to another and to organize its three-dimensional structure in different physiological or pathological situations.

4. Materials and Methods

4.1. Reagents

MG149 (Axon MedChem, Groningen, The Netherlands), C646 (SelleckChem, Houston, TX, USA), KU55933 (Tocris Bioscience, Bristol, UK) were dissolved in dimethyl sulfoxide. All other reagents were from Sigma-Aldrich-Merck (Darmstadt, Germany).

4.2. Plasmids

Human VRK1 was expressed from plasmid pCEFL-HA-VRK1 [18,20,74]. Human Tip60 was expressed from plasmid pcDNA3.1-TIP60-V5-His obtained from D. Maurer [63]. Murine VRK1 (mVRK1) was expressed from plasmid pCMV6-mVRK1-myc-DKK (OriGene, Rockville, MD, USA). A kinase-dead construct of the murine VRK1(K179E) was generated with the Quick-Mutagenesis system (Stratagene, San Diego, CA, USA) [74]. Murine VRK1, wild-type and kinase dead (K179E) were also made in lentiviral construct, plasmids pLenti-C-HA-IRES-BSD-mVRK1 and pLenty-C-HA-IRES-BSD-mVRK(K179E) were used to make A549-derived stable cell lines that were selected with blasticidine.

For in vitro kinase assays of the human protein, the following plasmids were used, PGEX-4T-VRK1 and pGEX-4T-VRK1-K179E [24,55,75] for expression and purification of the fusion proteins expressed in *Escherichia coli* DH5α and the GST-fusion proteins were purified as previously reported [26,75]. Human Tip60 cloned in vector pET28a-LIC (HTATIP-2OU2) with a hexahistidine tag for bacterial expression was a gift from Cheryl Arrowsmith (Addgene reference 33338). Mutations introduced in human of murine were confirmed by Sanger sequencing and reported in previous studies [19,20].

4.3. Cell Lines, Culture and Transfections

The following cell lines were used and obtained from the ATCC (Teddington, Middlesex, UK) A549 (CCL-185) and HT144 (*ATM−/−*) (HTB-63). Cell lines were mycoplasma free. Cells were grown in 100 mm dishes with DMEM medium (GIBCO) supplemented with 10% inactivated fetal bovine serum (GIBCO), 1% L-Glutamine (GIBCO) and 0.5% Pen Strep (GIBCO). Twenty-four hours later, cells were transfected with the corresponding expression plasmid. Transfections were performed mixing the amount of plasmid with two volumes of polyethylenimine (PEI) reagent (Polysciences, Inc., Warrington, PA, USA) following manufacturer's instructions in 1 mL of 150 mM NaCl, incubated for 30 min at room temperature, and added to the cell culture [18,74]. Cell lysis was performed with mild lysis buffer (50 mM Tris–HCl (pH 8.0), 1 mM EDTA, 150 mM NaCl, and 1% triton X-100). At the time of the lysis, the buffer was complemented with phosphatases inhibitors (1 mM NaF and 1 mM sodium orthovanadate) and proteases inhibitors (1 mM PMFS, 10 μg/mL aprotinin and 10 μg/mL (leupeptin).

In all experiments involving induction of DNA damage by doxorubicin treatment, cells were placed in 0.5% FBS for 48 h before doxorubicin addition to the culture. Serum deprivation was used to remove mitogenic signals from growth factors, and to accumulate cell in G0/G1, which was checked by flow cytometry and the lack of cyclin D1and phosho-Rb [17,19].

A549 cells lines were infected with lentiviral particles containing the vector pLentiC-HA-IRES-BSD (OriGene Technologies, Rockville, MD, USA) expressing murine VRK1 or kinase-dead murine VRK1 (K179E) were cloned and selected with blasticidine [76].

In all time course experiments, the reference value is the one corresponding to the starting time point (0 min), and the sequential time points were compared with it after normalization by the levels of endogenous and transfected protein, where applicable. The inhibitors MG149 (2 μM) or C646 (10 μM) were added 10 h before addition of doxorubicin. All experiments were repeated three times.

4.4. VRK1 Depletion by siRNA

Specific silencing of VRK1 was performed using two different siRNA from Dharmacon (DHARMACON RNA Technologies). The VRK1 sequences targeted by these siRNA oligonucleotides were siVRK1-02 (siV1-02), CAAGGAACCTGGTGTTGAA; and siVRK1 03 (siV1-03): ThAt GGAAUGG AAAGUAGGAUUA. As negative control, the "ON-TARGETplus siCONTROL Non-targeting siRNA" from DHARMACON was used and is indicated as siCt in experiments. The efficiency of RNAi transfection was determined with "siGLO RISC-free siRNA" (DHARMACON). Briefly, cells were transfected with the indicated siRNA at a concentration of 20 nM using Lipofectamine 2000 Reagent (Invitrogen) or Lipotransfectin (Nivorlab) [18,34,74]. After transfection, cells were processed at the times indicated in specific experiments that were performed as previously reported [19,77]. The depletion of VRK1 by siRNA has been previously reported for A549 [18,21,36] and HT144 [20,21] cell lines.

4.5. Antibodies

The primary and secondary antibodies, applications and conditions used in this work are listed in Tables S1 and S2 respectively.

4.6. Immunoblots

Protein extracts from cell lysates were quantified using the Protein assay (Bio-Rad; Hercules, CA, USA). Forty micrograms of protein extracts were used for immunoblots. Protein samples were fractionated in a 7.5%, 10%, or 12.5% SDS polyacrylamide gel and transferred to a PVDF Immobilon-FL membrane (Millipore), at 90 V, 4 °C, for 90 min. PVDF membranes were blocked for 1 h at room temperature with 5% defatted milk in TBS-T buffer (25 mM Tris-HCl pH 8.50 mM NaCl, 2.5 mM KCl, 0.1% Tween-20) or, alternatively, with 5% of BSA in TBS-T buffer when phosphorylated state of proteins was analyzed [20,34,36]. Membranes were washed in TBS-T buffer 3 times for 10 min each time and incubated with the primary antibody for 8 h, or overnight, at 4 °C. Next, PVDF membranes were extensively washed in TBS-T buffer and incubated with the corresponding secondary antibody (Goat Anti-Mouse IgG, Dylight 680 -red colored- or Goat Anti-Rabbit IgG, DyLight 800 -green colored-) at 1:10,000 for 1 h at room temperature (in darkness). Membranes were washed in TBS-T buffer for 10 min three times. Finally, fluorescence signals were detected, and quantified, using a LI-COR Odyssey Infrared Imaging System (LI-COR Biosciences, Lincoln, NE, USA).

4.7. Immunoprecipitations

Cells were lysed at a density of seventy percent confluence. Cell lysates (1–2 mg of protein) were incubated with the corresponding antibody for each experiment for 8 h, or overnight, at 4 °C with agitation. Subsequently, the protein-antibody immune complexes were precipitated with 80 μL of Protein G–Agarose Resin 4 Rapid Run (4RRPG, Agarose Bead Technologies) for 8 h at 4 °C in agitation [18,34,74] and the immunoprecipitate was collected by centrifugation (2200 rpm, 2 min) and washed three times with lysis buffer. Next, 10 μL of buffer 5× (250 mM Tris-HCl, 10% SDS, 50% glycerol, 0.5% bromophenol blue) were added to the samples, boiled for 5 min and subjected to electrophoresis, followed by immunoblot analysis. Specific antibodies for immunoblot analysis are listed in Table S1.

4.8. In Vitro VRK1-Tip60 Protein Interaction and Kinase Assay

The kinase assay contained, either 10 μg of purified GST-VRK1 wild-type or 10 μg of purified GST-VRK1-K179E (kinase-dead) with 6 μg of purified His-Tip60 as substrate, to maintain an equimolar ratio. The protein mix was incubated in a specific buffer for casein kinases (20 mM Tris-HCl pH 7.5, 5 mM $MgCl_2$, 0.5 mM DTT and 150 mM KCl) and 2 mM of cold ATP during 1 h at 30 °C. The proteins fractionated in SDS-polyacrylamide gels, and transferred to an Inmobilon-FL membrane (Millipore). Tip60 phosphorylation was detected with monoclonal anti-phosphoserine antibody (clone 4A4). The proteins on the membrane were detected by Western blot.

To study the interaction between human VRK1 and Tip60 a binding assay was performed using bacterially expressed and purified GST-VRK1 and His-Tip60 in the amounts indicated in the experiment [74,75]. The proteins were incubated in a buffer containing 20 mM Tris-HCl pH 7.5, 5 mM $MgCl_2$, 0.5 mM DTT and 150 mM KCl in a volume of 25 μL at 35 °C and gentle agitation for 1 h, followed by the addition of 80 μL of Gutathione-sepharose 4 Fast Flow (Merck, ref: GE17-5132-01) equilibrated with lysis buffer. The mix was incubated at 4 °C for eight hours. Finally, a pull-down was performed by centrifugation at 2800 rpm for 5 min at 4 °C. The resin was washed three times in the same pull-down buffer, and finally 10 μL of buffer were added and loaded in a 10% polyacrylamide-SDS gel. The proteins were transferred to a PVDF Immobilon-FL membrane that were used for immunoblot analysis.

4.9. Immunofluorescence and Confocal Microscopy

Cells were cultured in coverslips placed in 60-mm dishes. Forty-eight or ninety-six hours after corresponding transfections of expression plasmids and/or siRNAs, coverslips were placed into T24 single wells and cells were fixed with 3% paraformaldehyde (MERCK) in 1× PBS during 30 min at room temperature. Next, cells were treated with 200 mM glycine during 15 min and permeabilized with 0.2% Triton X-100 in PBS for 30 min. Finally, cells were blocked with 1% BSA in PBS 1× for, at least, 1 h. Once permeabilized, coverslips were incubated with the corresponding first primary antibody in 1% BSA in PBS for 8 h, or overnight, at 4 °C. Afterwards, cells were washed 3 times with PBS, and the secondary antibody was added and incubated and washed in a similar manner. The specific antibodies and dilutions used for this technique are indicated in Table S1. The secondary antibodies (Table S2) were incubated together in 1% BSA in PBS for 1 h at room temperature. Finally, cell nuclei were stained with 0.1% DAPI (SIGMA) in 1× PBS for 15 min at room temperature and washed 3 times with PBS. Coverslips were mounted with Mowiol (Calbiochem-Merck), and images were captured with a LEICA SP5 DMI-6000B confocal microscope. The lasers used in this microscope were: Argon (488 nm) for detecting green fluorescence, DPSS (561 nm) for detecting red fluorescence, and UV Diode (405 nm) for DAPI detection. Images were captured with a 63.0× lens zoomed in 2× with a 1024 × 1024 frame and 600 Hz scanning speed. Images were analyzed with the ImageJ program (NIH).

4.10. Nucleoplasm-Chromatin Fractionation

Fractionation of nucleoplasm and chromatin fraction was performed as reported for Tip60 [64]. Briefly, cells were lysed and incubated on ice for 8 min in cytosol lysis buffer (10 mM HEPES; 10 mM KCl, 1.5 mM MgCl$_2$, 0.34 mM sucrose, 10% glycerol, 20 µM MG132, 0.1% Triton X-100, 1:100 PMSF, 1:1000 aprotinin, 1:1000 leupeptin, 1:500 sodium orthovanadate and 1:500 NaF). Subsequently, cell lysate was centrifuged at 1300× g for 5 min in order to separate cytoplasm fraction (supernatant), which was discarded, and whole nuclei extract (pellet). Nuclei fraction was taken up in nucleoplasm extracting buffer (400 mM NaCl, 3 mM EDTA, 0.2 mM EGTA, 1 mM DTT, 20 µM MG132, 1:100 PMSF, 1:1000 aprotinin, 1:1000 leupeptin, 1:500 sodium orthovanadate and 1:500 NaF) and incubated at 4 °C for 20 min. To precipitate chromatin from nucleoplasm (supernatant) an additional centrifugation at 1000× g for 2 min was performed. The chromatin fraction was washed three times in nucleoplasm extracting buffer. After that, the chromatin fraction was resuspended in nuclei lysis buffer (50 mM Tris-HCl, pH 8.1, 10 mM EDTA, 0.5% SDS, 1:100 PMSF, 1:1000 aprotinin, 1:1000 leupeptin, 1:500 sodium orthovanadate and 1:500 NaF) and sonicated 5 times for 30 seconds, waiting 30 seconds between each sonication to break DNA. Nucleoplasm and chromatin-associated proteins were quantified by Bradford assay, and analyzed by Western blotting.

4.11. Statistical Analysis

Statistical results were analyzed using the SPSS23 statistical package. Quantitative experiments were performed at least three times, the number of cells is indicated and statistical analysis was performed by the non-parametric Mann–Whitney U test after confirming samples did not adjust to a normal distribution according to two-tailed Kolmogorov test using the IBM SPSS 23 statistics package. Results are presented as box plots with the median, first and third quartiles and standard deviations [78].

4.12. TUNEL Assay

TUNEL (TdT-mediated dUTP Nick-End Labeling) was performed to analyze the DNA free ends of DNA breaks associated to doxorubicin treatments following the indications of the provider (In Situ Cell Death Detection Kit, Fluorescein; Ref: 11684795910; Roche). Cells were cultured in coverslips placed in 60-mm dishes under the specific conditions of the experiments and, subsequently, they were fixed and permeabilized as indicated for immunofluorescence assays. Simultaneously, 50 µL of enzyme solution, containing terminal deoxynucleotidyl transferase (TdT), were mixed with 550 µL of label solution, which contains nucleotide mixture in reaction buffer. The coverslips were incubated with 50 µL of the TUNEL reaction mixture in a humidified atmosphere for 60 min at 37 °C in the dark. Later, coverslips were rinse 3 times with PBS and samples were analyzed in the confocal microscope using an excitation wavelength of 488 nm and detection in the range of 515–565 nm (green).

4.13. Database Submission

The protein interactions from this publication have been submitted to the IMEx (http://www.imexconsortium.org) consortium through IntAct [79], and assigned the identifier IM-27878.

5. Conclusions

We have identified that VRK1 regulates the phosphorylation of Tip60 in the absence of ATM and in the presence of ATM inhibitors, indicating that VRK1 is an upstream component needed for the H4K16ac associated to the aberrant relaxation of damaged DNA and required for initiation of the specific sequential steps in DDR.

Supplementary Materials: The following are available online at http://www.mdpi.com/2072-6694/12/10/2986/s1, Figure S1. Induction of DNA damage by doxorubicin and triggering a DNA-Damage response (DDR) by the NHEJ pathway in A549 cells. Figure S2. Effect of acetyl transferase inhibitors on the basal level of endogenous H4K16 acetylation. Figure S3. Phosphorylation of ATM is lost by either depletion of VRK1 or inhibition of Tip60 in A549 (ATM+/+) cells. Field images. Figure S4. Uncropped Western Blotting figures. Table S1. Primary antibodies, conditions of applications. Table S2. Secondary antibodies, conditions of applications.

Author Contributions: R.G.-G. performed most of the experiments. P.M.-G. performed recue experiments. I.C.-M. and M.S. performed initial experiments on histone acetylation. P.A.L. planned the work, designed experiments and wrote the manuscript with input from all authors. All authors have read and approved the manuscript.

Funding: This work was supported by grants from Agencia Estatal de Investigación-Ministerio de Economía y Competitividad-FEDER [SAF2016-75744-R; RED2018-102801-T, PID2019-105610RB-I00] Consejería de Educación de la Junta de Castilla y León-ERDF [CLC-2017-01, and UIC-258] to P.A.L., R.G.-G, P.M.-G. and I.C.-M. were supported by Consejería de Educación-Junta de Castilla y León-Fondo Social Europeo (ESF), Ministerio de Educación y Universidades [FPU-16-01883] and MINECO-FPI [BES-2014-067729] predoctoral fellowships respectively.

Acknowledgments: We acknowledge support of the publication fee by the CSIC Open Access Publication Support Initiative through its Unit of Information Resources for Research (URICI).

Conflicts of Interest: The authors declare no conflict of interest.

References

1. Smith, E.; Shilatifard, A. The chromatin signaling pathway: Diverse mechanisms of recruitment of histone-modifying enzymes and varied biological outcomes. *Mol. Cell* **2010**, *40*, 689–701. [CrossRef] [PubMed]
2. Bannister, A.J.; Kouzarides, T. Regulation of chromatin by histone modifications. *Cell Res.* **2011**, *21*, 381–395. [CrossRef] [PubMed]
3. Dawson, M.A.; Kouzarides, T. Cancer epigenetics: From mechanism to therapy. *Cell* **2012**, *150*, 12–27. [CrossRef] [PubMed]
4. Tessarz, P.; Kouzarides, T. Histone core modifications regulating nucleosome structure and dynamics. *Nat. Rev. Mol. Cell. Biol.* **2014**, *15*, 703–708. [CrossRef] [PubMed]
5. Ting, A.H.; McGarvey, K.M.; Baylin, S.B. The cancer epigenome—components and functional correlates. *Genes Dev.* **2006**, *20*, 3215–3231. [CrossRef] [PubMed]
6. Beekman, R.; Chapaprieta, V.; Russinol, N.; Vilarrasa-Blasi, R.; Verdaguer-Dot, N.; Martens, J.H.A.; Duran-Ferrer, M.; Kulis, M.; Serra, F.; Javierre, B.M.; et al. The reference epigenome and regulatory chromatin landscape of chronic lymphocytic leukemia. *Nat. Med.* **2018**, *24*, 868–880. [CrossRef] [PubMed]
7. Mazor, T.; Pankov, A.; Song, J.S.; Costello, J.F. Intratumoral Heterogeneity of the Epigenome. *Cancer Cell* **2016**, *29*, 440–451. [CrossRef] [PubMed]
8. Wysocka, J.; Swigut, T.; Xiao, H.; Milne, T.A.; Kwon, S.Y.; Landry, J.; Kauer, M.; Tackett, A.J.; Chait, B.T.; Badenhorst, P.; et al. A PHD finger of NURF couples histone H3 lysine 4 trimethylation with chromatin remodelling. *Nature* **2006**, *442*, 86–90. [CrossRef]

9. Xhemalce, B.; Kouzarides, T. A chromodomain switch mediated by histone H3 Lys 4 acetylation regulates heterochromatin assembly. *Genes Dev.* **2010**, *24*, 647–652. [CrossRef]
10. Murata, K.; Kouzarides, T.; Bannister, A.J.; Gurdon, J.B. Histone H3 lysine 4 methylation is associated with the transcriptional reprogramming efficiency of somatic nuclei by oocytes. *Epigenet. Chromatin* **2010**, *3*, 4. [CrossRef]
11. Kouzarides, T. Chromatin modifications and their function. *Cell* **2007**, *128*, 693–705. [CrossRef] [PubMed]
12. Dawson, M.A.; Kouzarides, T.; Huntly, B.J. Targeting epigenetic readers in cancer. *N. Engl. J. Med.* **2012**, *367*, 647–657. [CrossRef] [PubMed]
13. Cantarero, L.; Moura, D.S.; Salzano, M.; Monsalve, D.M.; Campillo-Marcos, I.; Martín-Doncel, E.; Lazo, P.A. VRK1 (vaccinia-related kinase 1). In *Encyclopedia of Signaling Molecules*, 2nd ed.; Choi, S., Ed.; Springer Science: Berlin, Germany, 2017. [CrossRef]
14. Aihara, H.; Nakagawa, T.; Mizusaki, H.; Yoneda, M.; Kato, M.; Doiguchi, M.; Imamura, Y.; Higashi, M.; Ikura, T.; Hayashi, T.; et al. Histone H2A T120 Phosphorylation Promotes Oncogenic Transformation via Upregulation of Cyclin D1. *Mol. Cell* **2016**, *64*, 176–188. [CrossRef] [PubMed]
15. Varjosalo, M.; Sacco, R.; Stukalov, A.; van Drogen, A.; Planyavsky, M.; Hauri, S.; Aebersold, R.; Bennett, K.L.; Colinge, J.; Gstaiger, M.; et al. Interlaboratory reproducibility of large-scale human protein-complex analysis by standardized AP-MS. *Nat. Methods* **2013**, *10*, 307–314. [CrossRef]
16. Santos, C.R.; Rodriguez-Pinilla, M.; Vega, F.M.; Rodriguez-Peralto, J.L.; Blanco, S.; Sevilla, A.; Valbuena, A.; Hernandez, T.; van Wijnen, A.J.; Li, F.; et al. VRK1 signaling pathway in the context of the proliferation phenotype in head and neck squamous cell carcinoma. *Mol. Cancer Res.* **2006**, *4*, 177–185. [CrossRef]
17. Valbuena, A.; Lopez-Sanchez, I.; Lazo, P.A. Human VRK1 is an early response gene and its loss causes a block in cell cycle progression. *PLoS ONE* **2008**, *3*, e1642. [CrossRef]
18. Moura, D.S.; Fernández, I.F.; Marín-Royo, G.; López-Sánchez, I.; Martín-Doncel, E.; Vega, F.M.; Lazo, P.A. Oncogenic Sox2 regulates and cooperates with VRK1 in cell cycle progression and differentiation. *Sci. Rep.* **2016**, *6*, 28532. [CrossRef]
19. Sanz-Garcia, M.; Monsalve, D.M.; Sevilla, A.; Lazo, P.A. Vaccinia-related Kinase 1 (VRK1) is an upstream nucleosomal kinase required for the assembly of 53BP1 foci in response to ionizing radiation-induced DNA damage. *J. Biol. Chem.* **2012**, *287*, 23757–23768. [CrossRef]
20. Monsalve, D.M.; Campillo-Marcos, I.; Salzano, M.; Sanz-Garcia, M.; Cantarero, L.; Lazo, P.A. VRK1 phosphorylates and protects NBS1 from ubiquitination and proteasomal degradation in response to DNA damage. *Biochim. Biophys. Acta Mol. Cell Res.* **2016**, *1863*, 760–769. [CrossRef]
21. Salzano, M.; Sanz-Garcia, M.; Monsalve, D.M.; Moura, D.S.; Lazo, P.A. VRK1 chromatin kinase phosphorylates H2AX and is required for foci formation induced by DNA damage. *Epigenetics* **2015**, *10*, 373–383. [CrossRef]
22. Campillo-Marcos, I.; Lazo, P.A. Implication of the VRK1 chromatin kinase in the signaling responses to DNA damage: A therapeutic target? *Cell Mol. Life Sci.* **2018**, *75*, 2375–2388. [CrossRef] [PubMed]
23. Lopez-Borges, S.; Lazo, P.A. The human vaccinia-related kinase 1 (VRK1) phosphorylates threonine-18 within the mdm-2 binding site of the p53 tumour suppressor protein. *Oncogene* **2000**, *19*, 3656–3664. [CrossRef] [PubMed]
24. Vega, F.M.; Sevilla, A.; Lazo, P.A. p53 Stabilization and accumulation induced by human vaccinia-related kinase 1. *Mol. Cell. Biol.* **2004**, *24*, 10366–10380. [CrossRef] [PubMed]
25. Valbuena, A.; Vega, F.M.; Blanco, S.; Lazo, P.A. p53 downregulates its activating vaccinia-related kinase 1, forming a new autoregulatory loop. *Mol. Cell. Biol.* **2006**, *26*, 4782–4793. [CrossRef] [PubMed]
26. Sevilla, A.; Santos, C.R.; Barcia, R.; Vega, F.M.; Lazo, P.A. c-Jun phosphorylation by the human vaccinia-related kinase 1 (VRK1) and its cooperation with the N-terminal kinase of c-Jun (JNK). *Oncogene* **2004**, *23*, 8950–8958. [CrossRef]
27. Sevilla, A.; Santos, C.R.; Vega, F.M.; Lazo, P.A. Human vaccinia-related kinase 1 (VRK1) activates the ATF2 transcriptional activity by novel phosphorylation on Thr-73 and Ser-62 and cooperates with JNK. *J. Biol. Chem.* **2004**, *279*, 27458–27465. [CrossRef]
28. Kang, T.H.; Park, D.Y.; Kim, W.; Kim, K.T. VRK1 phosphorylates CREB and mediates CCND1 expression. *J. Cell. Sci.* **2008**, *121*, 3035–3041. [CrossRef]
29. Jamin, A.; Wiebe, M.S. Barrier to Autointegration Factor (BANF1): Interwoven roles in nuclear structure, genome integrity, innate immunity, stress responses and progeria. *Curr. Opin. Cell Biol.* **2015**, *34*, 61–68. [CrossRef]

30. Wiebe, M.S.; Jamin, A. The Barrier to Autointegration Factor: Interlocking Antiviral Defense with Genome Maintenance. *J. Virol.* **2016**, *90*, 3806–3809. [CrossRef]
31. Samwer, M.; Schneider, M.W.G.; Hoefler, R.; Schmalhorst, P.S.; Jude, J.G.; Zuber, J.; Gerlich, D.W. DNA Cross-Bridging Shapes a Single Nucleus from a Set of Mitotic Chromosomes. *Cell* **2017**, *170*, 956–972.e923. [CrossRef]
32. Kang, T.H.; Park, D.Y.; Choi, Y.H.; Kim, K.J.; Yoon, H.S.; Kim, K.T. Mitotic histone H3 phosphorylation by vaccinia-related kinase 1 in mammalian cells. *Mol. Cell. Biol.* **2007**, *27*, 8533–8546. [CrossRef] [PubMed]
33. Vazquez-Cedeira, M.; Barcia-Sanjurjo, I.; Sanz-Garcia, M.; Barcia, R.; Lazo, P.A. Differential Inhibitor Sensitivity between Human Kinases VRK1 and VRK2. *PLoS ONE* **2011**, *6*, e23235. [CrossRef] [PubMed]
34. Moura, D.S.; Campillo-Marcos, I.; Vazquez-Cedeira, M.; Lazo, P.A. VRK1 and AURKB form a complex that cross inhibit their kinase activity and the phosphorylation of histone H3 in the progression of mitosis. *Cell. Mol. Life Sci.* **2018**, *76*, 2591–2611. [CrossRef]
35. Aihara, H.; Nakagawa, T.; Yasui, K.; Ohta, T.; Hirose, S.; Dhomae, N.; Takio, K.; Kaneko, M.; Takeshima, Y.; Muramatsu, M.; et al. Nucleosomal histone kinase-1 phosphorylates H2A Thr 119 during mitosis in the early Drosophila embryo. *Genes Dev.* **2004**, *18*, 877–888. [CrossRef] [PubMed]
36. Campillo-Marcos, I.; Lazo, P.A. Olaparib and ionizing radiation trigger a cooperative DNA-damage repair response that is impaired by depletion of the VRK1 chromatin kinase. *J. Exp. Clin. Cancer Res.* **2019**, *38*, 203. [CrossRef]
37. Choi, Y.H.; Lim, J.K.; Jeong, M.W.; Kim, K.T. HnRNP A1 phosphorylated by VRK1 stimulates telomerase and its binding to telomeric DNA sequence. *Nucleic Acids Res.* **2012**, *40*, 8499–8518. [CrossRef]
38. Shin, J.; Chakraborty, G.; Bharatham, N.; Kang, C.; Tochio, N.; Koshiba, S.; Kigawa, T.; Kim, W.; Kim, K.T.; Yoon, H.S. NMR solution structure of human vaccinia-related kinase 1 (VRK1) reveals the C-terminal tail essential for its structural stability and autocatalytic activity. *J. Biol. Chem.* **2011**, *286*, 22131–22138. [CrossRef]
39. Kim, W.; Chakraborty, G.; Kim, S.; Shin, J.; Park, C.H.; Jeong, M.W.; Bharatham, N.; Yoon, H.S.; Kim, K.T. Macro Histone H2A1.2 (MacroH2A1) Protein Suppresses Mitotic Kinase VRK1 during Interphase. *J. Biol. Chem.* **2012**, *287*, 5278–5289. [CrossRef]
40. Sanz-Garcia, M.; Lopez-Sanchez, I.; Lazo, P.A. Proteomics identification of nuclear Ran GTPase as an inhibitor of human VRK1 and VRK2 (vaccinia-related kinase) activities. *Mol. Cell. Proteom.* **2008**, *7*, 2199–2214. [CrossRef]
41. Robinson, P.J.; An, W.; Routh, A.; Martino, F.; Chapman, L.; Roeder, R.G.; Rhodes, D. 30 nm chromatin fibre decompaction requires both H4-K16 acetylation and linker histone eviction. *J. Mol. Biol.* **2008**, *381*, 816–825. [CrossRef]
42. Murr, R.; Loizou, J.I.; Yang, Y.G.; Cuenin, C.; Li, H.; Wang, Z.Q.; Herceg, Z. Histone acetylation by Trrap-Tip60 modulates loading of repair proteins and repair of DNA double-strand breaks. *Nat. Cell. Biol.* **2006**, *8*, 91–99. [CrossRef] [PubMed]
43. Stante, M.; Minopoli, G.; Passaro, F.; Raia, M.; Vecchio, L.D.; Russo, T. Fe65 is required for Tip60-directed histone H4 acetylation at DNA strand breaks. *Proc. Natl. Acad. Sci. USA* **2009**, *106*, 5093–5098. [CrossRef]
44. Krishnan, V.; Chow, M.Z.; Wang, Z.; Zhang, L.; Liu, B.; Liu, X.; Zhou, Z. Histone H4 lysine 16 hypoacetylation is associated with defective DNA repair and premature senescence in Zmpste24-deficient mice. *Proc. Natl. Acad. Sci. USA* **2011**, *108*, 12325–12330. [CrossRef]
45. Ikura, M.; Furuya, K.; Matsuda, S.; Matsuda, R.; Shima, H.; Adachi, J.; Matsuda, T.; Shiraki, T.; Ikura, T. Acetylation of Histone H2AX at Lys 5 by the TIP60 Histone Acetyltransferase Complex Is Essential for the Dynamic Binding of NBS1 to Damaged Chromatin. *Mol. Cell. Biol.* **2015**, *35*, 4147–4157. [CrossRef] [PubMed]
46. Jacquet, K.; Fradet-Turcotte, A.; Avvakumov, N.; Lambert, J.P.; Roques, C.; Pandita, R.K.; Paquet, E.; Herst, P.; Gingras, A.C.; Pandita, T.K.; et al. The TIP60 Complex Regulates Bivalent Chromatin Recognition by 53BP1 through Direct H4K20me Binding and H2AK15 Acetylation. *Mol. Cell* **2016**, *62*, 409–421. [CrossRef] [PubMed]
47. Renaud, E.; Barascu, A.; Rosselli, F. Impaired TIP60-mediated H4K16 acetylation accounts for the aberrant chromatin accumulation of 53BP1 and RAP80 in Fanconi anemia pathway-deficient cells. *Nucleic Acids Res.* **2016**, *44*, 648–656. [CrossRef] [PubMed]
48. Sun, Y.; Jiang, X.; Chen, S.; Fernandes, N.; Price, B.D. A role for the Tip60 histone acetyltransferase in the acetylation and activation of ATM. *Proc. Natl. Acad. Sci. USA* **2005**, *102*, 13182–13187. [CrossRef]
49. Chen, G.; Cheng, Y.; Tang, Y.; Martinka, M.; Li, G. Role of Tip60 in human melanoma cell migration, metastasis, and patient survival. *J. Investig. Dermatol.* **2012**, *132*, 2632–2641. [CrossRef]

50. Miyamoto, N.; Izumi, H.; Noguchi, T.; Nakajima, Y.; Ohmiya, Y.; Shiota, M.; Kidani, A.; Tawara, A.; Kohno, K. Tip60 is regulated by circadian transcription factor clock and is involved in cisplatin resistance. *J. Biol. Chem.* **2008**, *283*, 18218–18226. [CrossRef]
51. Finetti, P.; Cervera, N.; Charafe-Jauffret, E.; Chabannon, C.; Charpin, C.; Chaffanet, M.; Jacquemier, J.; Viens, P.; Birnbaum, D.; Bertucci, F. Sixteen-kinase gene expression identifies luminal breast cancers with poor prognosis. *Cancer Res.* **2008**, *68*, 767–776. [CrossRef]
52. Salzano, M.; Vazquez-Cedeira, M.; Sanz-Garcia, M.; Valbuena, A.; Blanco, S.; Fernandez, I.F.; Lazo, P.A. Vaccinia-related kinase 1 (VRK1) confers resistance to DNA-damaging agents in human breast cancer by affecting DNA damage response. *Oncotarget* **2014**, *5*, 1770–1778. [CrossRef] [PubMed]
53. Li, L.; Wang, Y. Cross-talk between the H3K36me3 and H4K16ac histone epigenetic marks in DNA double-strand break repair. *J. Biol. Chem.* **2017**, *292*, 11951–11959. [CrossRef] [PubMed]
54. Bowers, E.M.; Yan, G.; Mukherjee, C.; Orry, A.; Wang, L.; Holbert, M.A.; Crump, N.T.; Hazzalin, C.A.; Liszczak, G.; Yuan, H.; et al. Virtual ligand screening of the p300/CBP histone acetyltransferase: Identification of a selective small molecule inhibitor. *Chem. Biol.* **2010**, *17*, 471–482. [CrossRef]
55. Martin-Doncel, E.; Rojas, A.M.; Cantarero, L.; Lazo, P.A. VRK1 functional insufficiency due to alterations in protein stability or kinase activity of human VRK1 pathogenic variants implicated in neuromotor syndromes. *Sci. Rep.* **2019**, *9*, 13381. [CrossRef] [PubMed]
56. Sun, Y.; Xu, Y.; Roy, K.; Price, B.D. DNA damage-induced acetylation of lysine 3016 of ATM activates ATM kinase activity. *Mol. Cell. Biol.* **2007**, *27*, 8502–8509. [CrossRef]
57. Kozlov, S.V.; Graham, M.E.; Jakob, B.; Tobias, F.; Kijas, A.W.; Tanuji, M.; Chen, P.; Robinson, P.J.; Taucher-Scholz, G.; Suzuki, K.; et al. Autophosphorylation and ATM activation: Additional sites add to the complexity. *J. Biol. Chem.* **2011**, *286*, 9107–9119. [CrossRef]
58. Zhang, T.; Shen, Y.; Chen, Y.; Hsieh, J.T.; Kong, Z. The ATM inhibitor KU55933 sensitizes radioresistant bladder cancer cells with DAB2IP gene defect. *Int. J. Radiat. Biol.* **2015**, *91*, 368–378. [CrossRef]
59. Carruthers, R.; Ahmed, S.U.; Strathdee, K.; Gomez-Roman, N.; Amoah-Buahin, E.; Watts, C.; Chalmers, A.J. Abrogation of radioresistance in glioblastoma stem-like cells by inhibition of ATM kinase. *Mol. Oncol.* **2015**, *9*, 192–203. [CrossRef]
60. Sarkaria, J.N.; Busby, E.C.; Tibbetts, R.S.; Roos, P.; Taya, Y.; Karnitz, L.M.; Abraham, R.T. Inhibition of ATM and ATR kinase activities by the radiosensitizing agent, caffeine. *Cancer Res.* **1999**, *59*, 4375–4382.
61. Zhou, B.B.; Chaturvedi, P.; Spring, K.; Scott, S.P.; Johanson, R.A.; Mishra, R.; Mattern, M.R.; Winkler, J.D.; Khanna, K.K. Caffeine abolishes the mammalian G(2)/M DNA damage checkpoint by inhibiting ataxia-telangiectasia-mutated kinase activity. *J. Biol. Chem.* **2000**, *275*, 10342–10348. [CrossRef]
62. Roos, W.P.; Krumm, A. The multifaceted influence of histone deacetylases on DNA damage signalling and DNA repair. *Nucleic Acids Res.* **2016**, *44*, 10017–10030. [CrossRef] [PubMed]
63. Charvet, C.; Wissler, M.; Brauns-Schubert, P.; Wang, S.J.; Tang, Y.; Sigloch, F.C.; Mellert, H.; Brandenburg, M.; Lindner, S.E.; Breit, B.; et al. Phosphorylation of Tip60 by GSK-3 determines the induction of PUMA and apoptosis by p53. *Mol. Cell* **2011**, *42*, 584–596. [CrossRef] [PubMed]
64. Brauns-Schubert, P.; Schubert, F.; Wissler, M.; Weiss, M.; Schlicher, L.; Bessler, S.; Safavi, M.; Miething, C.; Borner, C.; Brummer, T.; et al. CDK9-mediated phosphorylation controls the interaction of TIP60 with the transcriptional machinery. *EMBO Rep.* **2018**, *19*, 244–256. [CrossRef] [PubMed]
65. Lemercier, C.; Legube, G.; Caron, C.; Louwagie, M.; Garin, J.; Trouche, D.; Khochbin, S. Tip60 acetyltransferase activity is controlled by phosphorylation. *J. Biol. Chem.* **2003**, *278*, 4713–4718. [CrossRef] [PubMed]
66. Sun, Y.; Jiang, X.; Price, B.D. Tip60: Connecting chromatin to DNA damage signaling. *Cell Cycle* **2010**, *9*, 930–936. [CrossRef]
67. Chailleux, C.; Tyteca, S.; Papin, C.; Boudsocq, F.; Puget, N.; Courilleau, C.; Grigoriev, M.; Canitrot, Y.; Trouche, D. Physical interaction between the histone acetyl transferase Tip60 and the DNA double-strand breaks sensor MRN complex. *Biochem. J.* **2010**, *426*, 365–371. [CrossRef] [PubMed]
68. Hsiao, K.Y.; Mizzen, C.A. Histone H4 deacetylation facilitates 53BP1 DNA damage signaling and double-strand break repair. *J. Mol. Cell. Biol.* **2013**, *5*, 157–165. [CrossRef]
69. Tang, J.; Cho, N.W.; Cui, G.; Manion, E.M.; Shanbhag, N.M.; Botuyan, M.V.; Mer, G.; Greenberg, R.A. Acetylation limits 53BP1 association with damaged chromatin to promote homologous recombination. *Nat. Struct. Mol. Biol.* **2013**, *20*, 317–325. [CrossRef] [PubMed]

70. Teufel, D.P.; Bycroft, M.; Fersht, A.R. Regulation by phosphorylation of the relative affinities of the N-terminal transactivation domains of p53 for p300 domains and Mdm2. *Oncogene* **2009**, *28*, 2112–2118. [CrossRef] [PubMed]
71. Lopez-Sanchez, I.; Valbuena, A.; Vazquez-Cedeira, M.; Khadake, J.; Sanz-Garcia, M.; Carrillo-Jimenez, A.; Lazo, P.A. VRK1 interacts with p53 forming a basal complex that is activated by UV-induced DNA damage. *FEBS Lett.* **2014**, *588*, 692–700. [CrossRef]
72. Kussie, P.H.; Gorina, S.; Marechal, V.; Elenbaas, B.; Moreau, J.; Levine, A.J.; Pavletich, N.P. Structure of the MDM2 oncoprotein bound to the p53 tumor suppressor transactivation domain. *Science* **1996**, *274*, 948–953. [CrossRef] [PubMed]
73. Toledo, F.; Wahl, G.M. Regulating the p53 pathway: In vitro hypotheses, in vivo veritas. *Nat. Rev. Cancer* **2006**, *6*, 909–923. [CrossRef] [PubMed]
74. Cantarero, L.; Sanz-Garcia, M.; Vinograd-Byk, H.; Renbaum, P.; Levy-Lahad, E.; Lazo, P.A. VRK1 regulates Cajal body dynamics and protects coilin from proteasomal degradation in cell cycle. *Sci. Rep.* **2015**, *5*, 10543. [CrossRef] [PubMed]
75. Lopez-Sanchez, I.; Sanz-Garcia, M.; Lazo, P.A. Plk3 interacts with and specifically phosphorylates VRK1 in Ser342, a downstream target in a pathway that induces Golgi fragmentation. *Mol. Cell. Biol.* **2009**, *29*, 1189–1201. [CrossRef]
76. Marcos, A.T.; Martin-Doncel, E.; Morejon-Garcia, P.; Marcos-Alcalde, I.; Gomez-Puertas, P.; Segura-Puimedon, M.; Armengol, L.; Navarro-Pando, J.M.; Lazo, P.A. VRK1 (Y213H) homozygous mutant impairs Cajal bodies in a hereditary case of distal motor neuropathy. *Ann. Clin. Transl. Neurol.* **2020**, *7*, 808–818. [CrossRef] [PubMed]
77. Valbuena, A.; Castro-Obregon, S.; Lazo, P.A. Downregulation of VRK1 by p53 in Response to DNA Damage Is Mediated by the Autophagic Pathway. *PLoS ONE* **2011**, *6*, e17320. [CrossRef]
78. Bremer, M.; Doerge, R.M. *Statistics at the Bench: A Step-By Step Handbook for Biologists*; Cold Spring Harbor Laboratory Press: New York, NY, USA, 2009.
79. Orchard, S.; Ammari, M.; Aranda, B.; Breuza, L.; Briganti, L.; Broackes-Carter, F.; Campbell, N.H.; Chavali, G.; Chen, C.; del-Toro, N.; et al. The MIntAct project–IntAct as a common curation platform for 11 molecular interaction databases. *Nucleic Acids Res.* **2014**, *42*, D358–D363. [CrossRef]

Publisher's Note: MDPI stays neutral with regard to jurisdictional claims in published maps and institutional affiliations.

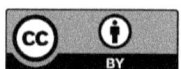

© 2020 by the authors. Licensee MDPI, Basel, Switzerland. This article is an open access article distributed under the terms and conditions of the Creative Commons Attribution (CC BY) license (http://creativecommons.org/licenses/by/4.0/).

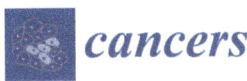

Article

GRK2-Dependent HuR Phosphorylation Regulates HIF1α Activation under Hypoxia or Adrenergic Stress

Clara Reglero [1,2,†], Vanesa Lafarga [1,3,†], Verónica Rivas [1,4], Ángela Albitre [1,4], Paula Ramos [1,4], Susana R. Berciano [1,4], Olga Tapia [5], María L. Martínez-Chantar [6,7], Federico Mayor Jr [1,4,8] and Petronila Penela [1,4,8,*,‡]

1. Department of Molecular Biology and Molecular Biology Centre Severo Ochoa (CMBSO), the Spanish National Research Council, the Autonomous University of Madrid (UAM-CSIC), 28049 Madrid, Spain; cr3023@cumc.columbia.edu (C.R.); vlafarga@cnio.es (V.L.); vrivas@cbm.csic.es (V.R.); angela.albitre@cbm.csic.es (A.A.); pramos@cbm.csic.es (P.R.); srberciano@cbm.csic.es (S.R.B.); fmayor@cbm.csic.es (F.M.J.)
2. Institute for Cancer Genetics, Columbia University Medical Center, New York, NY 10037, USA
3. Department of Molecular Oncology, Spanish National Cancer Research Centre (CNIO), 28029 Madrid, Spain
4. Department of Cellular and Molecular Mechanisms in Inflammatory and Autoimmune Diseases, Institute of Health Research La Princesa, 28006 Madrid, Spain
5. Department of Anatomy and Cell Biology, CIBER of Neurodegenerative Diseases (CIBERNED), University of Cantabria–IDIVAL, 39011 Santander, Spain; olga.tapia@unican.es
6. CIC bioGUNE, Center for Cooperative Research in Biosciences, Liver Disease and Liver Metabolism Lab, 48160 Derio, Spain; mlmartinez@cicbiogune.es
7. Biomedical Research Center Network of Hepatic and Digestive Diseases (CIBERehd), The Instituto de Salud Carlos III (ISCIII), 28029 Madrid, Spain
8. CIBER of Cardiovascular Diseases (CIBERCV), The Instituto de Salud Carlos III (ISCIII), 28029 Madrid, Spain
* Correspondence: ppenela@cbm.csic.es
† These authors contributed equally to this work.
‡ Lead contact.

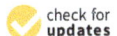

Received: 1 April 2020; Accepted: 11 May 2020; Published: 13 May 2020

Abstract: Adaptation to hypoxia is a common feature in solid tumors orchestrated by oxygen-dependent and independent upregulation of the hypoxia-inducible factor-1α (HIF-1α). We unveiled that G protein-coupled receptor kinase (GRK2), known to be overexpressed in certain tumors, fosters this hypoxic pathway via phosphorylation of the mRNA-binding protein HuR, a central HIF-1α modulator. GRK2-mediated HuR phosphorylation increases the total levels and cytoplasmic shuttling of HuR in response to hypoxia, and GRK2-phosphodefective HuR mutants show defective cytosolic accumulation and lower binding to HIF-1α mRNA in hypoxic Hela cells. Interestingly, enhanced GRK2 and HuR expression correlate in luminal breast cancer patients. GRK2 also promotes the HuR/HIF-1α axis and VEGF-C accumulation in normoxic MCF7 breast luminal cancer cells and is required for the induction of HuR/HIF1-α in response to adrenergic stress. Our results point to a relevant role of the GRK2/HuR/HIF-1α module in the adaptation of malignant cells to tumor microenvironment-related stresses.

Keywords: hypoxia; β-adrenergic signaling; breast cancer; mRNA regulation; nucleocytoplasmic shuttling; GRK2; HuR; HIF1α; VEGF

1. Introduction

Oxygen is a key factor in embryonic development and in normal tissue homeostasis, and its shortage triggers adaptive mechanisms required for cell survival [1,2]. Hypoxia is also a hallmark of solid tumors that results from a leaky vasculature within the tumor and the high proliferation rate of both cancerous cells and immune infiltrating cells [3]. Tumor-associated hypoxia correlates with cellular resistance to chemotherapy, metastasis, and poor patient survival, indicating that hypoxia acts as an extrinsic driver of tumor progression [4,5]. The hypoxia-inducible transcription factors HIF-1 and HIF-2 are the main coordinators of the cellular response to low oxygen tension in both normal and transformed cells [2,5]. HIF-1 is formed by two helix-loop-helix-PAS proteins, namely HIF-1α and HIF-1β or ARNT. Under normoxia, HIF-1α subunits are efficiently ubiquitinated and targeted for proteasome-dependent degradation by the multimeric SCF2 E3 ligase coupled with the von Hippel-Lindau tumor suppressor protein VHL, which recognizes HIF subunits only after their hidroxylation by PHD1-3, a family of oxygen-dependent prolyl-hidroxylases. In hypoxic conditions, HIF-1α subunits are stabilized as a result of PHD inhibition and translocated to the nucleus, where they dimerize with ARNT, in order to activate the transcription of hundreds of genes [5,6].

Interestingly, in cancerous cells, the HIF signaling pathway can also be regulated by other environmental and intracellular signaling factors in an oxygen-independent manner, via modulation of protein stability, gene transcription, or mRNA binding proteins such as YB-1 and HuR (Human antigen R), which are often up-regulated in tumor contexts thereby leading to enhanced translation of HIF-1α mRNA in normoxic and hypoxic conditions [7–9]. HIF-1α is often downstream of the activation of different plasma membrane receptors-triggered signaling pathways, thus linking HIF-1α status to the growth needs of cells [10–12].

Different G protein-coupled receptors (GPCRs) have been associated with the progression of several types of tumors [13,14]. Of note, activation of GPCRs by β-adrenergic, endothelin-1 or lysophosphatidic acid agonists has been shown to promote the stabilization of HIF proteins [12,15,16], thus mimicking hypoxic conditions. Cumulative evidence indicates that chronic neurosympathetic activity fosters the malignant growth and dissemination of tumor cells through direct stimulation of β2AR receptors [17]. Several processes appear to underlie the influence of βAR on tumor progression, including increased HIF-1α signaling and angiogenesis. Besides its role in GPCR desensitization, the G protein-coupled receptor kinase 2 (GRK2) is emerging as a key signaling hub. GRK2 can act as a positive effector of certain GPCR and receptor-tyrosine kinases (RTK) transduction cascades [18,19], and also directly interacts/phosphorylates components of signaling networks involved in cell transformation [20]. We have recently shown that GRK2 expression is up-regulated in different breast cancer contexts, playing a driving role in the acquisition of oncogenic features [21,22]. Concurrently, GRK2 downregulation takes place in the breast tumor vessels [23]. Such opposite and cellular-specific alterations in GRK2 expression seem to be causally related, promoting a marked increase of intra-tumoral hypoxia and of the tumor-associated macrophage-derived factor adrenomedullin, a known VHL-HIF-1 target gene.

In this report we unveil that GRK2 is a relevant modulator of the hypoxic pathway in transformed epithelial cells via phosphorylation-dependent modulation of the mRNA-binding protein HuR, leading to subsequent nuclear accumulation of the HIF-1α protein. Stimulation of GRK2 upon hypoxia or adrenergic receptor activation emerges as a novel mechanism of regulation of HIF signaling in physiological or pathological processes, such as cancer progression.

2. Results

Our previous results pointed to GRK2 as a common regulatory and transducing effector of diverse pathways that are altered in luminal and basal breast cancer [21,22]. Remarkably, the mRNA binding protein ELAV-like protein 1 (HuR), a key upstream modulator of HIF-1α and other targets, is also overexpressed in these tumor contexts [24,25]. Moreover, GRK2 upregulation alters the activity of several transcription factors in normal breast cells that are chronically stimulated with EGF [21], whereas HuR activity changes in response to EGF [26]. A subset of EGF- and GRK2-regulated transcription factors in such conditions can be linked to a GRK2-mediated gain-of-function of the prolyl isomerase Pin1 [21] (Figure S1). Interestingly, other subsets can be linked to HuR (Figure S1), since their mRNAs are either regulated or potentially targeted by this protein [27]. Altogether, these observations suggested a potential functional relationship between HuR and GRK2 in both tumor and non-tumor settings.

2.1. HuR Protein Levels Positively Correlate with GRK2 Activity

We analyzed the steady-state levels of HuR protein under different GRK2 expression and activation status contexts in Hela cells, a cellular model widely used in the functional characterization of HuR. The protein levels of HuR directly correlated with GRK2 abundance, being significantly upregulated in cells over-expressing the wild-type GRK2 (Hela-WT5), but down-modulated upon stable GRK2 silencing (Hela-shGRK2) (Figure 1A). Interestingly, HuR abundance remained unaltered compared to parental Hela cells, upon stable over-expression of the catalytically inactive GRK2-K220R mutant (Hela-K1 cells) or of GRK2-S670A, which lacks the ability to phosphorylate a subset of GRK2 substrates (Hela-A1 cells) [21,28]. These results suggested that GRK2-mediated phosphorylation of either HuR or an intermediate factor was involved in the regulation of HuR expression levels.

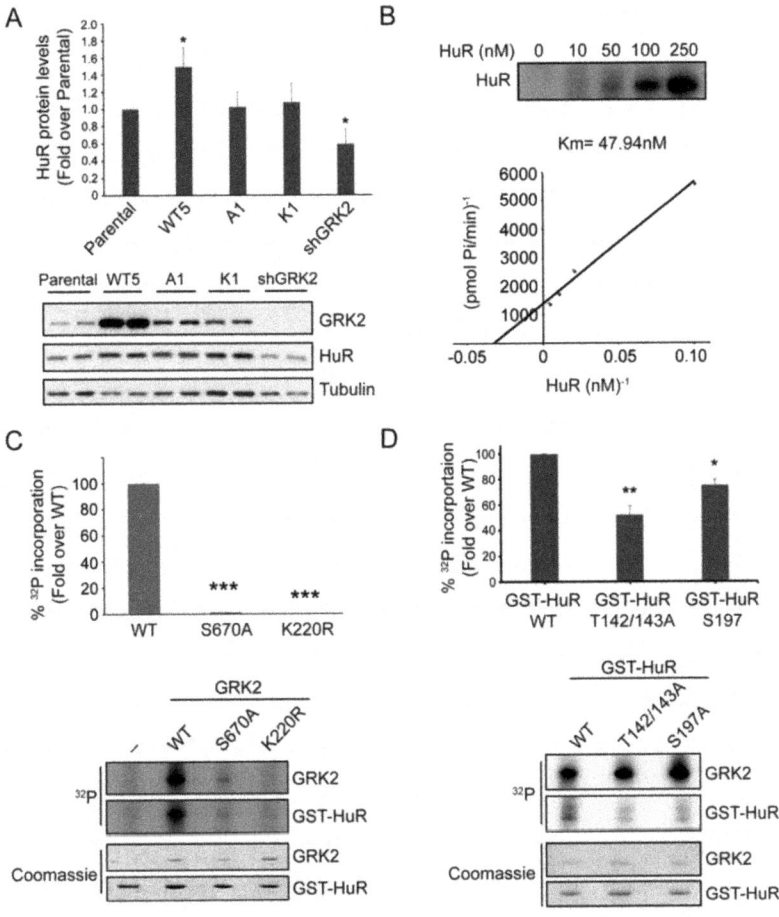

Figure 1. GRK2 phosphorylates and regulates HuR. (**A**) HuR total levels were analyzed by immunoblotting of the total lysates of parental and HeLa cell lines over-expressing wild-type GRK2

(Hela-WT5), a mutant lacking the ability to phosphorylate a subset of GRK2 substrates (Hela-A1), the catalytically inactive GRK2-K220R mutant (Hela-K1) or harboring stable GRK2 silencing (Hela-shGRK2). Values are mean ± SEM from four independent experiments. * $p < 0.05$ vs. parental (Student's t-test). (**B**) GRK2 and GST-HuR were incubated in the presence of [γ-^{32}P]-ATP, as detailed in Materials and Methods. Km was estimated by double-reciprocal plot analysis of three independent experiments. (**C**) Phosphorylation of GST-HuR was performed in the presence of [γ-^{32}P]-ATP using recombinant GRK2-WT, GRK2-S670A, or GRK2-K220R proteins, as described in Materials and Methods. Intensity of ^{32}P and the Coomassie bands were quantified by densitometry and plotted as a percentage of WT GRK2-triggered ^{32}P incorporation. Data representative of two independent experiments are shown. *** $p < 0.001$ vs. parental (Student's t-test). (**D**) GRK2 (50 nM) and GST-HuR, GST-HuR-T142/143A, or GST-HuR-S197A (100 nM) were incubated in the presence of [γ-^{32}P]-ATP, as detailed in Materials and Methods. Intensity of the ^{32}P and Coomassie bands was quantified by densitometry and plotted as a percentage of GRK2-triggered ^{32}P incorporation. The graph shows fold differences in two independent experiments. * $p < 0.05$ vs. WT ** $p < 0.01$ vs. WT (1-way ANOVA). Detailed information about the Western blots can be found in Figure S2.

2.2. HuR Is a GRK2 Phosphorylation Substrate

Purified GST-HuR was efficiently phosphorylated by recombinant GRK2 (Km of ~ 48 nM, Figure 1B), similar to the well-known physiological substrates of GRK2 [28,29], whereas no phosphorylation was observed in the recombinant GRK2-K220R (Figure 1C), indicating that HuR is a direct target of GRK2. Consistently, a direct and preferential binding of HuR to the catalytic domain of GRK2 was detected in the overlay assays (Figure S3A).

Akin to some GRK2 substrates such as HDAC6 [28], phosphorylation of GRK2 at the regulatory site Ser670 seems to be required to enable kinase activity towards HuR, since the recombinant GRK2-S670A mutant was incapable of phosphorylating HuR (Figure 1C), despite being able to fully phosphorylate other well-established GRK2 substrates [28]. These data and those obtained in Hela-A1 cells suggest that HuR belongs to the subset of 'phospho-Ser670-biased' GRK2 targets.

We identified three potential phosphorylation site(s) on the GRK2-phosphorylated GST-HuR, by using proteomic approaches (Figure S3B). Single or double site-directed mutagenesis to alanine of these candidate sites, followed by in vitro phosphorylation assays showed that GST-HuR-Thr-142/143A and GST-HuRS-197A purified proteins displayed a significantly reduced phosphorylation by GRK2, compared to the wild-type (Figure 1D), indicating that these residues are accounting for circa 75% of total GRK2-dependent HuR phosphorylation. Interestingly, these residues are located in two key functional and regulatory regions of the HuR protein, the second RNA-binding domain (RRM2) (residues Thr142 and 143) and the nucleocytoplasmic localization hinge region (residue Ser197) (Figure S3B). Phosphorylation of the hinge region and the RRM domains by different kinases has been shown to underlie changes in HuR subcellular localization, binding affinity with mRNA, and regulation of translational efficiency [30–34].

2.3. GRK2 Activity Modulates the Hypoxia-Induced Modulation of HuR Cellular Levels and Cytoplasmic Shuttling

Hypoxia is a well-characterized stress known to upregulate HuR protein levels, in order to foster HuR actions [35]. Interestingly, Hela-WT5 cells stably expressing GRK2, displayed an enhanced boost in HuR levels upon acute exposure to low oxygen, while such HuR upregulation was absent upon kinase downregulation (Hela-shGRK2 cells) (Figure 2A). A similar unresponsive pattern was observed in the hypoxic Hela cells expressing GRK2 mutants that are unable to phosphorylate HuR (Hela-A1 and Hela-K1 cells) (Figure 2A). These data supported the notion that regulation of HuR by GRK2 was strictly dependent on its kinase activity and on previous GRK2 phosphorylation at Ser670. Consistently, parallel to changes in the HuR levels, a clear up-regulation of S670-GRK2 phosphorylation was noted after 2 h of hypoxia, which was sustained afterwards in both parental and Hela-WT5 cells (Figure 2B), but not in Hela-A1 or Hela-K1 cells.

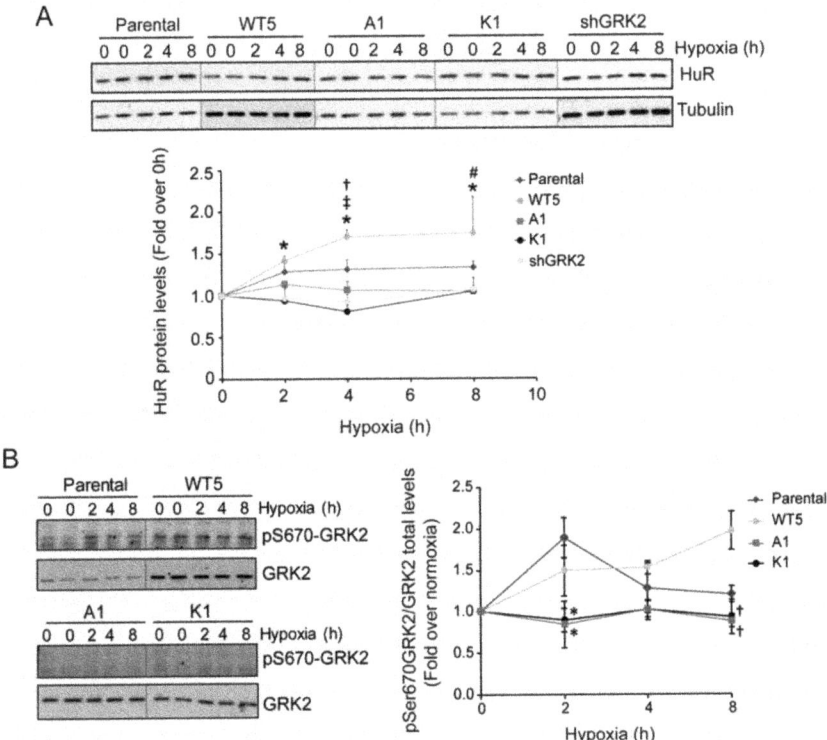

Figure 2. pS670-GRK2 modulates hypoxia-induced HuR upregulation. (**A,B**) HeLa stable cell lines were cultured under hypoxia and the pSer670 GRK2, GRK2, and HuR levels were analyzed by immunoblotting, at the indicated times. Values are mean ± SEM from 4–6 independent experiments. Upper panel: ‡ $p < 0.05$ wt5 vs. parental; # $p < 0.05$ A1 vs. parental; * $p < 0.05$ K1 vs. parental; † $p < 0.05$ shGRK2 vs. parental (Student's t-test). Lower panel: * $p < 0.05$ A1 and K1 vs. parental; † $p < 0.05$ A1 and K1 vs. WT5 (Student's t-test). Detailed information about the Western blots can be found in Figure S4.

HuR is mainly localized in the cell nucleus in basal conditions, whereas its activity in stress conditions is tightly linked to protein cytosolic shuttling [32,36]. Akin to stress conditions such as UV treatment [37], serum starvation [38], or heat shock [39], cytosolic translocation of the HuR protein occurs after prolonged $CoCl_2$ exposure, a condition mimicking hypoxic stress [35]. We observed that GRK2-mediated HuR phosphorylation markedly affects the HuR cytoplasmic accumulation in hypoxia. In parental Hela cells, HuR protein is mobilized from the nucleus as early as 2 h after low oxygen exposure, in line with previous reports [40], and enhanced cytoplasmic HuR levels are still noted 24 h afterwards (Figure 3A). Such a pattern of HuR mobilization was potentiated by over-expression of wild-type GRK2, whereas no shuttling was observed in the cells expressing a catalytically inactive GRK2 mutant (Hela-K1) or upon GRK2 downmodulation (Hela-shGRK2). Consistent with a relevant role for GRK2-mediated HuR phosphorylation in this process, the cytosolic redistribution of phospho-defective HuR mutants HuR-S197A or HuR-T142/143A was markedly reduced upon exposure to hypoxia for 3 h or 6 h (Figure 3B). The combination of these mutations in the triple HuR-T142/143/197A construct resulted in a stronger impairment of HuR shuttling (Figure 3B). None of these HuR mutations appear to disturb the localization of HuR in untreated cells, suggesting that GRK2 regulation specifically takes place under stress.

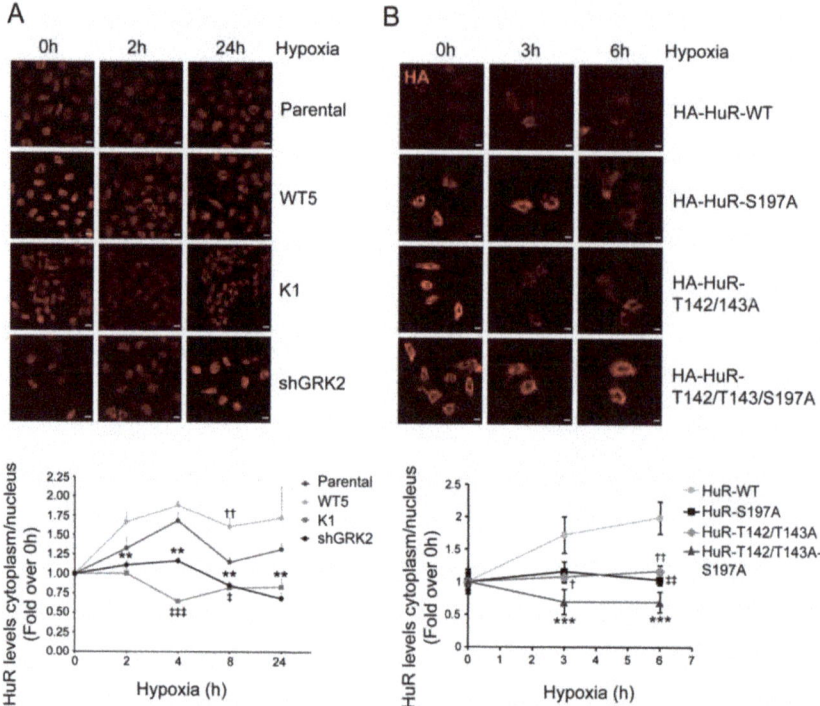

Figure 3. GRK2 affects hypoxia-dependent changes in HuR subcellular distribution. (**A**) The indicated HeLa stable cell lines were cultured under hypoxia, and HuR nuclear and cytosolic levels were analyzed by immunofluorescence, at the indicated times. Values are mean ± SEM from 3–4 independent experiments. †† $p < 0.01$ wt5 vs. parental; ‡ $p < 0.05$ ‡‡‡ $p < 0.001$ K1 vs. parental; ** $p < 0.01$ shGRK2 vs. parental (Student's *t*-test). Representative images are shown. Scale Bar = 10 µm. (**B**) HeLa cells were transiently transfected with HA-HuR WT, HA-HuR-S197A, HA-HuR-T142/143A, or HA-HuR-T142/143A-S197A, and was cultured under hypoxia for the indicated times. Localization of HA-tagged HuR was assessed by immunofluorescence and the nuclear and cytosolic levels were quantified. Values are mean ± SD from two independent experiments. ‡‡ $p < 0.01$ S197A vs. wt; † $p < 0.05$ †† $p < 0.01$ T142/142A vs. wt; *** $p < 0.001$ T142/143A-S197A vs. wt; (two-way ANOVA). Representative images are shown. Scale Bar = 7 µm.

Overall, these results indicated that GRK2-mediated phosphorylation at the residues located in the different domains of HuR can modulate the cellular levels and the cytoplasmic localization of HuR protein, in response to hypoxia.

2.4. GRK2 Phosphorylation of HuR Is Required for HIF-1α Upregulation in Response to Hypoxia

Central to cellular hypoxia is the upregulation of HIF-1α, which is in turn required for the transcriptional induction of genes involved in metabolism, angiogenesis, or survival [5,6,41]. In addition to protein stabilization, HuR-mediated translational control of HIF-1α mRNA is an important mechanism accounting for HIF-1α protein accumulation, in response to short-term hypoxia [42,43].

Interestingly, nuclear levels of HIF-1α after 4 h of hypoxia were markedly potentiated in the presence of extra GRK2 (HeLa-WT5 cells), compared to parental Hela cells. By contrast, such HIF-1α nuclear accumulation was impaired in the Hela cells overexpressing either GRK2-K220R or GRK2-S670A mutants, both unable to phosphorylate/mobilize the HuR protein (Figure 4A).

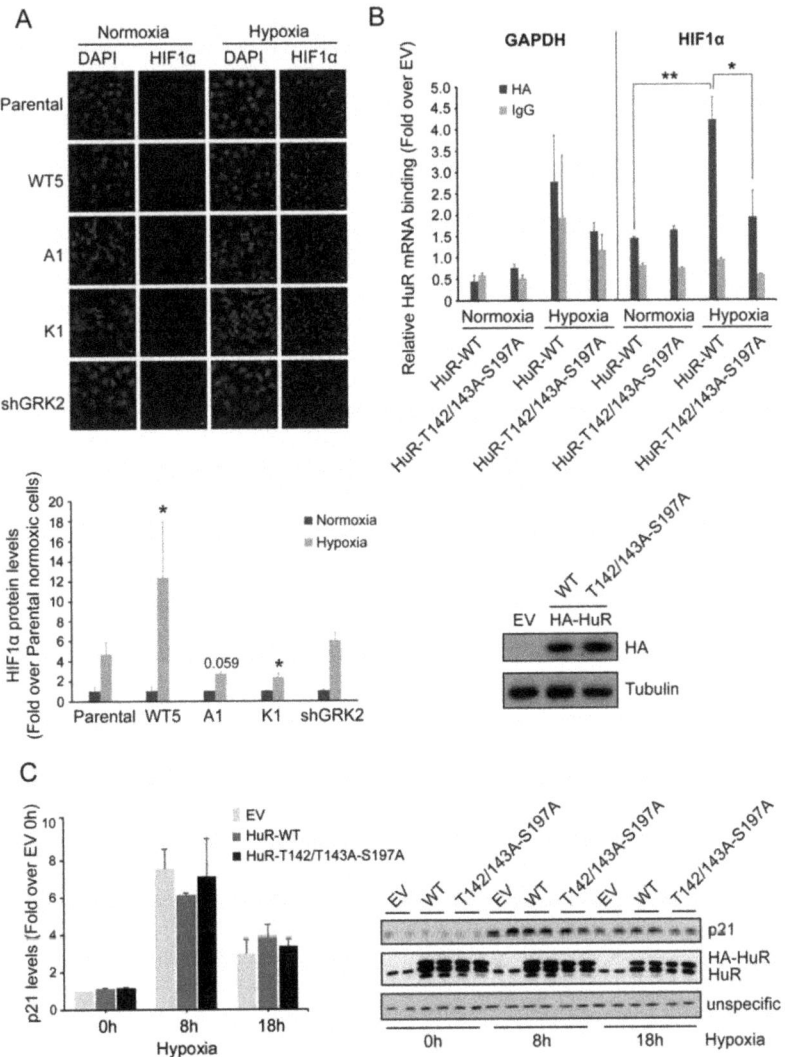

Figure 4. GRK2 kinase activity is required for HuR-induced upregulation of HIF1α. (**A**) HeLa stable cell lines were cultured under hypoxia for 2 h and HIF1α levels were analyzed by immunofluorescence. Values are mean ± SEM (fold-change over parental cells in normoxia) from 3–4 independent experiments. * $p < 0.05$ (Student's t-test) comparing the changes in hypoxic HIF1α levels in Hela stable cells lines, with those observed in hypoxic parental cells. Representative images are shown. Scale Bar = 10 μm. (**B**) HeLa cells were transiently transfected with pcDNA3 as empty vector (EV), HA-HuR WT, or

HA-HuR-T142/143A-S197A, and cultured for 4 h under hypoxia. Total lysates were then immunoprecipitated with either an HA antibody or control IgGs. RNA was purified from immunoprecipitates and used for qRT-PCRs. GAPDH was used as an endogenous control. The graph shows fold differences in transcript abundance (mean ± SEM in two independent experiments performed in triplicates). ** $p < 0.01$ hypoxic vs. normoxic WT; * $p < 0.05$ hypoxic triple mutant vs. hypoxic WT (two-way ANOVA). The expression levels of the different HA-HuR proteins analyzed by immunoblotting are shown below. (C) HeLa cells were transiently transfected with pcDNA3 as empty vector (EV), HA-HuR WT, or HA-HuR-T142/143A-S197A, and was cultured under hypoxia for the indicated times. p21 and endogenous and overexpressed HuR levels were analyzed by immunoblot. A non-specific band was used as the loading control. Values are mean ± SEM from two independent experiments. Detailed information about the Western blots can be found in Figure S5.

These results suggested that GRK2-phosphorylated HuR could be more efficient in binding to HIF-1α mRNA or in regulating its decay or translation rates.

Then, we performed RNA immunoprecipitation (RIP) assays to detect HuR-HIF-1α mRNA complexes in Hela cells that were overexpressing HA-tagged constructs of HuR. As shown in Figure 4B, circa 2.7-fold enrichment in HuR-bound HIF-1α mRNA was found in the hypoxic cells, as compared to the normoxic cells. In contrast, no significant hypoxia-induced increase in the binding of the HuR-T142/T143A-S197A mutant to HIF-1α mRNA was noted. The specificity of these responses was assessed using the non-HuR target GAPDH mRNA and control IgG immunoprecipitates, in parallel experiments (Figure 4B). These data strongly supported the importance of GRK2-mediated HuR modulation in the activation of the HuR/HIF-1α axis in hypoxia.

It has been proposed that stress-induced HuR might not bind with identical affinities to its mRNA targets [40], suggesting an HuR target "prioritization" in response to specific stress stimuli. Interestingly, the hypoxia-induced protein levels of p21, a well-known HuR target [34] was not altered by the HuR-T142/T143A-S197A expression (Figure 4C), thereby suggesting that phosphorylation of HuR by GRK2 alone or together with other hypoxia-induced kinases, does not necessarily affect other HuR targets.

2.5. GRK2 Fosters the HuR/HIF-1α Axis and a Pro-Lymphangiogenic Response in the Normoxic Breast Luminal Cancer Cells

Expression of the *ELAVL1* (HuR) and *ADRBK1* (GRK2) genes showed a direct correlation in breast cancer patients inspected with the web tool CANCERTOOL (Figure S6A). A significant positive association in hormone-stratified cohorts was found only in estrogen-positive tumors (Figure S6B). No association of *ELAVL1* and *ADRBK1* co-expression was evidenced with the molecular subtypes of breast cancer "basal-like", "normal-like" or "HER2-enriched" in the three independent cohorts, whereas a significant direct correlation was noted in the luminal subtype (Figure S6C).

Therefore, we used the cell line MCF7, a model of estrogen receptor (ER)-positive and luminal A human breast tumors engineered to express different dosages of GRK2 [21], and further characterized the effects on HuR. In basal conditions, cells overexpressing GRK2 (MCF7-GRK2) displayed a marked increase in total HuR protein levels, compared to parental MCF7 cells, whereas the opposite effect was observed upon GRK2 down-regulation in MCF7-shGRK2 cells (Figure 5A). Basal cytosolic translocation of HuR was higher in MCF7-GRK2 cells compared to parental cells, as inferred from the significant reduction of nuclear HuR levels, in spite of the global upregulation of the protein (Figure 5B).

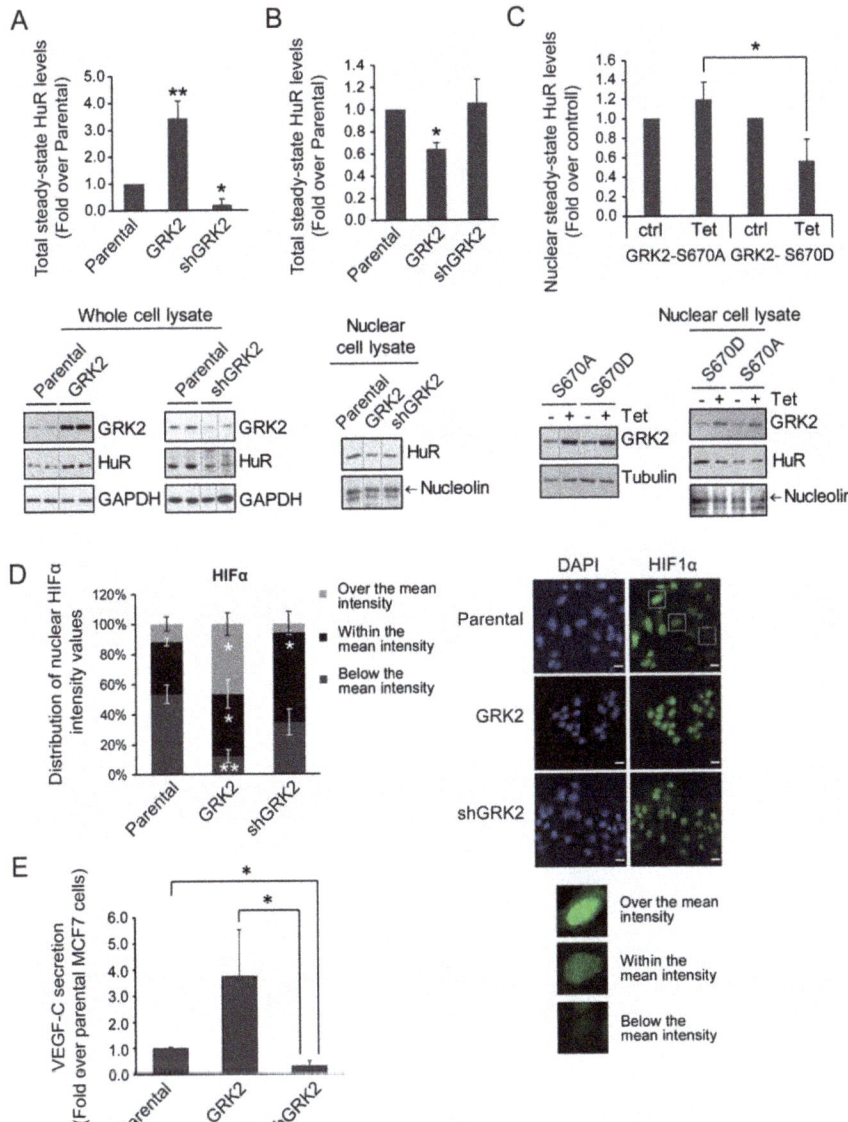

Figure 5. GRK2 modulates HuR levels and cytoplasmic shuttling, HIF1-α distribution, and VEGF-C secretion in luminal breast cancer cells. (**A**,**B**) Whole lysates or nuclear extracts from MCF7 cells stably expressing GRK2-wt or shGRK2 were used to analyze the HuR levels by immunoblot. Values are mean ± SEM from 3–4 independent experiments. * $p < 0.05$ ** $p < 0.01$ (Student's *t*-test). Representative blots with loading controls are shown. (**C**) MCF7 stable inducible cell lines were treated with tetracyclin (Tet) to induce the expression of the indicated GRK2 mutants. HuR nuclear levels were analyzed by immunoblot. Values are mean ± SEM from two independent experiments. * $p < 0.05$ (Student's *t*-test). Representative blots with loading controls are shown. (**D**,**E**) HIF1-α distribution and VEGF-C secretion levels were analyzed in parental MCF7 cells or in derived cells lines stably overexpressing GRK2 or

a silencing construct (shGRK2) of the kinase. (**D**) HIF1-α and DAPI staining was analyzed by immunofluorescence; distribution of intensity values is shown. Values are distribution percentages of cells with HIF1-α intensity values over, within, or below the mean intensity. Representative images are shown. * $p < 0.05$; ** $p < 0.01$ (Student's *t*-test) when each category (over, within, below) in MCF7-GRK2 and MCF7-shGRK2 cells is compared to parental ones. Scale Bar = 25 μm. (**E**) ELISA-measured VEGF-C secretion values are shown (mean ± SEM from 3 independent experiments). * $p < 0.05$ (Student's *t*-test). Detailed information about the Western blots can be found in Figure S7.

This effect depended on the GRK2-dependent phosphorylation of HuR, as the inducible over-expression of GRK2-S670A did not trigger a reduction in nuclear HuR levels, whereas a kinase mutant mimicking the positive regulatory S670 phosphorylation event (GRK2-S670D) decreased the nuclear HuR levels akin to the wild-type GRK2 protein (Figure 5C).

We next investigated whether GRK2-dependent HuR modulation in MCF7 cells might affect HIF-1α nuclear distribution. As expected in tumor cells [44], normoxic MCF7 cells had a constitutive elevation of HIF-1α protein in the nucleus. Levels of HIF-1α protein display cell-to-cell variations, with a Gaussian distribution when the cells were stratified in subgroups, according to staining intensity, ranging from no signal (0) to maximal signal (800), with steps of 100 arbitrary units, peaking at the average intensity of 364.40 ± 39 (mean ± SD) arbitrary units (mean gray value). We then grouped the stratified cell population according to the proportion of cells with intensities in the range of the average value (34.8 ± 2.4%), above the average value (11.7 ± 4.8%), or below the average value (53.5 ± 6.1%) (Figure 5D). Interestingly, the overexpression of GRK2 did not affect the average intensity of nuclear HIF-1α protein (382.58 ± 17 arbitrary units), but markedly altered the distribution of cells around this value. Thus, the proportion of cells with HIF-1α levels higher than the average value was increased circa 3-fold, while those with lower levels were reduced circa 5.5-fold. Conversely, in the MCF7-shGRK2 cells, the average intensity of the HIF-1α protein (422.25 ± 23) was within the range of the parental cells, but the proportion of cells with HIF-1α a level over this value was reduced 2-fold (Figure 5D). Altogether, these results suggested that the increased expression of GRK2 noted in the breast cancer cell lines and in patients, would also contribute to tumor progression by fostering the cellular mechanisms that induce and stabilize the HIF-1α protein in normoxia.

A main pro-carcinogenic effect of the HIF-1α factor is the induction of angiogenesis and lymphangiogenesis through the activation of transcription of the VEGF family members [41,45]. Of note, the secretion of VEGF-C, a potent inducer of lymphatic vessels through which breast cancer cells often disseminate [46,47] was strongly increased in the MCF7 cells overexpressing GRK2 as compared to the parental cells, and conversely secretion was reduced upon GRK2 downregulation (Figure 5E). Therefore, it is tempting to suggest that GRK2 might impact VEGF-C expression via pathways downstream of HuR phosphorylation to foster lymphangiogenesis and metastases of luminal breast cancer cells.

2.6. Adrenergic Stress Induces a HuR/HIF1-α Hypoxia-Like Response in MCF7 Breast Cancer Cells in a GRK2-Mediated Manner

The effects of GRK2 on the HuR/HIF1-α axis in MCF7 cells suggested that stressful or microenvironment conditions other than hypoxia might also contribute to foster this tumorigenic pathway. In this context, it is known that adrenergic stimulation promotes ERK-mediated phosphorylation of GRK2 on Ser670 in different cellular systems [48] and also strengths hypoxic signaling via HIF1-α accumulation in a GRK2-dependent manner in normoxic endothelial cells [12]. In addition, compelling evidence demonstrates that chronic adrenergic stress is involved in breast cancer progression [49,50].

Therefore, we addressed whether chronic β2-adrenergic receptor stimulation promoted HuR regulation by GRK2 in MCF7 breast cancer cells. Isoproterenol challenge upregulated total HuR protein levels in both parental and MCF7-GRK2 cells, but not in GRK2-silenced cells (Figure 6A). Isoproterenol also triggered parallel changes in GRK2 protein, suggesting that adrenergic effects on

HuR levels involve GRK2. In addition, isoproterenol stimulation also promoted a reduction of HuR nuclear protein levels in parental cells, and this effect was potentiated in the presence of extra kinase in MCF7-GRK2 cells (Figure 6B). However, isoproterenol treatment failed to promote the nuclear exit of HuR in MCF7-shGRK2 cells, indicating that GRK2 activity is required for HuR mobilization. Consistent with the increased mobilization of nuclear HuR, nuclear HIF1-α protein was upregulated after 48 h of βAR stimulation in cells overexpressing GRK2, compared to parental cells (Figure 6C).

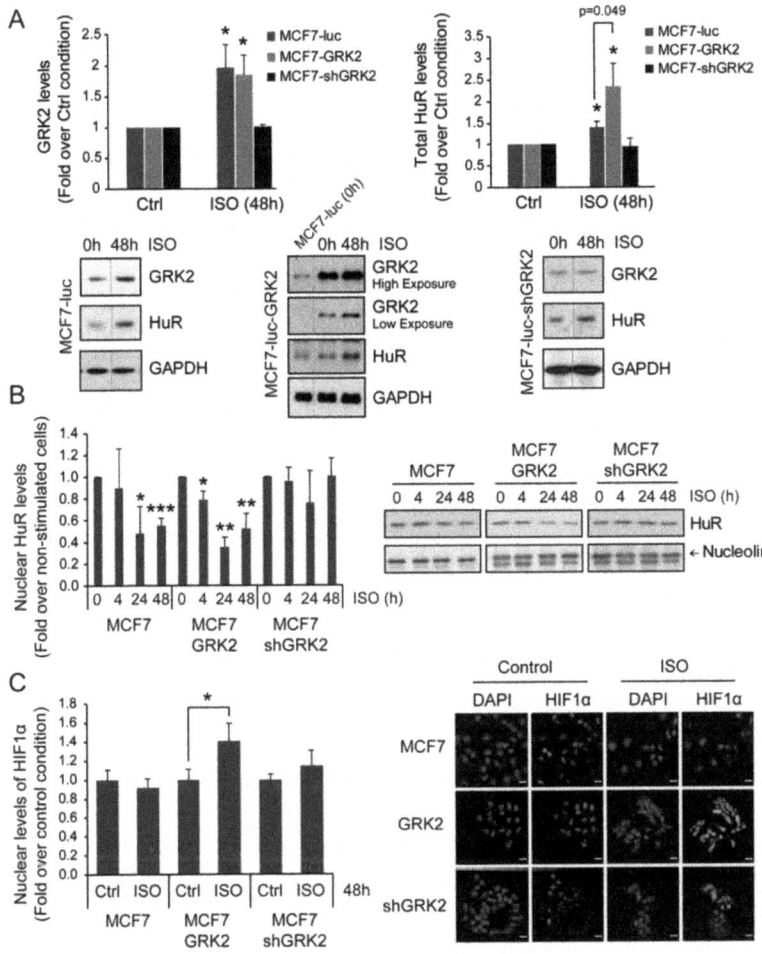

Figure 6. Chronic adrenergic stress leads to HIF1α accumulation through GRK2 and HuR upregulation in luminal breast cancer cells. Adrenergic signaling facilitates nuclear export of HuR in a GRK2-dependent manner. MCF7-luc (control MCF7 cells) and cells stably expressing GRK2-wt or shGRK2 were treated with 50 μM isoproterenol for the indicated times to induce adrenergic stress. Total GRK2 and HuR levels (**A**) and nuclear HuR levels (**B**) were analyzed by immunoblot with the indicated loading controls. (**C**) HIF1-α and DAPI nuclear marker levels were analyzed by immunofluorescence. Representative images are shown (scale bar, 25 μm). All values are mean ± SEM from three independent experiments. * $p < 0.05$, ** $p < 0.01$, *** $p < 0.001$ (Student's t-test). Detailed information about the Western blot can be found in Figure S8.

Overall, our results point that the GRK2/HuR/HIF-1α axis is potentiated in response to hypoxic and adrenergic stresses, thus emerging as a relevant pro-tumorigenic module.

3. Discussion

In this paper, we identified GRK2 as a modulator of the HuR/HIF-1α axis in relevant pathological settings. We uncovered that HuR is a GRK2 substrate, requiring prior phosphorylation of GRK2 at its Ser670 regulatory site. Phosphorylation by GRK2 enhances the HuR levels and the cytosolic shuttling of HuR upon hypoxic conditions, favoring its binding to HIF-1α mRNA and increased nuclear accumulation of this central modulator of hypoxia-driven pathways. In the MCF7 cells, a cellular model of luminal A breast cancer in which upregulation of GRK2 and HuR frequently concur, GRK2 increased the total and basal cytosolic HuR protein levels, which correlated with a higher nuclear distribution of HIF-1α and enhanced secretion of the lymphoangiogenic factor VEGF-C in normoxic conditions. Moreover, chronic adrenergic stimulation fosters the HuR/HIF1-α module in MCF7 cells through GRK2 (Figure 7), which could facilitate survival of malignant cells even before the expanding tumor mass become hypoxic, and could also improve the adaptation of tumor cells to the hypoxic environment of lymphatic vessels and to other tumor-related stresses.

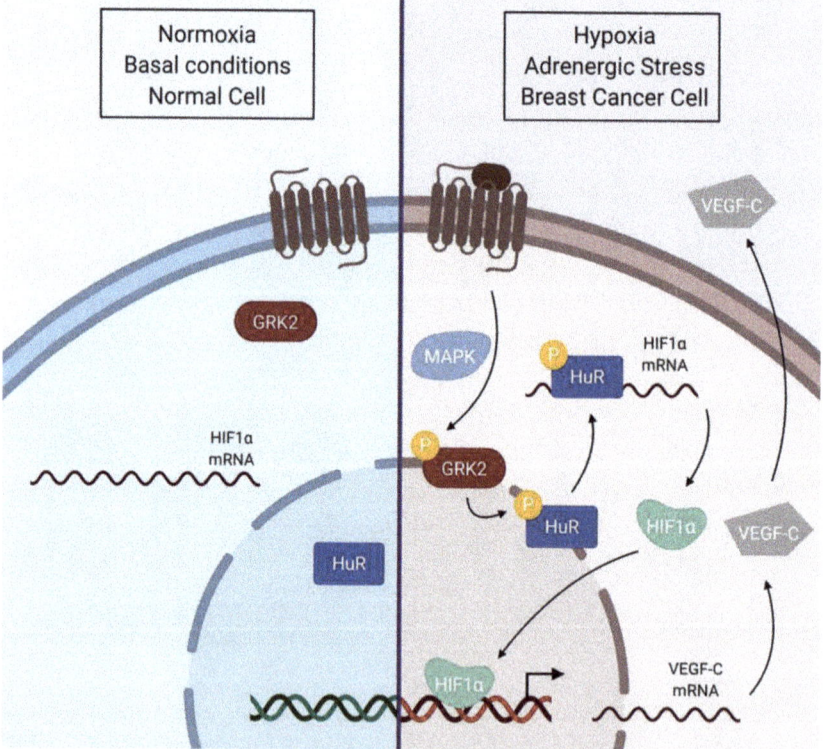

Figure 7. Model for the GRK2-dependent activation of the HuR/HIF1α axis. In basal conditions, the main HuR protein pool is located in the nucleus. Hypoxia or adrenergic signaling facilitates GRK2 phosphorylation at Ser670, enabling HuR phosphorylation by GRK2, thus increasing HuR nuclear export. Cytosolic HuR protein binds to and stabilizes HIF1-α mRNA, increasing protein translation and HIF-1α function as a transcription factor. As a consequence, transcription and protein secretion of the VEGF-C angiogenic factor would be enhanced (scheme created with BioRender).

Ser670 phosphorylation is an emerging regulatory switcher in GRK2 substrate specificity and partner association [18]. Context-specific ERK1/2-dependent GRK2 Ser670 phosphorylation is necessary for GRK2 to phosphorylate HDAC6 [21,28], to disrupt its interaction with GIT1 [51], or to allow its HSP90-mediated localization to the mitochondrial membrane [52]. A variety of stimuli, including growth factors [28,29], adrenergic and other GPCR ligands [53], ischemia [54], or hypoxic conditions (this manuscript) can trigger GRK2 phosphorylation at this residue via ERK1/2 stimulation, which is also triggered by hypoxic mimetics [55]. Therefore, it is likely that enhanced ERK1/2 activity in response to different environmental factors would switch on the ability of GRK2 to phosphorylate and modulate HuR.

We have identified residues within the hinge region (S197) and the RRM2 domain (T142/T143) as the main targets of GRK2-mediated HuR phosphorylation, and mutations preventing such modifications specifically impair hypoxia-induced HuR cytoplasmic shuttling in HeLa cells, without altering its basal localization. Moreover, the triple HuR-T142/143/197A mutant also displays reduced binding to HIF-1α mRNA in hypoxic conditions.

Several mechanisms might underlie the observed effects of GRK2 on HuR functionality. Enhanced cytosolic levels of GRK2-phosphorylated HuR might be a consequence of increased nuclear export/decreased nuclear import or fostered cytoplasmic retention. The long hinge region (aa 187–243) includes the HuR Nucleocytoplasmic Shuttling (HNS) sequence (aa 205–237) containing both nuclear localization and nuclear export determinants [30–33,56]. This HNS resembles a consensus bipartite Nuclear Localization Signal, NLS sequence, with two clusters of the basic residues near the N-terminus (aa 205–206 and aa217–219), being the first of the ones critical for nuclear targeting [57]. Introduction of a negative charge by phosphorylation at S197 might reduce the electrostatic potential of the neighboring basic lysine residues (aa 205–206), which are key for the interaction with the import machinery and favors the nuclear exit. Additionally, phosphorylation of HuR on S197 might inhibit its interaction with trans-acting factors that facilitate its translocation through the nuclear pore complex [30,56], thus favoring cytoplasmic retention. The hinge region of HuR (aa 190–243) is involved in the interaction with the nuclear protein ligands pp32 and April [58], in turn recognized by the export receptor CRM1 [39], thereby making it feasible for the phosphorylation of S197 to improve its association to pp32/April. Our results showing a cytoplasmic localization of HuR phosphorylated on S197 adds complexity to these HuR trafficking regulatory mechanisms.

GRK2-mediated phosphorylation at T142/143 within the RRM2, the second HuR RNA binding domain also fosters HuR cytoplasmic localization. It has been reported that interaction of HuR with nuclear importin TNR2 is reduced by binding of ARE-containing RNA to HuR [56]. Since GRK2 phosphorylation increases the formation of HuR/HIF1 mRNA complexes, this could hamper the interaction with the nuclear import machinery. In addition to TNR2 and the transporting homologue TNR1 [56,59], the importing α/β pathway is required for nuclear import of HuR [60]. We cannot rule out that the mechanisms whereby GRK2 regulates HuR shuttling include interference of HuR/importin α/β complexes.

The subcellular location in which the phosphorylation of HuR by GRK2 takes place could shed light on the GRK2-mediated modulation of HuR trafficking. HuR and GRK2 display opposite canonical subcellular distribution at the basal conditions. Although GRK2 was initially described as a cytoplasmic protein, its nuclear presence has also been reported [61], thus allowing HuR phosphorylation at this location and regulation of nuclear export. Alternatively, or in addition, since HuR moves to the cytosol under hypoxia, this would facilitate GRK2-mediated phosphorylation and decreased nuclear import or fostered cytoplasmic retention.

Preventing HuR modification by GRK2 also results in a defective interaction with HIF1-α mRNA. HuR phosphorylation has a notable impact on the binding of HuR to mRNA targets [24]. Conformational changes occurring on RRM1 and RRM2 regions are crucial for mRNA-binding [62,63]. Tandem RRM1-RRM2 displays prominent inter-domain flexibility, particularly affecting residues in the linker and in the loops of RRM [63]. This flexibility allows HuR to fit around low affinity strands with high efficiency, enabling the recognition of many different mRNA substrates. Interestingly, Thr142 is one of the positions in the RRM2 loop showing large chemical shift perturbations [63]. Thus, phosphorylation of Thr142 by GRK2 could favor structural flexibility in the close-bound state of HuR by preventing some stabilizing interaction in the proximity of the inter-domain linker. It has been proposed that binding of mRNAs bearing shorter 3′UTR with lower AU content could be more influenced by the flexibility of RRM1-2 domains [63]. Remarkably, with 8 AU-rich motifs throughout the 3′UTR (AREsite2 database, http://rna.tbi.univie.ac.at/AREsite), HIF1α mRNA could fit in the group of mRNAs with greater dependence on HuR conformations. Therefore, it is tempting to suggest that GRK2 might favor recognition of a subset of mRNAs displaying lower intrinsic affinities for HuR.

Furthermore, although we have not analyzed in-depth the mechanism whereby HuR phosphorylation by GRK2 impacts its total protein levels, it is worth noting that phosphorylation of RRM2 residues has been linked to HuR stabilization. Phosphorylation of Thr118 by CHK2 protects HuR from proteasomal degradation upon heat shock [64]. Modifications at this site alter the extent of HuR polyubiquitination, mainly assembled on Lys182, a RRM2 residue key for protein stability. Whether phosphorylation of Thr142/143 by GRK2 has similar effects remains to be investigated.

The role of HuR in breast cancer development is well-documented in model cell lines, in vivo animal models, and clinical studies [24,25]. The increased levels of HuR in MCF7 cells compared to non-tumoral cells is implicated in the regulation of many genes involved in the cell cycle, survival, and angiogenesis [38,65,66]. Our data put forward that in this luminal A breast cancer model GRK2 would foster HuR/HIF-1α pathways even in normoxic conditions. In MCF7 cells, GRK2 dosage positively correlated with the total HuR protein levels, cytoplasmic HuR translocation, higher nuclear distribution of HIF-1α, and increased VEGF-C secretion. Upregulation of HIF-1α in normoxia is a feature of tumor cells [44] and different non-canonical modalities of HIF-1α modulation have been identified [8]. We have previously shown that in MCF7 cells the activation of estrogen and growth factor pathways converge for promoting an enhanced GRK2 expression and fostering GRK2 phosphorylation at Ser670 [21], which would enable GRK2-meditaed HuR phosphorylation and enhanced functionality and, thus, cooperate with other pathways in upregulating HIF-1α cascades.

HuR can modulate HIF1α mRNA via the 3′UTR region for transcript stabilization or via 5′UTR for translation, depending on the cellular context [67,68]. It seems that the 5′UTR-based mechanism predominates in highly malignant cells, while those based on 3′UTR-mediated stabilization do so in less aggressive ones (such as MCF7) [69]. Thus, it is feasible that GRK2 phosphorylation of HuR in MCF7 cells would foster the latter mechanism. Our results also point that the GRK2/HuR/HIF1α axis is involved in modulating the expression of VEGF-C, a critical factor for remodeling the lymphatic network and tumor cell dissemination [45–47]. It is well-known that VEGF factors are transcriptional targets of HIF-1α but are also HIF-1-independent post-transcriptional targets of HuR itself [70,71]. Therefore, GRK2-phosphorylated HuR might also directly modulate the VEGF-C mRNA in breast tumor MCF7 cells.

Adrenergic stress is emerging as a relevant microenvironmental player in cancer progression [49,50]. Chronic emotional stressors increase the catecholamine levels and βAR activation in cancer cells and increases metastatic potential [72] and levels of pro-angiogenic factors [73]. We unravel that chronic adrenergic stimulation triggers the upregulation of both GRK2 and HuR protein levels, increases cytoplasmic HuR and fosters nuclear HIF-1α presence, thus, mimicking a pseudo-hypoxia situation that might contribute to tumor progression. Chronic adrenergic stimulation increases GRK2 expression by different transcriptional and post-transcriptional mechanisms [74,75], and also to promote HuR expression [76]. Normoxic HIF-1α accumulation in adrenergic-stimulated endothelial cells depends on the phosphorylation of β-AR by GRK2 [12]. Our data suggest a mechanism linking β-AR activation to a GRK2/HuR/HIF1α downstream axis (Figure 7). Upon agonist stimulation, GRK2-mediated phosphorylation of β-AR would enable β-arrestin-dependent MAPK activation and subsequent modification of GRK2 at S670, the key event allowing the targeting of HuR and the HIF1 cascade. β-adrenergic stimulation is known to activate the MAPK cascade [77,78], and prolonged and high-dose stimulation of the β2AR induces a switch in receptor coupling from Gs to Gi, shifting the signaling to MAPK pathways [79].

In sum, our data put forward a relevant role for the GRK2/HuR/HIF1α module in cancer cells and in response to the adrenergic overdrive, regardless of the oxygen status. Enhanced GRK2 expression and S670 phosphorylation status in the given tumor contexts would lead to enhanced HuR functionality, thus, counteracting the canonical HIF protein degradation driven by prolyl hydroxylases [7,9] and recapitulating a pseudo-hypoxic state in normoxia, as a consequence. Besides inducing the angiogenic remodeling of tumoral stroma, GRK2-induced pseudo-hypoxia might favor cancer cell de-differentiation and emergence of cancer stem-like cells. Pseudohypoxic cells are often observed at the tumor–stromal interface in locally invading tumors, providing growing advantages during tumor expansion, as these cells are more aggressive and resistant [4]. The coordinated regulation of key players in angiogenesis such as HuR, HIF-1α, and VEGF-C suggest that upregulation of GRK2 might be a relevant event for acquiring increased malignancy and invasiveness, and point that combined pharmacological inhibition of GRK2 might be useful in certain cancer therapy contexts. This mechanism reinforces the notion of GRK2 as a central oncomodulator influencing several hallmarks of cancer [22].

4. Methods

4.1. Cell Culture and Treatments

Cells were maintained in DMEM supplemented with 10% fetal bovine serum. Stable Hela (ATCC) cells were previously described [27]. MCF7luc-F5 cells stably expressing pcDNA3-GRK2-wt or pLKO-GRK2-shRNA (5′-GCAAGAAAGCCAAGAACAAGC-3′) and tetracycline-inducible expression (TET-on) system for mutant GRK2-S670A or GRK2-S670D in MCF7 cell, were also previously described [21]. GRK2 expression in the TET-on system was promoted by treating the cells with 1 µg/mL tetracyclin for 24 h. Hypoxia (1% O_2) was achieved in an Invivo2 400 hypoxia Workstation (Baker Ruskinn, USA). Isoproterenol (50 µM) was supplemented with 1 mM ascorbic acid and 20 mM HEPES pH 7.5.

4.2. Plasmids and Cell Transfection

Plasmids encoding HA-HuR WT were previously described [33]. HA-HuR-S197A, HA-HuR-T142/143A, or HA-HuR-T142/143A-S197A were generated using QuickChange® Lightning site-directed mutagenesis kit (Thermo Fisher, Waltham, MA, USA). HeLa cells (70%–80% confluent monolayers in 60 or 100 mm dishes) were transiently transfected using the lipofectamine/plus method.

4.3. Immunoprecipitation, Western Blot, Dot Blot, and ELISA

Whole cellular lysates were prepared in RIPA buffer (Tris-HCl 20 mM pH 7.5, 150 mM NaCl, 1% Triton X100, 0.1% SDS, 0.5% sodium deoxycholate, cocktail of protease, and phosphatase inhibitors), as described [28]. For the analysis of nuclear and cytoplasmic pools of HuR and HIF-1α, cells were collected in hypotonic lysis buffer (10 mM Tris–HCl, pH 7.4, 10 mM NaCl, 3 mM MgCl2, 0.3% (v/v) Nonidet P-40, 2 mM Na3V04, 10 mM NaF, and protease inhibitors), incubated on ice for 10 min and centrifuged at 500 ×g for 5 min to obtain the nuclear fraction. The cytoplasmic supernatant contains the extranuclear fraction (plasma membrane, microsomal vesicles, cytoskeleton, and cytosol). Pellets containing cell nuclei were washed in lysis buffer without Nonidet P-40 and again pelleted at 500 ×g. Both fractions were solubilized in Laemmli sample buffer and resolved by SDS–PAGE. Proteins were resolved in SDS–PAGE and transferred to nitrocellulose membranes. Cytosolic (GAPDH) and nuclear (Nucleolin) markers were used for control loading. For the dot-blot experiments, GST-tagged GRK2 fragments (2 µg) and recombinant GRK2 full-length protein were spotted on strips of nitrocellulose and incubated for 4 h at 37 °C, with GST-HuR (2 µg/mL) in the interaction buffer (20 mM Tris-HCl pH 7.5, 100 mM NaCl, 1 mM EDTA, 0.3% NP-40, 10% Glycerol, 0.5 mM NaF, and 1 mM Na3VO4). Membranes were incubated with the indicated primary antibodies—α-Actin (1:2000, Santa Cruz Biotechnology,

Santa Cruz, CA, USA), GAPDH (1:2000, Santa Cruz Biotechnology), (pSer670-GRK2 (1:500, GeneTex, Irvine, CA, USA), GRK2 (1:1000, Santa Cruz Biotechnology), HuR (1:000, Santa Cruz Biotechnology), Nucleolin (1:1000, Santa Cruz Biotechnology), p21 (1:500, Santa Cruz Biotechnology), and α-Tubulin (1:2000, Santa Cruz Biotechnology). Blots were developed using a chemiluminescent method (ECL, Amersham, Little Chalfont, UK). Band density was quantitated by laser densitometric analysis.

VEGF-C secretion was determined in cell-conditioned media of MCF7 cells incubated in DMEM 1% FCS for 48 h, by using a Human VEGF-C Quantikine ELISA Kit (R&D Systems, Minneapolis, MN, USA). Measurements in duplicates were normalized to the amount of the total protein in cell lysates quantified by the Lowry method.

4.4. Immunofluorescence and Confocal Microscopy

As described in [28], 4% PFA-fixed cells were processed and incubated O/N at 4 °C, with primary antibodies—HA (1:600, Cell Signaling, Leiden, The Netherlands), HIF1α (1:200, Novus Biologicals, Centennial, CO, USA) and HuR (1:200, Santa Cruz Biotechnology). Then, coverslips were incubated for 1 h RT with fluorescent secondary antibodies, and for 5 min with To-Pro3 (1:2000, ThermoFisher, Waltham, MA, USA) or DAPI (1 µg/mL, Merck, Darmstadt, Germany) to stain nuclei. Finally, samples were mounted using Mowiol-DABCO (Boston Bioproducts, Ashland, MA, USA), let to dry overnight at RT and then stored at 4 °C. Images were acquired using a confocal laser microscope LSM710 (Zeiss, Oberkochen, Germany) and the nucleus area and mean intensity values were analyzed using ImageJ (NIH, Bethesda, MD, USA). In both the basal and stress conditions, nuclear masks were drawn using the nuclear staining distribution pattern of HuR and were guided by the morphological features (nucleolus, euchromatin, speckles) (Figure S9). For each cell, three measurements were made within the nucleoplasm, excluding the HuR-negative areas corresponding to nucleoli and nuclear speckles, or indistinctly in the cytoplasm peripheral to the nucleus. Fluorescence intensity values were corrected for background staining. The ratio of the mean cytoplasmic (C) to nuclear (N) value was calculated for each cell. Average C/N values from all cells within a field were pooled for subsequent plotting and comparative analysis. Cells from 10 different randomly acquired fields (40× or 63×) were measured for each cell type and condition. Average values from all cells within a field were pooled for subsequent plotting and analysis.

4.5. Kinase Activity Assays

In vitro kinase assays with wild-type, S670A or K220R GRK2 full-length (50 nM); and WT, T142/143A or S197A GST-tagged HuR recombinant proteins (50–250 nM for Km value and 100 nM for the rest) were performed, as described [28]. The Michaelis constant (Km) was estimated by double-reciprocal plot analysis of three independent experiments.

4.6. Mass Spectrometry Analysis

GRK2 (50 nM) and GST-HuR (100 nM) were incubated in the presence of cold ATP, as detailed above and resolved by SDS–PAGE. The band corresponding to full-length GST-HuR was digested by trypsin and chymotrypsin, and the fragments were analyzed using LC–MS/MS in the 'CBMSO PROTEIN CHEMISTRY FACILITY' that belonged to the ProteoRed network, PRB2-ISCIII, supported by the grant PT13/0001.

4.7. RNA Immunoprecipitation

RNA Immunoprecipitation (RIP) assays were performed, as previously described [80]. Whole-cell lysates (500 µg) were incubated with a suspension of Protein A/G PLUS-Agarose, precoated with 15 µg of either IgG or anti-HA antibody-conjugated agarose beads (all from Santa Cruz Biotechnology). Bound mRNA was purified from immunoprecipitants, retrotranscribed by RT-PCR, and the HIFα mRNA content was measured by real-time PCR analysis and normalized to GAPDH mRNA bound in a nonspecific manner to IgG.

4.8. Bioinformatics Analysis of HuR and GRK2 Expression in Human Breast Tumors

Pairwise correlation of gene expression *ELAVL1* (HuR protein) and *ADRBK1* (GRK2 protein) levels in breast tumors was calculated and represented using the CANCERTOOL webtool [81]. Pearson correlation test was applied to analyze the relationship between paired genes, and the correlation coefficient and *p*-values were adjusted using the Benjamini–Hochberg method. Datasets with a correlation coefficient greater than 20% ($-0.2 < R < 0.2$) and a *p*-value lower than 0.05 were considered.

4.9. Statistical Analysis

Data analysis was performed using the GraphPad Prism for Windows. Means between groups were compared by two-way or one-way ANOVA with Bonferroni's or Tukey's post-hoc test, or with unpaired Student's *t*-test, as indicated in the figure legends. All results are expressed as mean ± SEM.

5. Conclusions

An active GRK2/HuR/ HIF-1α module, particularly in estrogen-positive luminal A breast tumors could facilitate survival of malignant cells, even before the expanding tumor mass becomes hypoxic, and also improves the adaptation of tumor cells to the hypoxic environment of lymphatic vessels and to other tumor-related stresses, such as chronic over-activation of the adrenergic system, in order to foster tumor progression.

Supplementary Materials: The following are available online at http://www.mdpi.com/2072-6694/12/5/1216/s1. Figure S1: GRK2 expression positively influences the activity of known and predicted HuR-regulated transcription factors in luminal mammary epithelial cells, Figure S2: Detailed information about the Western blot in Figure 1, Figure S3: GRK2 binds to and phosphorylates HuR, Figure S4: Detailed information about the Western blot in Figure 2, Figure S5: Detailed information about the Western blot in Figure 4, Figure S6: CANCERTOOL analysis of HuR and GRK2 expression in human breast cancers, Figure S7: Detailed information about the Western blot in Figure 5, Figure S8: Detailed information about the Western blot in Figure 6, Figure S9: Endogenous HuR or HA-HuR-WT fluorescent image analysis and quantitative data acquisition methodology.

Author Contributions: Conceptualization, V.L., C.R., P.P., F.M.J., and M.L.M.-C.; Methodology: C.R., V.L., and S.R.B.; Investigation: C.R., V.L., V.R., Á.A., O.T., and P.R.; Formal Analysis: C.R., V.L., and P.P.; Visualization: C.R., V.L., and P.P.; Resources: M.L.M.-C., P.P., and F.M.; Writing—Original Draft: P.P. with contributions from C.R.; Writing—Review & Editing: P.P. and F.M.; Funding acquisition: P.P. and F.M.; Supervision: P.P. and F.M. All authors have read and agreed to the published version of the manuscript.

Funding: This research was funded by the Instituto de Salud Carlos III: PI17-00576; Ministerio de Economía, Industria y Competitividad, Gobierno de España: SAF2017-84125-R; Ministerio de Economía, Industria y Competitividad, Gobierno de España: SAF2017-87301-R; Instituto de Salud Carlos III: CIBERCV CB16/11/00278; Instituto de Salud Carlos III: PI14-00435; Fundación Ramón Areces and the Comunidad de Madrid: B2017/BMD-3671-INFLAMUNE.

Acknowledgments: Our laboratories are supported by Instituto de Salud Carlos III, Spain, with FEDER cofinancing (grants PI14-00435 and PI17-00576 to PP); by Ministerio de Economía; Industria y Competitividad (MINECO) of Spain (grant SAF2017-84125-R to F.M. and SAF2017-87301-R (to M.L.M-C); by CIBERCV-Instituto de Salud Carlos III, Spain (grant CB16/11/00278 to F.M, co-funded with European Regional Development Fund-FEDER contribution); by Programa de Actividades en Biomedicina de la Comunidad de Madrid-B2017/BMD-3671-INFLAMUNE and Fundación Ramón Areces to F.M.); and by Asociación Española contra el Cáncer, Canceres raros, La Caixa Foundation, and Ayudas Fundación BBVA (to M.L.M-C). We also acknowledge institutional support to the CBMSO from Fundación Ramón Areces and MINECO (SEV-2016-0644) for the Severo Ochoa Excellence Accreditation.

Conflicts of Interest: The authors declare no competing interests.

References

1. Choudhry, H.; Harris, A.L. Advances in Hypoxia-Inducible Factor Biology. *Cell Metab.* **2018**, *27*, 281–298. [CrossRef] [PubMed]
2. Pugh, C.W.; Ratcliff, P.J. New horizons in hypoxia signaling pathways. *Exp. Cell Res.* **2017**, *356*, 116–121. [CrossRef] [PubMed]
3. Laitala, A.; Erler, J.T. Hypoxic Signalling in Tumour Stroma. *Front. Oncol.* **2018**, *29*, 189. [CrossRef]

4. Velaei, K.; Samadi, N.; Barazvan, B.; Soleimani, A.; Rad, J. Tumor microenvironment-mediated chemoresistance in breast cancer. *Breast* **2016**, *30*, 92–100. [CrossRef] [PubMed]
5. Schito, L.; Semenza, G.L. Hypoxia-Inducible Factors: Master Regulators of Cancer Progression. *Trends Cancer* **2016**, *2*, 758–770. [CrossRef] [PubMed]
6. Suzuki, N.; Gradin, K.; Poellinger, L.; Yamamoto, M. Regulation of hypoxia-inducible gene expression after HIF activation. *Exp. Cell Res.* **2017**, *356*, 182–186. [CrossRef] [PubMed]
7. Zhang, J.; Zhang, Q. VHL and Hypoxia Signaling: Beyond HIF in Cancer. *Biomedicines* **2018**, *6*, 35. [CrossRef]
8. Iommarini, L.; Porcelli, A.M.; Gasparre, G.; Kurelac, I. Non-Canonical Mechanisms Regulating Hypoxia-Inducible Factor 1 Alpha in Cancer. *Front. Oncol.* **2017**, *7*, 286. [CrossRef]
9. Hayashi, Y.; Yokota, A.; Harada, H.; Huang, G. Hypoxia/pseudohypoxia-mediated activation of hypoxia-inducible factor-1α in cancer. *Cancer Sci.* **2019**, *110*, 1510–1517. [CrossRef]
10. Masson, N.; Ratcliffe, P.J. Hypoxia signaling pathways in cancer metabolism: The importance of co-selecting interconnected physiological pathways. *Cancer Metab.* **2014**, *2*, 3. [CrossRef]
11. Laughner, E.; Taghavi, P.; Chiles, K.; Mahon, P.C.; Semenza, G.L. HER2 (neu) Signaling Increases the Rate of Hypoxia-Inducible Factor 1α (HIF-1α) Synthesis: Novel Mechanism for HIF-1-Mediated Vascular Endothelial Growth Factor Expression. *Mol. Cell. Biol.* **2001**, *21*, 3995–4004. [CrossRef] [PubMed]
12. Cheong, H.I.; Asosingh, K.; Stephens, O.R.; Queisser, K.A.; Xu, W.; Willard, B.; Erzurum, S.C. Hypoxia sensing through β-adrenergic receptors. *JCI Insight* **2016**, *1*, e90240. [CrossRef] [PubMed]
13. O'Hayre, M.; Degese, M.S.; Gutkind, J.S. Novel insights into G protein and G protein-coupled receptor signaling in cancer. *Curr. Opin. Cell Biol.* **2014**, *27*, 126–135. [CrossRef] [PubMed]
14. Liu, Y.; An, S.; Ward, R.; Yang, Y.; Guo, X.X.; Li, W.; Xu, T.R. G protein-coupled receptors as promising cancer targets. *Cancer Lett.* **2016**, *376*, 226–239. [CrossRef] [PubMed]
15. Gras, E.; Belaidi, E.; Briançon-Marjollet, A.; Pépin, J.L.; Arnaud, C.; Godin-Ribuot, D. Endothelin-1 mediates intermittent hypoxia-induced inflammatory vascularremodeling through HIF-1 activation. *J. Appl. Physiol.* **2016**, *120*, 437–443. [CrossRef]
16. Radhakrishnan, R.; Ha, J.H.; Jayaraman, M.; Liu, J.; Moxley, K.M.; Isidoro, C.; Dhanasekaran, D.N. Ovarian cancer cell-derived lysophosphatidic acid induces glycolytic shift and cancer-associated fibroblast-phenotype in normal and peritumoral fibroblasts. *Cancer Lett.* **2019**, *442*, 464–474. [CrossRef]
17. Cole, S.W.; Sood, A.K. Molecular pathways: Beta-adrenergic signaling in cancer. *Clin. Cancer Res.* **2012**, *18*, 1201–1206. [CrossRef]
18. Penela, P.; Ribas, C.; Sánchez-Madrid, F.; Mayor, F., Jr. G protein-coupled receptor kinase 2 (GRK2) as a multifunctional signaling hub. *Cell. Mol. Life Sci.* **2019**, *76*, 4423–4446. [CrossRef]
19. Evron, T.; Daigle, T.L.; Caron, M.G. GRK2: Multiple roles beyond G protein-coupled receptor desensitization. *Trends Pharmacol. Sci.* **2012**, *33*, 154–164. [CrossRef]
20. Han, C.C.; Ma, Y.; Li, Y.; Wang, Y.; Wei, W. Regulatory effects of GRK2 on GPCRs and non-GPCRs and possible use as a drug target. *Int. J. Mol. Med.* **2016**, *38*, 987–994. [CrossRef]
21. Nogués, L.; Reglero, C.; Rivas, V.; Salcedo, A.; Lafarga, V.; Neves, M.; Zhou, X.Z. G Protein-coupled Receptor Kinase 2 (GRK2) Promotes Breast Tumorigenesis through a HDAC6-Pin1 Axis. *EBioMedicine* **2016**, *13*, 132–145. [CrossRef] [PubMed]
22. Nogués, L.; Palacios-García, J.; Reglero, C.; Rivas, V.; Neves, M.; Ribas, C.; Mayor, F., Jr. G protein-coupled receptor kinases (GRKs) in tumorigenesis and cancer progression: GPCR regulators and signaling hubs. *Semin. Cancer Biol.* **2018**, *48*, 78–90. [CrossRef] [PubMed]
23. Rivas, V.; Carmona, R.; Muñoz-Chápuli, R.; Mendiola, M.; Nogués, L.; Reglero, C.; Mayor, F. Developmental and tumoral vascularization is regulated by G protein-coupled receptor kinase 2. *J. Clin. Investig.* **2013**, *123*, 4714–4730. [CrossRef] [PubMed]
24. Abdelmohsen, K.; Gorospe, M. Posttranscriptional regulation of cancer traits by HuR. *WIREs RNA* **2010**, *1*, 214–229. [CrossRef] [PubMed]
25. Kotta-Loizou, I.; Vasilopoulos, S.N.; Coutts, R.H.; Theocharis, S. Current Evidence and Future Perspectives on HuR and Breast Cancer Development, Prognosis, and Treatment. *Neoplasia* **2016**, *18*, 674–688. [CrossRef] [PubMed]
26. Giles, K.M.; Daly, J.M.; Beveridge, D.J.; Thomson, A.M.; Voon, D.C.; Furneaux, H.M.; Leedman, P.J. The 3'-untranslated region of p21WAF1 mRNA is a composite cis-acting sequence bound by RNA-binding

proteins from breast cancer cells, including HuR and poly(C)-binding protein. *J. Biol. Chem.* **2003**, *278*, 2937–2946. [CrossRef] [PubMed]
27. López de Silanes, I.; Zhan, M.; Lal, A.; Yang, X.; Gorospe, M. Identification of a target RNA motif for RNA-binding protein HuR. *Proc. Natl. Acad. Sci. USA* **2004**, *101*, 2987–2992. [CrossRef] [PubMed]
28. Lafarga, V.; Aymerich, I.; Tapia, O.; Mayor, F., Jr.; Penela, P. A novel GRK2/HDAC6 interaction modulates cell spreading and motility. *EMBO J.* **2012**, *31*, 856–869. [CrossRef] [PubMed]
29. Peregrin, S.; Jurado-Pueyo, M.; Campos, P.M.; Sanz-Moreno, V.; Ruiz-Gomez, A.; Crespo, P.; Murga, C. Phosphorylation of p38 by GRK2 at the docking groove unveils a novel mechanism for inactivating p38MAPK. *Curr. Biol.* **2006**, *16*, 2042–2047. [CrossRef] [PubMed]
30. Kim, H.H.; Abdelmohsen, K.; Lal, A.; Pullmann, R., Jr.; Yang, X.; Galban, S.; Gorospe, M. Nuclear HuR accumulation through phosphorylation by Cdk1. *Genes Dev.* **2008**, *22*, 1804–1815. [CrossRef] [PubMed]
31. Kim, H.H.; Yang, X.; Kuwano, Y.; Gorospe, M. Modification at HuR(S242) alters HuR localization and proliferative influence. *Cell Cycle* **2008**, *7*, 3371–3377. [CrossRef]
32. Doller, A.; Pfeilschifter, J.; Eberhardt, W. Signalling pathways regulating nucleo-cytoplasmic shuttling of the mRNA-binding protein HuR. *Cell Signal* **2008**, *20*, 2165–2173. [CrossRef] [PubMed]
33. Doller, A.; Schlepckow, K.; Schwalbe, H.; Pfeilschifter, J.; Eberhardt, W. Tandem phosphorylation of serines 221 and 318 by protein kinase Cdelta coordinates mRNA binding and nucleocytoplasmic shuttling of HuR. *Mol. Cell. Biol.* **2010**, *30*, 1397–1410. [CrossRef] [PubMed]
34. Lafarga, V.; Cuadrado, A.; Lopez de Silanes, I.; Bengoechea, R.; Fernandez-Capetillo, O.; Nebreda, A.R. p38 Mitogen-activated protein kinase- and HuR-dependent stabilization of p21(Cip1) mRNA mediates the G(1)/S checkpoint. *Mol. Cell. Biol.* **2009**, *29*, 4341–4351. [CrossRef] [PubMed]
35. Talwar, S.; Jin, J.; Carroll, B.; Liu, A.; Gillespie, M.B.; Palanisamy, V. Caspase-mediated cleavage of RNA-binding protein HuR regulates c-Myc protein expression after hypoxic stress. *J. Biol. Chem.* **2011**, *286*, 32333–32343. [CrossRef]
36. Grammatikakis, I.; Abdelmohsen, K.; Gorospe, M. Posttranslational control of HuR function. *WIREs RNA* **2017**, *8*, e1372. [CrossRef]
37. Wang, W.; Furneaux, H.; Cheng, H.; Caldwell, M.C.; Hutter, D.; Liu, Y.; Gorospe, M. HuR regulates p21 mRNA stabilization by UV light. *Mol. Cell. Biol.* **2000**, *20*, 760–769. [CrossRef]
38. De, S.; Das, S.; Sengupta, S. Involvement of HuR in the serum starvation induced autophagy through regulation of Beclin1 in breast cancer cell-line, MCF-7. *Cell Signal* **2019**, *61*, 78–85. [CrossRef]
39. Gallouzi, I.E.; Brennan, C.M.; Steitz, J.A. Protein ligands mediate the CRM1-dependent export of HuR in response to heat shock. *RNA* **2001**, *7*, 1348–1361. [CrossRef]
40. Blanco, F.F.; Jimbo, M.; Wulfkuhle, J.; Gallagher, I.; Deng, J.; Enyenihi, L.; Risbud, M.V. The mRNA-binding protein HuR promotes hypoxia-induced chemoresistance through posttranscriptional regulation of the proto-oncogene PIM1 in pancreatic cancer cells. *Oncogene* **2016**, *35*, 2529–2541. [CrossRef]
41. Pezzuto, A.; Carico, E. Role of HIF-1 in Cancer Progression: Novel Insights. A Review. *Curr. Mol. Med.* **2018**, *18*, 343–351. [CrossRef] [PubMed]
42. Hui, A.S.; Bauer, A.L.; Striet, J.B.; Schnell, P.O.; Czyzyk-Krzeska, M.F. Calcium signaling stimulates translation of HIF-alpha during hypoxia. *FASEB J.* **2006**, *20*, 466–475. [CrossRef] [PubMed]
43. Schulz, K.; Milke, L.; Rübsamen, D.; Menrad, H.; Schmid, T.; Brüne, B. HIF-1α protein is upregulated in HIF-2α depleted cells via enhanced translation. *FEBS Lett.* **2012**, *586*, 1652–1657. [CrossRef] [PubMed]
44. Doe, M.R.; Ascano, J.M.; Kaur, M.; Cole, M.D. Myc posttranscriptionally induces HIF1 protein and target gene expression in normal and cancer cells. *Cancer Res.* **2012**, *72*, 949–957. [CrossRef] [PubMed]
45. Alitalo, K. The lymphatic vasculature in disease. *Nat. Med.* **2011**, *17*, 1371–1380. [CrossRef]
46. Pérez, D.; Rohde, A.; Callejón, G.; Pérez-Ruiz, E.; Rodrigo, I.; Rivas-Ruiz, F.; Zarcos, I. Correlation between serum levels of vascular endothelial growth factor-C and sentinel lymph node status in early breast cancer. *Tumour. Biol.* **2015**, *36*, 9285–9293. [CrossRef]
47. Ni, X.; Zhao, Y.; Ma, J.; Xia, T.; Liu, X.; Ding, Q.; Zha, X.; Wang, S. Hypoxia-induced factor-1 alpha upregulates vascular endothelial growth factor C to promote lymphangiogenesis and angiogenesis in breast cancer patients. *J. Biomed. Res.* **2013**, *27*, 478–485.
48. Penela, P. Chapter Three—Ubiquitination and Protein Turnover of G-Protein-Coupled Receptor Kinases in GPCR Signaling and Cellular Regulation. *Prog. Mol. Biol. Transl. Sci.* **2016**, *141*, 85–140.

49. Obeid, E.I.; Conzen, S.D. The role of adrenergic signaling in breast cancer biology. *Cancer Biomark.* **2013**, *13*, 161–169. [CrossRef]
50. Childers, W.K.; Hollenbeak, C.S.; Cheriyath, P. β-Blockers Reduce Breast Cancer Recurrence and Breast Cancer Death: A Meta-Analysis. *Clin. Breast Cancer* **2015**, *15*, 426–431. [CrossRef]
51. Penela, P.; Ribas, C.; Aymerich, I.; Eijkelkamp, N.; Barreiro, O.; Heijnen, C.J.; Mayor, F. G protein-coupled receptor kinase 2 positively regulates epithelial cell migration. *EMBO J.* **2008**, *27*, 1206–1218. [CrossRef] [PubMed]
52. Chen, M.; Sato, P.Y.; Chuprun, J.K.; Peroutk, R.J.; Otis, N.J.; Ibetti, J.; Koch, W.J. Prodeath signaling of G protein-coupled receptor kinase 2 in cardiac myocytes after ischemic stress occurs via extracellular signal-regulated kinase-dependent heat shock protein 90-mediated mitochondrial targeting. *Circ. Res.* **2013**, *112*, 1121–1134. [CrossRef]
53. Penela, P.; Elorza, A.; Sarnago, S.; Mayor, F., Jr. Beta-arrestin- and c-Src-dependent degradation of G-protein-coupled receptor kinase 2. *EMBO J.* **2001**, *20*, 5129–5138. [CrossRef] [PubMed]
54. Penela, P.; Inserte, J.; Ramos, P.; Rodriguez-Sinovas, A.; Garcia-Dorado, D.; Mayor, F., Jr. Degradation of GRK2 and AKT is an early and detrimental event in myocardial ischemia/reperfusion. *EBioMedicine* **2019**, *48*, 605–618. [CrossRef] [PubMed]
55. Yang, S.J.; Pyen, J.; Lee, I.; Lee, H.; Kim, Y.; Kim, T. Cobalt chloride-induced apoptosis and extracellular signal-regulated protein kinase 1/2 activation in rat C6 glioma cells. *J. Biochem. Mol. Biol.* **2004**, *37*, 480–486. [CrossRef] [PubMed]
56. Güttinger, S.; Mühlhäusser, P.; Koller-Eichhorn, R.; Brennecke, J.; Kutay, U. Transportin2 functions as importin and mediates nuclear import of HuR. *Proc. Natl. Acad. Sci. USA* **2004**, *101*, 2918–2923. [CrossRef] [PubMed]
57. Fan, X.C.; Steitz, J.A. HNS, a nuclear-cytoplasmic shuttling sequence in HuR. *Proc. Natl. Acad. Sci. USA* **1998**, *95*, 15293–15298. [CrossRef]
58. Brennan, C.M.; Gallouzi, I.E.; Steitz, J.A. Protein ligands to HuR modulate its interaction with target mRNAs in vivo. *J. Cell Biol.* **2000**, *151*, 1–14. [CrossRef]
59. Rebane, A.; Aab, A.; Steitz, J.A. Transportins 1 and 2 are redundant nuclear import factors for hnRNP A1 and HuR. *RNA* **2004**, *10*, 590–599. [CrossRef]
60. Wang, W.; Yang, X.; Kawai, T.; López de Silanes, I.; Mazan-Mamczarz, K.; Chen, P.; Gorospe, M. AMP-activated protein kinase-regulated phosphorylation and acetylation of importin alpha1: Involvement in the nuclear import of RNA-binding protein HuR. *J. Biol. Chem.* **2004**, *279*, 48376–48388. [CrossRef]
61. Bychkov, E.; Zurkovsky, L.; Garret, M.B.; Ahmed, M.R.; Gurevich, E.V. Distinct cellular and subcellular distributions of G protein-coupled receptor kinase and arrestin isoforms in the striatum. *PLoS ONE* **2012**, *7*, e48912. [CrossRef] [PubMed]
62. Wang, H.; Zeng, F.; Liu, Q.; Liu, H.; Liu, Z.; Niu, L.; Li, X. The structure of the ARE-binding domains of Hu antigen R (HuR) undergoes conformational changes during RNA binding. *Acta Crystallogr. D Biol. Crystallogr.* **2013**, *69*, 373–380. [CrossRef] [PubMed]
63. Lal, P.; Cerofolini, L.; D'Agostino, V.G.; Zucal, C.; Fuccio, C.; Bonomo, I.; Preet, R. Regulation of HuR structure and function by dihydrotanshinone-I. *Nucleic Acids Res.* **2017**, *45*, 9514–9527. [CrossRef] [PubMed]
64. Abdelmohsen, K.; Srikantan, S.; Yang, X.; Lal, A.; Kim, H.H.; Kuwano, Y.; Gorospe, M. Ubiquitin-mediated proteolysis of HuR by heat shock. *EMBO J.* **2009**, *28*, 1271–1282. [CrossRef] [PubMed]
65. Zhang, Z.; Huang, A.; Zhang, A.; Zhou, C. HuR promotes breast cancer cell proliferation and survival via binding to CDK3 mRNA. *Biomed. Pharmacother.* **2017**, *91*, 788–795. [CrossRef]
66. Calaluce, R.; Gubin, M.M.; Davis, J.W.; Magee, J.D.; Chen, J.; Kuwano, Y.; Atasoy, U. The RNA binding protein HuR differentially regulates unique subsets of mRNAs in estrogen receptor negative and estrogen receptor positive breast cancer. *BMC Cancer* **2010**, *10*, 126. [CrossRef]
67. Galbán, S.; Kuwano, Y.; Pullmann, R., Jr.; Martindale, J.L.; Kim, H.H.; Lal, A.; Lewis, S.M. RNA-binding proteins HuR and PTB promote the translation of hypoxia-inducible factor 1alpha. *Mol. Cell. Biol.* **2008**, *28*, 93–107. [CrossRef]
68. Sheflin, L.G.; Zou, A.P.; Spaulding, S.W. Androgens regulate the binding of endogenous HuR to the AU-rich 3'UTRs of HIF-1alpha and EGF mRNA. *Biochem. Biophys. Res. Commun.* **2004**, *322*, 644–651. [CrossRef]
69. Yasuda, M.; Hatanaka, T.; Shirato, H.; Nishioka, T. Cell type-specific reciprocal regulation of HIF1A gene expression is dependent on 5'- and 3'-UTRs. *Biochem. Biophys. Res. Commun.* **2014**, *447*, 638–643. [CrossRef]

70. Mitsunari, K.; Miyata, Y.; Asai, A.; Matsuo, T.; Shida, Y.; Hakariya, T.; Sakai, H. Human antigen R is positively associated with malignant aggressiveness via upregulation of cell proliferation, migration, and vascular endothelial growth factors and cyclooxygenase-2 in prostate cancer. *Transl. Res.* **2016**, *175*, 116–128. [CrossRef]
71. Morfoisse, F.; Kuchnio, A.; Frainay, C.; Gomez-Brouchet, A.; Delisle, M.B.; Marzi, S.; Bousquet, C. Hypoxia induces VEGF-C expression in metastatic tumor cells via a HIF-1α-independent translation-mediated mechanism. *Cell Rep.* **2014**, *6*, 155–167. [CrossRef]
72. Choy, C.; Raytis, J.L.; Smit, D.D.; Duenas, M.; Neman, J.; Jandial, R.; Lew, M.W. Inhibition of β2-adrenergic receptor reduces triple-negative breast cancer brain metastases: The potential benefit of perioperative β-blockade. *Oncol. Rep.* **2016**, *35*, 3135–3142. [CrossRef]
73. Lutgendorf, S.K.; Cole, S.; Costanzo, E.; Bradley, S.; Coffin, J.; Jabbari, S.; Sood, A.K. Stress-related mediators stimulate vascular endothelial growth factor secretion by two ovarian cancer cell lines. *Clin. Cancer Res.* **2003**, *9*, 4514–4521.
74. Jafferjee, M.; Reyes Valero, T.; Marrero, C.; McCrink, K.A.; Brill, A.; Lymperopoulos, A. GRK2 Up-Regulation Creates a Positive Feedback Loop for Catecholamine Production in Chromaffin. *Cells Mol. Endocrinol.* **2016**, *30*, 372–381.
75. Aluja, D.; Inserte, J.; Penela, P.; Ramos, P.; Ribas, C.; Iñiguez, M.Á.; Garcia-Dorado, D. Calpains mediate isoproterenol-induced hypertrophy through modulation of GRK2. *Basic Res. Cardiol.* **2019**, *114*, 21. [CrossRef] [PubMed]
76. Yin, Q.; Yang, C.; Wu, J.; Lu, H.; Zheng, X.; Zhang, Y.; Li, Z. Downregulation of β-Adrenoceptors in Isoproterenol-Induced Cardiac Remodeling through HuR. *PLoS ONE* **2016**, *11*, e0152005. [CrossRef] [PubMed]
77. Shenoy, S.K.; Drake, M.T.; Nelson, C.D.; Houtz, D.A.; Xiao, K.; Madabushi, S.; Lefkowitz, R.J. β-Arrestin-dependent, G protein-independent ERK1/2 activation by the beta2 adrenergic receptor. *J. Biol. Chem.* **2006**, *281*, 1261–1273. [CrossRef] [PubMed]
78. O'Hayre, M.; Eichel, K.; Avino, S.; Zhao, X.; Steffen, D.J.; Feng, X.; Inoue, A. Genetic evidence that β-arrestins are dispensable for the initiation of β2-adrenergic receptor signaling to ERK. *Sci. Signal* **2017**, *10*, eaal3395. [CrossRef]
79. Sun, Y.; Huang, J.; Xiang, Y.; Bastepe, M.; Jüppner, H.; Kobilka, B.K.; Huang, X.Y. Dosage-dependent switch from G protein-coupled to G protein-independent signaling by a GPCR. *EMBO J.* **2007**, *26*, 53–64. [CrossRef]
80. Keene, D.; Komisarow, J.M.; Friedersdorf, M.B. RIP-Chip: The isolation and identification of mRNAs, microRNAs and protein components of ribonucleoprotein complexes from cell extracts. *Nat. Protoc.* **2006**, *1*, 302. [CrossRef]
81. Cortazar, A.R.; Torrano, V.; Martín-Martín, N.; Caro-Maldonado, A.; Camacho, L.; Hermanova, I.; Apaolaza, I. CANCERTOOL: A Visualization and Representation Interface to Exploit Cancer Datasets. *Cancer Res.* **2018**, *78*, 6320–6328. [CrossRef] [PubMed]

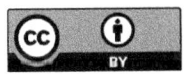

© 2020 by the authors. Licensee MDPI, Basel, Switzerland. This article is an open access article distributed under the terms and conditions of the Creative Commons Attribution (CC BY) license (http://creativecommons.org/licenses/by/4.0/).

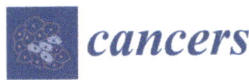

Article

Uncovering Tumour Heterogeneity through PKR and nc886 Analysis in Metastatic Colon Cancer Patients Treated with 5-FU-Based Chemotherapy

María Belén Ortega-García [1,2,3,4], Alberto Mesa [5], Elisa L.J. Moya [1], Beatriz Rueda [6], Gabriel Lopez-Ordoño [7], Javier Ángel García [2], Verónica Conde [2], Eduardo Redondo-Cerezo [8], Javier Luis Lopez-Hidalgo [6], Gema Jiménez [1,3,4], Macarena Peran [4,9], Luis J. Martínez-González [10], Coral del Val [1,5,11], Igor Zwir [1,5,11,12], Juan Antonio Marchal [1,3,4,13,*] and María Ángel García [1,3,4,14,*]

1. Instituto de Investigación Biosanitaria ibs.GRANADA, 18012 Granada, Spain; bgorteg@correo.ugr.es (M.B.O.-G.); elisajimenezmoya@correo.ugr.es (E.L.J.M.); gemajg@ugr.es (G.J.); delval@decsai.ugr.es (C.d.V.); jorgezwir@wustl.edu (I.Z.)
2. Department of Oncology, Virgen de las Nieves University Hospital, 18014 Granada, Spain; javier.garcia.garcia.sspa@juntadeandalucia.es (J.Á.G.); veronica.conde.sspa@juntadeandalucia.es (V.C.)
3. Biopathology and Regenerative Medicine Institute (IBIMER), Centre for Biomedical Research, (CIBM) University of Granada, 18100 Granada, Spain
4. Excellence Research Unit "Modelling Nature" (MNat), University of Granada, 18071 Granada, Spain; mperan@ujaen.es
5. Andalusian Research Institute in Data Science and Computational Intelligence (DaSCI Institute), 18014 Granada, Spain; alber12@correo.ugr.es
6. Department of Pathology, San Cecilio University Hospital, 18016 Granada, Spain; beatriz.rueda.sspa@juntadeandalucia.es (B.R.); javierl.lopez.sspa@juntadeandalucia.es (J.L.L.-H.)
7. Department of Gastroenterology, Torrecardenas Hospital, 04009 Almería, Spain; gabriel.lopez.sspa@juntadeandalucia.es
8. Department of Gastroenterology, Virgen de las Nieves University Hospital, 18014 Granada, Spain; Eduardo.redondo.sspa@juntadeandalucia.es
9. Department of Health Sciences, University of Jaén, 23071 Jaen, Spain
10. GENYO: Centre for Genomics and Oncological Research: Pfizer/University of Granada/Andalusian Regional Government, PTS, 18007 Granada, Spain; luisjavier.martinez@genyo.es
11. Department of Computer Science and Artificial Intelligence, University of Granada, 18071 Granada, Spain
12. Department of Psychiatry, Washington University School of Medicine, St Louis, MO 63110, USA
13. Department of Human Anatomy and Embryology, University of Granada, 18016 Granada, Spain
14. Department of Biochemistry and Molecular Biology III, University of Granada, 18016 Granada, Spain
* Correspondence: jmarchal@ugr.es (J.A.M.); mangelgarcia@ugr.es (M.Á.G.)

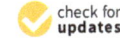

Received: 15 January 2020; Accepted: 4 February 2020; Published: 7 February 2020

Abstract: Colorectal cancer treatment has advanced over the past decade. The drug 5-fluorouracil is still used with a wide percentage of patients who do not respond. Therefore, a challenge is the identification of predictive biomarkers. The protein kinase R (PKR also called EIF2AK2) and its regulator, the non-coding pre-mir-nc886, have multiple effects on cells in response to numerous types of stress, including chemotherapy. In this work, we performed an ambispective study with 197 metastatic colon cancer patients with unresectable metastases to determine the relative expression levels of both nc886 and PKR by qPCR, as well as the location of PKR by immunohistochemistry in tumour samples and healthy tissues (plasma and colon epithelium). As primary end point, the expression levels were related to the objective response to first-line chemotherapy following the response evaluation criteria in solid tumours (RECIST) and, as the second end point, with survival at 18 and 36 months. Hierarchical agglomerative clustering was performed to accommodate the heterogeneity and complexity of oncological patients' data. High expression levels of nc886 were related to the response to treatment and allowed to identify clusters of patients. Although the PKR mRNA expression was not associated with chemotherapy response, the absence of PKR location in the nucleolus was correlated with first-line chemotherapy response. Moreover, a relationship between survival and the expression of both PKR and nc886 in healthy tissues was found. Therefore, this work evaluated the best way to analyse the potential biomarkers PKR and nc886 in order to establish clusters of patients depending on the cancer outcomes using algorithms for complex and heterogeneous data.

Keywords: colorectal cancer; 5-fluorouracil-based chemotherapy; protein kinase PKR; non-coding nc886; ambispective study; cluster of patients; biomarkers

1. Introduction

Colorectal cancer (CRC) is one of the most common forms of cancer worldwide, being the third most commonly diagnosed malignancy and the second leading cause of cancer death in recent years [1]. Although CRC treatment has advanced over the past decades, treatment outcomes depend, in part, on tumour- and patient-specific molecular characteristics [2]. Even though many novel drugs have been developed for patients with advanced CRC, 5-fluorouracil (5-FU) is still widely used as the classic and basic drug in adjuvant chemotherapy and palliative care. 5-FU is used as an infusion, taken orally (capecitabine), or used in combination with different drugs (FOLFOX, FOLFIRI) but its efficacy is limited by numerous factors including tumour cell genetics, epigenetics, and proteomics, which promote chemoresistance and metastasis [2]. In the last decade, the efficacy of these regimens has been increased by incorporating new biological therapies based on the use of monoclonal antibodies [3]. Despite the fact of the considerable improvement in the efficacy, there are still a wide percentage of patients who do not benefit from 5-FU-based treatments. Therefore, the identification of biomarkers that associate or predict the benefit of an appropriate selection of candidates for 5-FU-based therapies and combined therapies constitutes a broad area in clinical and translational research.

The protein kinase R (PKR, also called EIF2AK2) is an interferon-inducible double-stranded RNA protein kinase with multiple effects on cells. This protein kinase plays an active part in the cellular response to numerous types of stress mediating in several biological pathways and with a potent role in the induction of apoptosis in response to numerous compounds [4]. PKR is a serine-threonine kinase, composed by the kinase domain shared by the other eukaryotic initiation factor 2 alpha (eIF2α) kinases, and two dsRNA binding domains (dsRBD) that regulate its activity. PKR autophosphorylation represents the activation reaction that leads to the phosphorylation of eIF-2α, impairing eIF-2 activity, which results in the inhibition of protein synthesis [5]. In addition to its translational regulatory function, PKR has a role in signal transduction and transcriptional control through the IκB inhibitor/ nuclear transcription factor NF-κB pathway [6]. Although the primary PKR activator is dsRNA—produced during infection by several viruses and detected at low levels in mammalian cells—PKR is also activated by a variety of cellular stresses including cytokines, calcium stress, oxidative stress, endoplasmic reticulum stress, lipo-stress, amyloid-β (Aβ) peptide accumulation, polyanions such as heparin, and several drugs, or through the PKR-associated activator (PACT) [7]. PKR, which is expressed constitutively in mammalian cells, has also been implicated in the control of cell growth and differentiation with debated antitumor role and as an important antiviral agent [7]. Recently, the role of PKR related to metabolism, inflammatory processes, cancer, and neurodegenerative diseases has gained great interest [7,8].

The importance of PKR function in cell growth, differentiation, stress response, and immunomodulation is further noted by the existence of numerous modulators. Therefore, it has been identified that several PKR regulators are involved in cancer outcome, where the non-coding RNA pre-miR-886, also called nc886 or vault vtRNA 2-1, has been described as a potent regulator of PKR [9–11]. Nc886 binds to PKR with an affinity comparable to dsRNA and prevents PKR from being activated, in contrast to the PKR-activating ligand dsRNA [9–11]. Although nc886 was initially discovered as a PKR inhibitor, recently researchers have demonstrated that nc886 can adopt two structurally distinct conformers that are functionally opposing regulators of PKR [12,13].

We have previously identified PKR as a molecular target of 5-FU in several colon and breast cancer cells lines, playing an important role in the cytotoxic effect of 5-FU at least, in part, through the induction of cell death by apoptosis [14]. Because PKR has also been implicated in the anti-tumour activity of chemotherapeutic drugs such as doxorubicin (DOX) and etoposide [15,16], and nc886 has been identified as an interesting tumour suppressor [17–19], we consider the analysis of PKR and the nc886 in patients as potential predictive biomarkers to be of clinical importance. For this reason, the aim of this work was to carry out an ambispective study in 197 metastatic colon cancer patients to evaluate the expression levels of PKR and its pre-microRNA-nc886 by qPCR in colon tumour samples and their respective healthy tissues and plasma, analysing its relation with the patient's clinical evolution. The primary end point was the evaluation of these variables with the objective response (OR) to first-line of 5-FU-based chemotherapy determined by the response evaluation criteria in solid tumours (RECIST). As the second end point, we also analysed the relationship of these variables with overall survival (OS) at 18 and 36 months in those patients when the information was available. In addition, we analysed the PKR location by immunohistochemistry in 76 colon tumours and its respective colon healthy tissues. For all of this study, novel bioinformatic analyses have been included in order to distinguish parameters and signals for the identification of different profiles in patients, who have the same diagnostic and disease. Hence, clustering analyses were done using hierarchical agglomerative clustering (Statistical Toolbox, Matlab 2007, Spotfire Decision Site 9.1.2) [20], with the objective of improving the quality and specificity of the results considering the heterogeneity between samples and the genetic and proteomic background of oncologic patients.

2. Materials and Methods

2.1. Patients and Samples

The study was approved by the Biomedical Research Ethics Committee of Granada (Cod Peiba. 0170-N-16) and informed patient consent was obtained. The process of recruitment, traceability of samples, and informed consent was regulated and controlled by the Andalusian Public Health System Biobank (BBSSPA), according to the World Medical Association Declaration of Helsinki.

The study included a total of 197 colon metastatic cancer patients with unresectable lung or liver metastases from September 2014 through to September 2018 who were treated with 5-FU-based therapy as first-line treatment using the standard treatment schedule. To avoid discarding as few samples as possible, the missing values were approximated to the median value established for each variable analysed (see the supplementary Excel document with available data in Figure S1). Criteria of the RECIST guidelines were used to characterize the response to this treatment [21,22]. According to these criteria, after the first restaging assessment that was generally performed around 3–4 months after the initiation of 5-FU-based treatment, patients with progressive disease were considered as non-responders with primary resistance and those patients with partial response or stable disease under the 5-FU treatment for at least 3–4 months were considered as responders. Survival was considered after 18 months and 36 months in those patients where the data were available (see the supplementary Excel document with available data in Figure S1).

Tumours were classified according to the 2002 tumour, node, metastasis (TNM) classification and the Fuhrman grading system by experienced pathologists (B.R. and J.L.L.-H.) [23]. Archived formalin-fixed paraffin-embedded (FFPE) tissue samples from colon tumour and their corresponding surrounding healthy colon tissues obtained for routine diagnostic purposes were used in this study.

Peripheral blood samples of subjects were collected prospectively with one tube for EDTA anticoagulant (3 mL). Samples were centrifuged at 3000 rpm for 10 min and, then, aliquoted and frozen at −80 °C until use. The flow diagram shown in Figure 1 outlines the steps performed in this ambispective study.

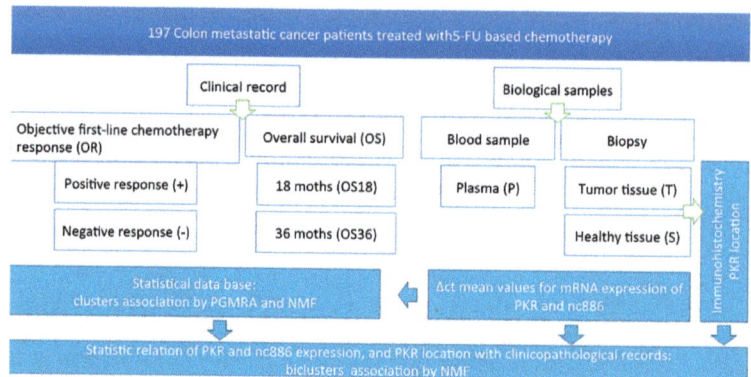

Figure 1. Flowchart of the ambispective study.

2.2. RNA Extraction from FFPE Tissue and from Plasma Sample

Haematoxylin and eosin-stained histological FFPE sections were prepared to identify areas of normal and tumour tissue. These regions of interest were biopsied by macrodissection after the xylene-alcohol dewaxing performed by specialist pathologists (Atrys Health S.A., Gr, SP). The tissue of interest was scraped with a scalpel and dipped in lysis buffer (ATL) (Qiagen, Hi, GE). Only tumour samples with more than 80% cancer cells were considered for further analysis. Non-malignant tissue with a distance of >100 mm to the cancer tissue was collected from all patients of the study cohort for comparison purposes. Total RNA was isolated from the dissected FFPE tissue samples using an miRNeasy FFPE Kit (Qiagen, Hi, Ge) and from plasma using the miRNeasy Serum-Plasma Kit (Qiagen, Hi, Ge) following the recommended protocol by previous concentration of 300 µL of cold plasma using the Vacufuge Concentrator system (Eppendorf, GE). Both RNA isolations were automated using the QIAcube (Qiagen, Hi, GE). Integrity and quality of RNA (RIN) was tested with Bioanalyzer (Agilent, CA) and diluted to a maximum concentration of 500 ng in 14 µL. The reverse transcription was performed with the SuperScript VILO cDNA Synthesis Kit (Invitrogen-Thermo Fisher Scientific, USA) on all samples (4 µL 5X VILO Reaction Mix, 2 µL 10X SuperScript Enzyme Mix, 14 µL RNA, 10 min at 25 °C, 60 min at 42 °C, and 5 min at 85 °C).

2.3. RT qPCR Assay

The determination of the expression of PKR gene and nc886 element was carried out in plasma, tumours, and healthy colon tissues from patients enrolled in this ambispective study. To determine the expression of the PKR (EIF2AK2) gene and nc886 (VTRNA2) element, specific fluorescent hydrolysis probes TaqMan-MGB (Thermo Fisher Scientific, MA, USA) were used (Hs01091582_m1, Hs04273370_s1, respectively) by real-time qPCR and by digital dPCR in different samples (Figures S2 and S3). To select the most appropriate endogenous control, we analysed the endogenous classic Glyceraldehyde 3-phosphate dehydrogenase (GADPH), Hypoxanthine-guanine phosphoribosyltransferase (HPRT), and β2 microglobulin (B2M) genes [24] by several tests to assess their stability in different types of tissue by qPCR (Figure S4). Due to the results obtained, B2M (Hs00187842_m1) was considered as the endogenous control for plasma and FFPE tissue samples. For the amplification of the samples, the "TaqMan Gene Expression Master Mix" protocol was adapted to a final volume of 10 µL in the QuantStudio 12K Flex system (Thermo Fisher Scientific, MA, USA). The mean Ct-values were technically normalized using the endogenous B2M, and the expression level was considered as $2^{-\Delta Ct}$ ($\Delta Ct = Ct_{targetgene} - Ct_{B2M}$) [25–27]. The missing values were approximated to the median value established for each variable analysed (see the supplementary Excel document in Figure S1).

2.4. Immunohistochemistry Analysis

Formalin-fixed paraffin-embedded samples ($n = 76$) were cut at 2.5 µm in thickness and placed on a slide. The antigenic retrieval was carried out by incubating the antibody for 30 min with hydrogen peroxide (H_2O_2) at pH 8. The immunohistochemical technique was carried out on the Lab Vision Autostainer 480S (Thermo Fisher Scientific, MA, USA). For the development of the technique, the Commercial Kit Detection System Master Polymer Plus (Peroxidase) was used. The polyclonal anti-PKR antibody was administered by Santa Cruz Biotechnology, and it was used with a 1:50 dilution in 30 min of incubation. The development of the technique was carried out with diaminobenzidine (DAB) and after, with hematoxylin and eosin staining. The immunohistochemical location of the PKR protein was determined by two pathologists that considered the presence of the PKR protein in the nucleolus or outside of nucleolus (mostly located in cytoplasm).

2.5. Machine Learning and Statistical Analysis

PGMRA is a deep unsupervised [28,29] and data-driven machine learning method that combines model-based, consensus, fuzzy, possibilistic, relational, optimization, and conceptual clustering techniques into a single method (see the supplementary material in [30] for a review, [20,31]). The model-based approach uses non-negative matrix factorization to identify candidates for functional clusters [20,32] represented as tensors or flattened biclusters (e.g., subjects × symptoms). Biclusters can be learned independently of the number of clusters, and thus, from different granularity partitions (consensus). The method separately searches for biclusters in distinct domains of knowledge (e.g., genetics, clinical symptoms) without regard for their calculations in other domains of knowledge [33]. Then, the approach agnostically co-clusters the inter-domain biclusters and identifies natural relationships (associations) among them. Associations result from optimizing the probability of the intersection among biclusters using hypergeometric statistics or Fisher's exact test [34,35] evaluated by a posterior permutation test instead of using typical inter/intra clustering metrics among dots in the n-dimensional space (model-based). Biclusters in one domain of knowledge or associations of biclusters from different domains of knowledge can be reorganized into networks at different levels of granularity, connected by sharing observations (subjects) and/or features (Δct mean values, objective first-line chemotherapy response). This framework constitutes a knowledge base and characterizes architecture of the disease. The methodological basis of PGMRA is available in [20,31,34–36], and its web server application is online at http://phop.ugr.es/fenogeno [20]. Fast parallel software implementations were run at the Centre for High Performance Computing (CHPC) facility at Washington University School of Medicine (WUSM).

2.6. Derivation of the Empirical Index

First, we calculated a purely empirical (i.e., agnostic and data-driven) indicator of character functioning. We clustered subjects corresponding to the two expression variables and assigned each subject the number of the cluster to which they belonged (as described in the next paragraph). The result was a single empirical index of cluster membership that served as a comprehensive measure of variability in the RNA expression.

To calculate the cluster rankings, we applied hierarchical agglomerative clustering (Statistical Toolbox, Matlab 2007b) [20] with a complete linkage method and correlation similarity measurement to group value phenotypic or environmental sets by their shared subjects using hypergeometric statistics. The function that controls the vertical order in which a row is plotted (Spotfire Decision Site 9.1.2) in a hierarchical clustering is defined as follows.

Given two sub-clusters within a cluster (there are always exactly two sub-clusters considered at each step), both sub-clusters are weighted and the sub-cluster with the highest weight is placed above the other sub-cluster. This function is systematically applied until a single cluster containing all rows is obtained. To calculate the weight w_3 of a new cluster, C_3 is formed from two sub-clusters C_1 and C_2 with a weight of w_1 and w_2, and each containing n_1 and n_2 rows, and the following expression is used:

$$w3 = \frac{n_1 \times w_1 + n_2 \times w_2}{(n_1 + n_2)} \qquad (1)$$

The weight of a sub-cluster with a single row is calculated as the average value of its columns.

2.7. Feature Selection Process Using Non-Negative Matrix Factorization (NMF) in PGMRA

We use non-negative matrix factorization (NMF) method as a deep autoencoder [29] in a particular domain of knowledge (qPCR data, clinical data) to identify candidates for functional clusters [20,32], represented as tensors or flattened biclusters (e.g., unknown relationships embedded in the data (subjects × non-coding RNA differential expression)). Our implementation of the NMF, termed fuzzy NMF method (FNMF), learns [20,30] biclusters independently of the number of clusters, and thus, from different granularity partitions (consensus). The method separately searches for biclusters in distinct domains of knowledge without regard for their calculations in other domain of knowledge [33]. Then, the approach agnostically co-clusters the inter-domain biclusters and identifies natural relationships (associations) among them. Associations result from optimizing the probability of the intersection among biclusters using hypergeometric statistics instead of using typical inter/intra clustering metrics among dots in the ndimensional space (model-based). These associations are learned regardless of any status of the observations (e.g., cases and controls, unsupervised) and are optimized on the basis of multiobjective and multimodal optimization techniques [37]. By incorporating a posteriori, a "supervised" status, the method is able to calculate the risk of the association by the frequency of one status vs. another. Once it occurs, the method becomes semi-supervised, and posterior statistical significance of the association is calculated using kernel-based and multivariate statistical analyses [20,38].

3. Results

3.1. Normalized Values of Non Coding nc886 in Plasma and Tumor Tissues Predicted the Objective First-Line Chemotherapy Response

We tested first the association of the expression level of the PKR gene and the nc886 RNA molecule determined by the Δct mean values identified by qPCR in tumour (T), plasma (P), and healthy (S) tissues (see the supplementary Excel document in Figure S1) with the OR to first-line chemotherapy. The response was encoded as a Boolean (positive/responders, negative/non-responders) tested after 3–4 months of starting the treatment as indicated in the Material and Methods section.

We identified two biclusters (subjects sharing subsets of features) composed of subjects sharing P-nc886 Δct mean and T-nc886 Δct mean values (Figure 2A). These biclusters exhibited significantly different values of their composite features (Figure 2B, $p < 2.44655 \times 10^{-77}$ ANOVA statistics).

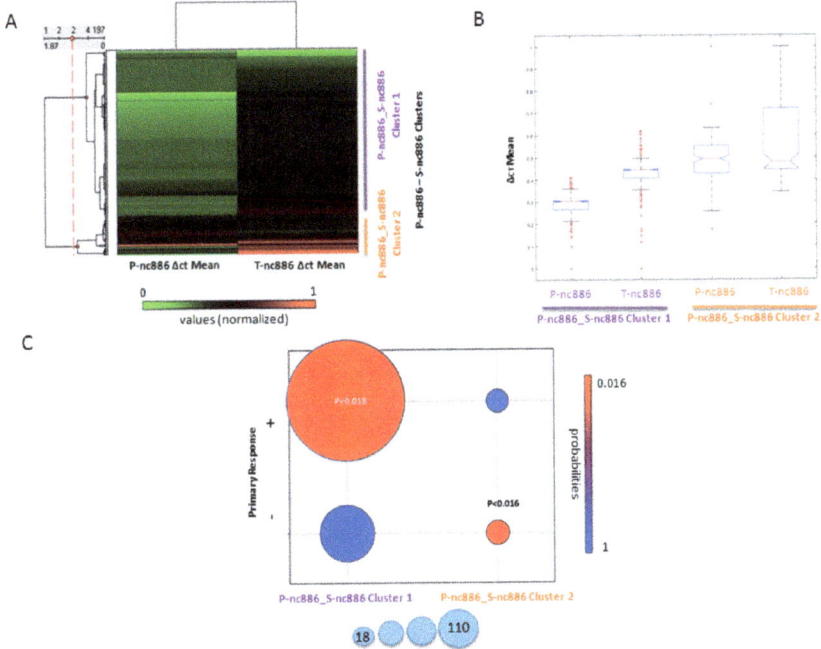

Figure 2. Association of the expression level of protein kinase R (PKR) and nc886 determined by the Δct mean values identified by RT qPCR in tumour (T), plasma (P), and healthy (S) tissues with the objective response to first-line chemotherapy. (**A**) P-T_nc886 clusters: Biclusters of subjects sharing Δct mean values of nc886 in P and T. Δct mean values are normalized between 0 (green) and 1 (red). (**B**) Boxplot of Δct mean values of nc886 in P and T for each cluster. (**C**) Correlation between the objective first-line chemotherapy response and the nc886 Δct mean clusters (Figure 2A). p-values were calculated with hypergeometric statistics. Colour code for p-values' statistical significance is indicated from high (red) to low (blue). The size of the circles indicates the number of individuals in the relationship.

Those subjects were significantly associated with the objective first-line chemotherapy response (Figure 2C). The first bicluster displayed low P-nc886 and mid/low T-nc886 Δct mean values and was associated with a positive response (Figure 2C, $p < 0.018$, hypergeometric statistics/Fisher's tests). The second bicluster exhibited high T-nc886 Δct mean values, and was associated with a negative response (Figure 2C, $p < 0.016$, hypergeometric statistics/Fisher's tests). The other studied variables that involved the expression of PKR in the different samples were not included in any bicluster significantly associated with the objective first-line chemotherapy response (see non-negative matrix factorization (NMF) in PGMRA as a feature selection process in the Materials and Methods section).

Once we detected the two highly associated variables, we independently validated the former results by performing a regression analysis between the cluster order (ranking, see the Materials and Methods section) and the individual features with respect to the OR to first-line chemotherapy. Δct values were normalized between [0,1] due to PGMRA requirements. We determined that the clusters, represented by the order of their observations, were better associated with the objective first-line chemotherapy response ($p < 0.00012$, F statistics) than the individual T-nc886 Δct mean values ($p < 0.0028$) and P-nc886 Δct mean values ($p < 0.013$) (data not shown). Moreover, all other variables involved in similar regressions were non-significantly associated with the OR.

Furthermore, because the relative level of gene expression is inversely proportional to the Δct mean value following the $2^{-\Delta Ct}$ method [26], our data suggest for cluster 1 a significant association between patients who showed high level of expression of nc886 in both plasma and tumour samples with a significant positive response to treatments based on the use of 5-FU. In contrast, cluster 2 included patients who mostly and significantly showed lower levels of nc886 expression in the tumour and a negative response to treatment. However, the levels of expression of the PKR gene were not related to the OR to first-line chemotherapy.

3.2. PKR Location Predicted the Objective First-Line Chemotherapy Response

Because the relative levels of expression of the PKR gene mRNA in the colon tumour could not be related to the patient's response to the treatment, we decided to analyse the location of PKR in the tumour and healthy colon tissue cells by immuhistochemistry ($n = 76$). Although PKR was located in all healthy tissues analysed at the level of the cytoplasm of the cells, in tumour samples its location could be restricted to the nucleolus in some cases (Figure 3). Therefore, we considered the two variables of presence or absence (located in the cytoplasm) of PKR in the nucleolus.

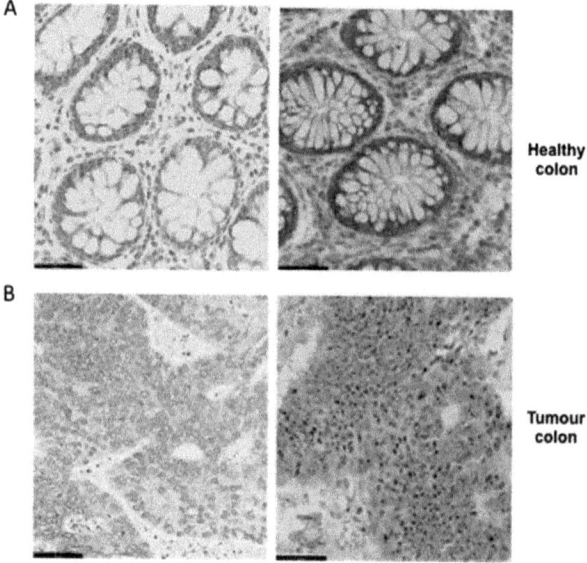

Figure 3. Different locations of PKR in healthy colon tissues and tumour tissues. (**A**) Representative immunohistochemical detection of total PKR in healthy colon tissues. PKR immunostaining was weak (first panel) or strong (second panel), but was mostly located in the cytoplasm of cells. Scale bar, 50 μm. (**B**) Representative immunohistochemical detection of total PKR in tumour colon tissues. PKR immunostaining was mostly located in the cytoplasm of cells (first panel); however, in several tumours, PKR was located heavily in the nucleolus (second panel). Scale bar, 50 μm.

To test the predictive value of the PKR location, we analysed the patients for which this information was available. Two biclusters were obtained by PGMRA when including PKR Δct mean values in P, T, and S (P-PKR, T-PKR, S-PKR) and the Δct mean values of nc886 in P, T, and S (T-nc886, P-nc886, S-nc886) (Figure 4A). The first bicluster displayed variable Δct mean values (high S-PKR, medium P-PKR, low or medium T-PKR and T-nc886, high or medium S-nc886, and medium P-nc886 values). A second bicluster was composed also of variable Δct mean values (high P-nc886 and T-nc886, medium S-PKR and T-PKR, and low P-PKR and S-nc886 values). These biclusters exhibited significant different values of their composite features (Figure 4B, $p < 2.05581 \times 10^{-204}$ ANOVA statistics). The main differences between clusters included variables in colon tumour and colon healthy tissues (Figure 4B). The first bicluster matched with the absence of PKR in the nucleolus (Figure 4C, $p < 0.00001$, hypergeometric statistics/Fisher's tests). The second bicluster was associated with a presence of PKR in the nucleolus (Figure 4C, $p < 0.00005$, hypergeometric statistics/Fisher's tests).

We independently validated the former results by calculating using ANOVA statistics with the six variables previously selected. We determined that the clusters were significantly better associated with the presence of PKR in the nucleolus ($p < 0.000002$) than the individual values ($p < 0.035$). The bicluster lacking PKR location in the nucleolus showed a relation to the positive first-line chemotherapy response (Figure 4D, $p < 0.006$, hypergeometric statistics), and the bicluster with PKR location in the nucleolus showed a relation to the negative first-line chemotherapy response (Figure 4D, $p < 0.03$, hypergeometric statistics).

Therefore, the analysis was able to group patients whose PKR location in the cytoplasm of the tumour cells corresponded with a positive response to the treatment, and in contrast, patients with PKR restricted to the nucleolus could be grouped in clusters that corresponded with the negative response to treatment. Although the expression levels of PKR and nc886 in the different tissues analysed were necessary to determine these significant clusters, these levels were highly variable.

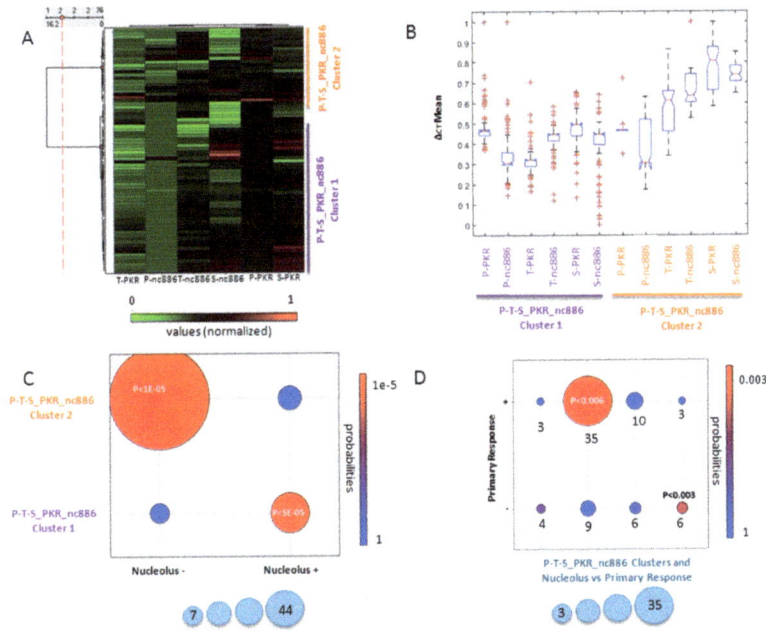

Figure 4. Association of the PKR location with Δct mean values identified by RT qPCR in tumor (T), plasma (P), and healthy (S) tissues and the objective response to first-line chemotherapy. (**A**) Clusters P-T-S_PKR_nc886: Biclusters of subjects sharing Δct mean values of PKR determined in the analysed tissues (P-PKR, T-PKR, S-PKR) and Δct mean values of nc886 determined in the analysed tissues (T-nc886, P-nc886, S-nc886). Δct Mean values are normalized between 0 (green) and 1 (red). (**B**) Boxplot of Δct mean values of PKR determined in the analysed tissues (P-PKR, T-PKR, S-PKR) and Δct mean values of nc886 determined in the analysed tissues (T-nc886, P-nc886, S-nc886) for each cluster P-T-S_PKR_nc886. (**C**) Co-clustering between the PKR location in the nucleolus and the clusters P-T-S_PKR_nc886. *p*-values were calculated with hypergeometric statistics. Colour code for *p*-values' statistical significance is indicated from high (red) to low (blue). The size of the circles indicates the number of individuals in the relationship. (**D**) Co-clustering occurred between the objective first-line chemotherapy response and the co-clusters identified in (**C**). *p*-values were calculated with hypergeometric statistics. Colour code for *p*-values' statistical significance is indicated from high (red) to low (blue). The size of the circles indicates the number of individuals in the relationship.

3.3. Final Outcome Was Predicted by the Expression Level of PKR and nc886 in Healthy Tissues

Finally, we raised the question about the correlation between the OR to first-line chemotherapy and the time-range patient survival after 18 and 36 months. To test the predictability effect of the measured variables, we first applied the PGMRA method to separately factorize these three measurements using NMF and we uncovered three biclusters, now called "survival clusters" (Figure 5A). Survival cluster 1 involved patients who mostly showed a negative response to the first line of treatment and died before 18 months (Figure 5A). Survival cluster 2 included patients who mostly showed a positive response to the first line of treatment and were alive after 18 months; however, they died before reaching 36 months (Figure 5A). Survival cluster 3 involved all patients who mostly showed a positive response to the first line of treatment and were alive after 18 and 36 months (Figure 5A).

On the other hand, independently, PGMRA selected the expression values of PKR and the nc886 in P, T, and S for two biclusters (Figure 5B). We found two clusters based on colon healthy tissue values from PKR and nc886, from now on called S-PKR_S-nc886 clusters. S-PKR_S-nc886 cluster 1 included a large number of patients mostly with low Δct mean values for nc886 and PKR. S-PKR_S-nc886 cluster 2 included fewer number of patients mostly with high Δct mean values for nc886 and PKR (Figure 5B). These S-PKR_S-nc886 biclusters exhibited significantly different values of their composite features (Figure 5C, $p < 2,48689 \times 10^{-136}$ ANOVA statistics).

Finally, we co-clustered the S-PKR_S-nc886 clusters with the survival clusters, identifying two significant associations. The most representative bicluster displayed low nc886 Δct mean values and medium PKR Δct mean values in healthy tissues (Figure 5D). This cluster was associated with a positive objective first-line chemotherapy response, and a long time-range patient survival (Figure 5D, $p < 0.014$, hypergeometric statistics/Fisher's tests). Therefore, higher expression levels of nc886 once again selected patients with better disease outcomes. The other significant bicluster exhibited high Δct mean values in healthy colon tissue of the two variables PKR and nc886 (Figure 5D), and was associated with negative objective first-line chemotherapy response and short survival (Figure 5D, $p < 0.016$, hypergeometric statistics/Fisher's tests). Therefore, lower expression levels of nc886 and PKR in healthy colon tissue selected patients with worst disease outcomes. A non-significant survival bicluster exhibiting a mixture survival values was not significantly associated with nc886 and PKR Δct mean values in healthy tissues (Figure 5D).

The three survival classes were independently validated using regression analysis with the clusters (rankings, see the Materials and Methods section) of healthy tissue nc886 Δct mean values and the healthy tissue PKR Δct mean values ($p < 0.0053$, F statistics).

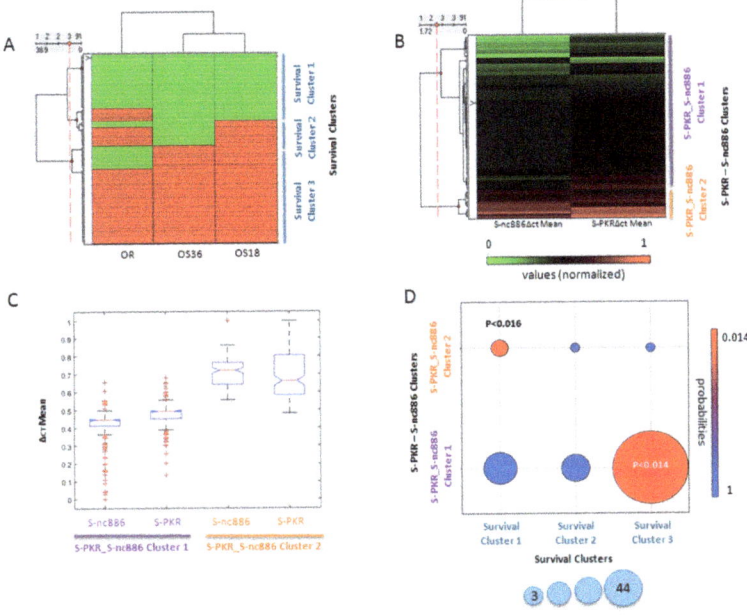

Figure 5. Correlation between the objective first-line chemotherapy response and the time-range patient survival with the Δct mean values identified by RT qPCR in colon healthy (S) tissue. (**A**) Survival clusters: Biclusters of subjects according to their objective first-line chemotherapy response, and survival after 18 and 36 months. Values are coded as follows: negative response in green and positive response in red. (**B**) S-PKR-S-nc886 clusters: Biclusters of patients according to their Δct mean values of nc886 and PKR in healthy tissue (S-nc886 Δct mean, S-PKR). Δct mean values are normalized between 0 (green) and 1 (red). (**C**) Boxplot of S-PKR and S-nc886 Δct mean values in healthy tissue for each S-PKR-S-nc886 cluster. (**D**) Co-clustering between survival clusters and the S-PKR-S-nc886 clusters. p-values were calculated with hypergeometric statistics. Colour code for p-values' statistical significance is indicated from high (red) to low (blue). The size of the circles indicates the number of individuals in the relationship.

4. Discussion

The identification of biomarkers that associate or predict the benefit of an appropriate selection of patient candidates for both 5-FU-based and combined therapies constitutes a broad area useful in clinical and translational research of CRC disease. However, the low specificity of chemotherapy and the great heterogeneity of the patients and samples analysed make the search for predictive biomarkers very complex [2]. Tests for microsatellite instability (MSI) and for the detection of loss of heterozygosity for chromosome 18q (18qLOH) in the early stage of the disease are beginning to be evaluated for guiding therapeutic decisions regarding the administration of 5-FU-based treatments; however, these are still under investigation. Thus, it is necessary to explore new biomarkers that can increase the portfolio to the oncologists and facilitate taking better decisions in the treatment of CRC patients. In many cancers, mutation or abnormal expression or activity of protein kinases is correlated with tumorigenesis, metastasis, and resistance to chemotherapy [39]. This study identified clusters of metastatic colon cancer patients on the basis of the kinase PKR and its modulator nc886 after the analysis of tumours and healthy samples in relation to the response to chemotherapy based on the use of the 5-FU drug (Table 1).

Table 1. Clusters of patients associated with objective first-line chemotherapy response and with overall survival at 18 and 36 months.

Metastatic Colon Cancer Patients		Total	Sex		Age (Mean Years), SD	
			Male	Female		
		197	127	70	65.1 ± 10.5	
Firs-line Chemotherapy Response clusters (OR)		Total	Responders(+)	Non-Responders(-)	Δct mean values, SD	
		197	128	69		
P-nc886_S-nc886					T-nc886	P-nc886
	Cluster 1	160	110	50	0.427 ± 0.09	0.289 ± 0.05
	Cluster 2	37	18	19	0.567 ± 0.17	0.495 ± 0.14
S-PKR_S-nc886					S-nc886	S-PKR
	Cluster 1	77	45	32	0.386 ± 0.12	0.465 ± 0.09
	Cluster 2	14	6	8	0.682 ± 0.09	0.703 ± 0.16
Survival clusters (OS)			First-line Response		OS 18 m	OS 36 m
Survival			+	−	Survival Exitus	Survival Exitus
	Cluster 1	26	0	26	0 26	0 26
	Cluster 2	18	15	3	12 6	0 18
	Cluster 3	47	36	11	47 0	47 0

In order to group patients sharing similar features within the existing heterogeneity, we approached this ambispective study using NMF techniques encoded into the PGMRA system [20]. This system was successfully used to identify complex genotypic–phenotypic architecture of mental disorders and personality traits [40], which has now been customized for cancer phenotypes. In contrast to classical clustering techniques, not all features are included in such associations, but only those that provide a multifaceted description of groups of patients at risk. These meaningful associations are termed biclusters [20,34].

When analysing the Δct mean values of nc886 in P and T, we identified two biclusters composed of subjects sharing Δct mean values of T-nc886 and P-nc886 that were associated with the OR to first-line chemotherapy. We found a significant association between patients with high levels of nc886 expression in both P and T, as well as a positive primary response to treatments based on 5-FU. Our results are consistent with previous results that show that nc886, as a Pol III transcript, is expressed abundantly and ubiquitously in all normal human tissues [41] and that its expression is increased in cancer cells [42]. In fact, most patients in our study expressed high levels of nc886 when considering the Δct mean values obtained in tumours (Table 1). The tumour suppressor role of nc886 has been already previously related to a better prognosis of the disease in several neoplasia such as lung, ovarian, and breast cancer, among others [17,19,43–45], but this study was the first time that has been related to CRC.

Moreover, we identified a smaller second significant cluster associating patients that showed a negative response to first-line treatment with lower levels of nc886 expression in the tumour. This result agrees with the previous results, where the expression of nc886 was found to be diminished or silenced in a subset of malignant cells by the DNA hypermethylation of its promoter's CpG island [17–19,44,45]. Although we did not analyse the level of silencing of nc886, our results are consistent with the poor outcome detected during nc886 epigenetic repression in several neoplasms, supporting the role of tumour suppressor of nc886 also in colon cancer disease.

The levels of PKR mRNA expression could not be associated to chemotherapy response in our analysis. The Ser/Thr kinase PKR is a non-canonical kinase involved in many cellular pathways exerting various functions on cell growth and tumorigenesis [4,7,8]. Although there have been multiple studies of PKR, the exact role in cancer biology remains controversial. This is due on one hand to its ability to induce eIF2α-mediated apoptosis and on the other hand to NF-κB-mediated pro-survival effect, involved in both tumour-suppressive or oncogenic roles [6–8,11,14]. Because we previously identified PKR as a molecular target of 5-FU in several colon cancer cells lines [14] playing an important role in the cytotoxic effect of 5-FU, through the induction of apoptosis, in a PKR expression-dependent manner, we expected a high expression level of the PKR gene in responder patients. However, the high level of post-translational modifications and regulation of the protein indicated that PKR activity does not necessarily have to correspond to the amount of its messenger RNA. In fact, numerous proteins have been described as regulating their activity (e.g., PACT, trans-activation response (TAR) RNA binding protein (TRBP), nucleophosmin (NPM)) [4,7,8,46–48] and several post-translational modifications have been showed by SUMOylation and ISGylation, among others [49,50]. Nc886 has been described as a PKR inhibitor, being the inhibition of PKR/NF-kB in correlation with its tumour suppressor activity. However, recently researchers have demonstrated that nc886 can adopt two structurally distinct conformers that are functionally opposing regulators of PKR that have a second conformation able to activate PKR [12]. Therefore, whether a high level of nc886 is related to a best response to 5-FU treatment that corresponds with a high ability of PKR to induce apoptosis is still unknown and needs further investigation. In addition, a different location of PKR in the nucleus and nucleolus has been demonstrated with different forms that also suggest differences in its activity [51,52]. It has been described that PKR localizes in the cytoplasm, strongly in the nucleolus, and diffusely throughout the nucleoplasm [52]. Our analysis of total PKR expression by immunohistochemistry in 76 samples of colon tumour and their respective healthy colon tissues showed expression in the cytoplasm in all healthy tissues and in most of the colon tumour analysed. However, a smaller group of tumours were shown diffuse staining in the nucleus and, above all, staining was restricted exclusively to the nucleolus. The PGMRA analysis considering the presence or absence of PKR in the nucleolus found a bicluster where patients with PKR located in tumour cytoplasm (and absent in the nucleolus) were related with OR to first-line chemotherapy. A cluster included patients whose PKR location in the cytoplasm of the tumour cells corresponded with a positive response to the treatment, and although the levels of expression of PKR and nc886 analysed were variable between samples, they were necessary to establish statistically significant clusters. In contrast, patients with PKR restricted to the nucleolus in the tumour could be grouped significantly in a cluster that corresponded with the negative response to treatment. Therefore, an increase in the number of samples to be analysed would be convenient in future research to specifically relate the levels of nc886 with the location of PKR and the response to treatment. Although the role that PKR activity may have in the nucleus/nucleolus is not yet known, it has been suggested that PKR exists in leukaemia cell lines and patient samples in diverse molecular weight forms in the nucleus as result of several post-translational modifications. Although cytoplasmic location was detected in leukaemia low-risk patients, nuclear location was restricted to high-risk patients [51]. In addition, intrahepatic PKR nucleolar labelling was observed in human blood PBMCs and liver biopsies, with a suggested ribosome biogenesis role [53].

Finally, we found different survival clusters in those patients for which information was available (Table 1), allowing for the grouping of patients according to the expression of nc886 and PKR in healthy colon tissue. Interestingly we found two clusters significantly related to the outcome of the patients; the most representative cluster included patients with higher expression levels of nc886 and medium expression levels of PKR in the healthy colon tissues who were alive after 3 years of the first-line treatment. In contrast, lower levels of expression of both PKR and nc886 in healthy colon tissue were related with patients who died at a year and a half after the first-line treatment. Although PKR levels did not appear to be related to their activity, as we have previously discussed, for tumour cells, they interestingly remained average in healthy tissue in the cluster of patients with the best outcome, and showed less expression in healthy tissue for the cluster with worse outcome. The role of PKR as a cellular stress response protein is widely known, as PKR intervenes against numerous and varied infections, also eliminating damaged cells inducing apoptosis. In addition, PKR is able to allow the cells to live via NF-kB activation once the stress has been resolved on time [4,7,8,13]. Moreover, PKR also regulates some tumour suppressors and protein kinases involved in cancer pathways such as the signal transducers and activators of transcription factors (STATs), activating transcription factors (ATFs), tumour suppressor p53 (Tp53), the phosphatase and tensin homologue tumour suppressor (PTEN), the mitogen-activated protein kinases (MAPKs), and the toll-like receptors (TLRs), among others [4,7,8,13]. All these data suggest how important it is that PKR is expressed at adequate levels in normal tissue where it would be slightly regulated, as well as the importance that PKR would have in tumours where, regardless of its expression, its regulation can be critical.

5. Conclusions

In summary, although it would be convenient to increase the "n", especially for studies where we have had less available data, we can consider that PGMA is a useful system for working with heterogeneous diseases such as cancer. PGMA analysis allowed us to identify clusters where the levels of expression of nc886 can be suggested as a potential biomarker for both the first-line response to chemotherapy and the survival of patients for at least 18 or 36 months. The higher levels of expression of nc886 in tumours, plasma, and healthy tissues were found in those patients with a better outcome. Although it is necessary to analyse a greater number of subjects to know the role of PKR as a biomarker, our data suggest that its location in the tumour cell compartments, but not its mRNA expression level, could predict the response to treatment based on the use of 5-FU in metastatic colon cancer patients.

Supplementary Materials: The following are available online at http://www.mdpi.com/2072-6694/12/2/379/s1: Figure S1: Excel document with data. Figure S2: Study of digital dPCR expression. Figure S3: Study of EIF2AK2 expression by dPCR and qPCR. Figure S4: Study of endogenous selection in qPCR.

Author Contributions: Conception and study design: M.Á.G., J.A.M., I.Z.; investigation: M.B.O.-G., G.J., M.P.; data curation: J.Á.G., V.C., G.L.-O., M.B.O.-G., E.R.-C., B.R., J.L.L.-H.; methodology: M.B.O.-G., A.M., E.L.J.M., L.J.M.-G.; software: C.d.V., I.Z.; writing—original draft: M.A.G., C.d.V., I.Z., J.A.M.; funding acquisition: M.A.G., J.A.M. All authors have read and agreed to the published version of the manuscript.

Funding: This research was funded by the Instituto de Salud Carlos III (DTS15/00174; PIE16-00045), by the Consejería de Economía, Conocimiento, Empresas y Universidad de la Junta de Andalucía and European Regional Development Fund (ERDF), references SOMM17/6109/UGR (UCE-PP2017-3) and (PI-0441-2014), and by the Chair "Doctors Galera-Requena in cancer stem cell research" (CMC-CTS963). This research was also funded partially by RTI2018-098983-B-I00.

Conflicts of Interest: The authors declare no conflict of interest.

References

1. Keum, N.; Giovannucci, E. Global burden of colorectal cancer: Emerging trends, risk factors and prevention strategies. *Nat. Rev. Gastroenterol. Hepatol.* **2019**, *16*, 713–732. [CrossRef] [PubMed]
2. Vacante, M.; Borzì, A.M.; Basile, F.; Biondi, A. Biomarkers in colorectal cancer: Current clinical utility and future perspectives. *World J. Clin. Cases* **2018**, *6*, 869–881. [CrossRef] [PubMed]
3. Van Cutsem, E.; de Haas, S.; Kang, Y.K.; Ohtsu, A.; Tebbutt, N.C.; Xu, J.M.; Yong, W.P.; Langer, B.; Delmar, P.; Scherer, S.J.; et al. Bevacizumab in Combination With Chemotherapy as First-Line Therapy in Advanced Gastric Cancer: A Biomarker Evaluation From the AVAGAST Randomized Phase III Trial. *J. Clin. Oncol.* **2012**, *30*, 2119–2127. [CrossRef] [PubMed]
4. Garcia, M.A.; Gil, J.; Ventoso, I.; Guerra, S.; Domingo, E.; Rivas, C.; Esteban, M. The impact of protein kinase PKR in cell biology: From antiviral to antiproliferative action. *Microbiol. Mol. Biol. Rev.* **2006**, *70*, 1032–1060. [CrossRef]
5. Der, S.D.; Yang, Y.L.; Weissmann, C.; Williams, B.R. A double stranded RNA-activated protein kinase-dependent pathway mediating stress-induced apoptosis. *Proc. Natl. Acad. Sci. USA* **1997**, *94*, 3279–3283. [CrossRef] [PubMed]
6. Gil, J.; Alcami, J.; Esteban, M. Activation of NFkappa B by the dsRNA-dependent protein kinase, PKR, involves the I kappa B kinase complex. *Oncogene* **2000**, *19*, 1369–1378. [CrossRef] [PubMed]

7. Marchal, J.A.; Lopez, G.J.; Peran, M.; Comino, A.; Delgado, J.R.; García-García, J.A.; Conde, V.; Aranda, F.M.; Rivas, C.; Esteban, M.; et al. The Impact of PKR activation:from Neurodegeneration to Cancer. *FASEB J.* 2014, *28*, 1965–1974. [CrossRef]
8. Garcia-Ortega, M.B.; Lopez, G.J.; Jimenez, G.; Garcia-Garcia, J.A.; Conde, V.; Boulaiz, H.; Carrillo, E.; Perán, M.; Marchal, J.A.; Garcia, M.A. Clinical and therapeutic potential of protein kinase PKR in cancer and metabolism. *Expert Rev. Mol. Med.* 2017, *19*, e9. [CrossRef]
9. Kunkeaw, N.; Jeon, S.H.; Lee, K.; Johnson, B.H.; Tanasanvimon, S.; Javle, M.; Pairojkul, C.; Chamgramol, Y.; Wongfieng, W.; Gong, B.; et al. Cell death/proliferation roles for nc886, a non-coding RNA, in the protein kinase R pathway in cholangiocarcinoma. *Oncogene* 2013, *32*, 3722–3731. [CrossRef]
10. Jeon, S.H.; Lee, K.; Lee, K.S.; Kunkeaw, N.; Johnson, B.H.; Holthauzen, L.M.; Gong, B.; Leelayuwat, C.; Lee, Y.S. Characterization of the direct physical interaction of nc886, a cellular non-coding RNA, and PKR. *FEBS Lett.* 2012, *586*, 3477–3484. [CrossRef]
11. Lee, Y.S. A Novel Type of Non-coding RNA, nc886, Implicated in Tumor Sensing and Suppression. *Genom. Inf.* 2015, *13*, 26–30. [CrossRef] [PubMed]
12. Calderon, B.M.; Conn, G.L. Human noncoding RNA 886 (nc886) adopts two structurally distinct conformers that are functionally opposing regulators of PKR. *RNA* 2017, *23*, 557–566. [CrossRef] [PubMed]
13. Lee, Y.S.; Kunkeaw, N.; Lee, Y.S. Protein kinase R and its cellular regulators in cancer: An active player or a surveillant? *Wiley Interdiscip. Rev. RNA* 2019, e1558. [CrossRef] [PubMed]
14. Garcia, M.A.; Carrasco, E.; Aguilera, M.; Alvarez, P.; Rivas, C.; Campos, J.M.; Prados, J.C.; Calleja, M.A.; Esteban, M.; Marchal, J.A.; et al. The Chemotherapeutic Drug 5-Fluorouracil Promotes PKR-Mediated Apoptosis in a p53-Independent Manner in Colon and Breast Cancer Cells. *PLoS ONE* 2011, *6*, e23887. [CrossRef] [PubMed]
15. Peidis, P.; Papadakis, A.I.; Muaddi, H.; Richard, S.; and Koromilas, A.E. Doxorubicin bypasses the cytoprotective effects of eIF2alpha phosphorylation and promotes PKR mediated cell death. *Cell Death Differ.* 2011, *18*, 145–154. [CrossRef] [PubMed]
16. Yoon, C.H.; Lee, E.S.; Lim, D.S.; Bae, Y.S. PKR, a p53 target gene, plays a crucial role in the tumor-suppressor function of p53. *Proc. Natl. Acad. Sci. USA* 2009, *106*, 7852–7857. [CrossRef] [PubMed]
17. Lee, K.S.; Park, J.L.; Lee, K.; Richardson, L.E.; Johnson, B.H.; Lee, H.S.; Lee, J.S.; Kim, S.B.; Kwon, O.H.; Song, K.S.; et al. nc886, a non-coding RNA of anti-proliferative role, is suppressed by CpG DNA methylation in human gastric cancer. *Oncotarget* 2014, *5*, 3944–3955. [CrossRef]
18. Lee, H.S.; Lee, K.; Jang, H.J.; Lee, G.K.; Park, J.L.; Kim, S.Y.; Kim, S.B.; Johnson, B.H.; Zo, J.I.; Lee, J.S.; et al. Epigenetic silencing of the non-coding RNA nc886 provokes oncogenes during human esophageal tumorigenesis. *Oncotarget* 2014, *5*, 3472–3481. [CrossRef]
19. Fort, R.S.; Matho, C.; Geraldo, M.V.; Ottati, M.C.; Yamashita, A.S.; Saito, K.C.; Leite, K.R.; Méndez, M.; Maedo, N.; Méndez, L.; et al. Nc886 is epigenetically repressed in prostate cancer and acts as a tumor suppressor through the inhibition of cell growth. *BMC Cancer* 2018, *18*, 127. [CrossRef]
20. Arnedo, J.; del Val, C.; de Erausquin, G.A.; Romero-Zaliz, R.; Svrakic, D.; Cloninger, C.R.; Zwir, I. PGMRA: A web server for (phenotype x genotype) many-to-many relation analysis in GWAS. *Nucleic Acids Res.* 2013, *41*, W142–W149. [CrossRef]
21. Therasse, P.; Arbuck, S.G.; Eisenhauer, E.A.; Wanders, J.; Kaplan, R.S.; Rubinstein, L.; Verweij, J.; Van, G.M.; van Oosterom, A.T.; Christian, M.C.; et al. New guidelines to evaluate the response to treatment in solid tumors. European Organization for Research and Treatment of Cancer, National Cancer Institute of the United States, National Cancer Institute of Canada. *J. Natl. Cancer Inst.* 2000, *92*, 205–216. [CrossRef] [PubMed]
22. Eisenhauer, E.A.; Therasse, P.; Bogaerts, J.; Schwartz, L.H.; Sargent, D.; Ford, R.; Dancey, J.; Arbuck, S.; Gwyther, S.; Mooney, M.; et al. New response evaluation criteria in solid tumours: Revised RECIST guideline (version 1.1). *Eur. J. Cancer* 2009, *45*, 228–247. [CrossRef] [PubMed]
23. Brierley, J.D.; Gospodarowicz, M.K.; Wittekind, C. *TNM Classification of Malignant Tumours*, 8th ed.; Wiley-Blackwell: New York, NY, USA, 2016; pp. 1–272.
24. Huggett, J.; Dheda, K.; Bustin, S.; Zumla, A. Real-time RT-PCR normalisation; strategies and considerations. *Genes Immun.* 2005, *6*, 279–284. [CrossRef] [PubMed]

25. Demes, M.; Bartsch, H.; Scheil-Bertram, S.; Mücke, R.; Fisseler-Eckhoff, A. Real-Time PCR Data Processing Shown by the Analysis of Colorectal Specific Candidate Genes, ERCC1, RRM1 and TS in Relation to β2M as Endogenous Control. *Appl. Sci.* **2012**, *2*, 139–159. [CrossRef]
26. Rao, X.; Huang, X.; Zhou, Z.; Lin, X. An improvement of the 2ˆ(-delta delta CT) method for quantitative real-time polymerase chain reaction data analysis. *Biostat. Bioinforma. Biomath.* **2013**, *3*, 71–85.
27. Schmittgen, T.D.; Livak, K.J. Analyzing real-time PCR data by the comparative C (T) method. *Nat. Protoc.* **2008**, *3*, 1101–1108. [CrossRef]
28. Geiger, J.T.; Weininger, F.; Gemmeke, J.F.; Wollmer, M.; Schuller, B.; Rigoll, G. Memory-enhanced neural networks and NMF for robust ASR. *IEEE/ACM Trans. Audio Speech Lang. Process.* **2014**, *22*, 1037–1046. [CrossRef]
29. Hinton, G.E.; Salakhutdinov, R.R. Reducing the dimensionality of data with neural networks. *Science* **2006**, *313*, 504–507. [CrossRef]
30. Arnedo, J.; Svrakic, D.M.; Del Val, C.; Romero-Zaliz, R.; Hernandez-Cuervo, H.; Fanous, A.H.; Pato, M.T.; Pato, C.N.; de Erausquin, G.A.; Cloninger, C.R.; et al. Uncovering the hidden risk architecture of the schizophrenias: Confirmation in three independent genome-wide association studies. *Am. J. Psychiatry.* **2015**, *172*, 139–153. [CrossRef]
31. Romero-Zaliz, R.C.; Rubio-Escudero, C.; Cobb, J.P.; Zwir, I. A Multiobjective Evolutionary Conceptual Clustering Methodology for Gene Annotation within Structural Databases: A Case of Study on the Gene Ontology Database. *IEEE Trans. Evol. Comput.* **2008**, *12*, 679–701. [CrossRef]
32. Arnedo, J.; Mamah, D.; Baranger, D.A.; Harms, M.P.; Barch, D.M.; Svrakic, D.M.; de Erausquin, G.A.; Cloninger, C.R.; Zwir, I. Decomposition of brain diffusion imaging data uncovers latent schizophrenias with distinct patterns of white matter anisotropy. *NeuroImage* **2015**, *120*, 43–54. [CrossRef] [PubMed]
33. Houle, D.; Govindaraju, D.R.; Omholt, S. Phenomics: The next challenge. *Nat. Rev. Genet.* **2011**, *11*, 855–866. [CrossRef] [PubMed]
34. Zwir, I.; Huang, H.; Groisman, E.A. Analysis of differentially-regulated genes within a regulatory network by GPS genome navigation. *Bioinformatics* **2005**, *21*, 4073–4083. [CrossRef] [PubMed]
35. Zwir, I.; Shin, D.; Kato, A.; Nishino, K.; Latifi, T.; Solomon, F.; Hare, J.M.; Huang, H.; Groisman, E.A. Dissecting the PhoP regulatory network of Escherichia coli and Salmonella enterica. *Proc. Natl. Acad. Sci. USA* **2005**, *102*, 2862–2867. [CrossRef] [PubMed]
36. Harari, O.; Park, S.Y.; Huang, H.; Groisman, E.A.; Zwir, I. Defining the plasticity of transcription factor binding sites by Deconstructing DNA consensus sequences: The PhoP-binding sites among gamma/enterobacteria. *PLoS Comput. Biol.* **2010**, *6*, e1000862. [CrossRef]
37. Arnedo, J.; Romero-Zaliz, R.; Zwir, I.; Del Val, C. A multiobjective method for robust identification of bacterial small non-coding RNAs. *Bioinformatics* **2014**, *30*, 2875–2882. [CrossRef]
38. Wu, M.C.; Kraft, P.; Epstein, M.P.; Taylor, D.M.; Chanock, S.J.; Hunter, D.J.; Lin, X. Powerful SNP-set analysis for case-control genome-wide association studies. *Am. J. Hum. Genet* **2010**, *86*, 929–942. [CrossRef]
39. Quan, C.; Xiao, J.; Liu, L.; Duan, Q.; Yuan, P.; Zhu, F. Protein Kinases as Tumor Biomarkers and Therapeutic Targets. *Curr. Pharm. Des.* **2017**, *23*, 4209–4225. [CrossRef]
40. Zwir, I.; Del-Val, C.; Arnedo, J.; Pulkki-Råback, L.; Konte, B.; Yang, S.S.; Romero-Zaliz, R.; Hintsanen, M.; Cloninger, K.M.; Garcia, D.; et al. Three genetic–environmental networks for human personality. *Mol. Psychiatry* **2019**, *21*. [CrossRef]
41. Lee, K.; Kunkeaw, N.; Jeon, S.H.; Lee, I.; Johnson, B.H.; Kang, G.Y.; Bang, J.Y.; Park, H.S.; Leelayuwat, C.; Lee, Y.S. Precursor miR-886, a novel noncoding RNA repressed in cancer, associates with PKR and modulates its activity. *RNA* **2011**, *17*, 1076–1089. [CrossRef]
42. Park, J.L.; Lee, Y.S.; Song, M.J.; Hong, S.H.; Ahn, J.H.; Seo, E.H.; Shin, S.P.; Lee, S.J.; Johnson, B.H.; Stampfer, M.R. Epigenetic regulation of RNA polymerase III transcription in early breast tumorigenesis. *Oncogene* **2017**, *36*, 6793–6804. [CrossRef]
43. Ahn, J.H.; Lee, H.S.; Lee, J.S.; Lee, Y.S.; Park, J.L.; Kim, S.Y.; Hwang, J.A.; Kunkeaw, N.; Jung, S.Y.; Kim, T.J.; et al. Nc886 is induced by TGF-beta and suppresses the micro-RNA pathway in ovarian cancer. *Nat. Commun.* **2018**, *9*, 1166. [CrossRef] [PubMed]
44. Cao, J.; Song, Y.; Bi, N.; Shen, J.; Liu, W.; Fan, J.; Sun, G.; Tong, T.; He, J.; Shi, Y.; et al. DNA methylation-mediated repression of miR-886-3p predicts poor outcome of human small cell lung cancer. *Cancer Res.* **2013**, *73*, 3326–3335. [CrossRef] [PubMed]

45. Treppendahl, M.B.; Qiu, X.; Sogaard, A.; Yang, X.; Nandrup-Bus, C.; Hother, C.; Andersen, M.K.; Kjeldsen, L.; Möllgård, L.; Hellström-Lindberg, E.; et al. Allelic methylation levels of the noncoding VTRNA2-1 located on chromosome 5q31.1 predict outcome in AML. *Blood* **2012**, *119*, 206–216. [CrossRef] [PubMed]
46. Burnett, S.B.; Vaughn, L.S.; Strom, J.M.; Francois, A.; Patel, R.C. A truncated PACT protein resulting from a frameshift mutation reported in movement disorder DYT16 triggers caspase activation and apoptosis. *J. Cell Biochem.* **2019**, *120*, 19004–19018. [CrossRef] [PubMed]
47. Chukwurah, E.; Patel, R.C. Stress-induced TRBP phosphorylation enhances its interaction with PKR to regulate cellular survival. *Sci. Rep.* **2018**, *8*, 1020. [CrossRef] [PubMed]
48. García, M.A.; Collado, M.; Muñoz-Fontela, C.; Matheu, A.; Marcos-Villar, L.; Arroyo, J.; Esteban, M.; Serrano, M.; Rivas, C. Antiviral action of the tumor suppressor ARF. *EMBO J.* **2006**, *25*, 4284–4292. [CrossRef]
49. De la Cruz-Herrera, C.F.; Campagna, M.; García, M.A.; Marcos-Villar, L.; Lang, V.; Baz-Martínez, M.; Gutiérrez, S.; Vidal, A.; Rodríguez, M.S.; Esteban, M. Activation of the double-stranded RNA-dependent protein kinase PKR by small ubiquitin-like modifier (SUMO). *J. Biol. Chem.* **2014**, *289*, 26357–26367. [CrossRef]
50. Villarroya-Beltri, C.; Guerra, S.; Sánchez-Madrid, F. ISGylation—A key to lock the cell gates for preventing the spread of threats. *J. Cell Sci.* **2017**, *130*, 2961–2969. [CrossRef]
51. Blalock, W.L.; Bavelloni, A.; Piazzi, M.; Tagliavini, F.; Faenza, I.; Martelli, A.M.; Follo, M.Y.; Cocco, L. Multiple forms of PKR present in the nuclei of acute leukemia cells represent an active kinase that is responsive to stress. *Leukemia* **2011**, *25*, 236–245. [CrossRef]
52. Tian, B.; Mathews, M.B. Functional characterization of and cooperation between the double-stranded RNA-binding motifs of the protein kinase PKR. *J. Biol. Chem.* **2001**, *276*, 9936–9944. [CrossRef] [PubMed]
53. Piazzi, M.; Bavelloni, A.; Gallo, A.; Faenza, I.; Blalock, W.L. Signal Transduction in Ribosome Biogenesis: A Recipe to Avoid Disaster. *Int. J. Mol. Sci.* **2019**, *20*, 2718. [CrossRef] [PubMed]

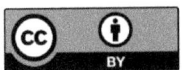 © 2020 by the authors. Licensee MDPI, Basel, Switzerland. This article is an open access article distributed under the terms and conditions of the Creative Commons Attribution (CC BY) license (http://creativecommons.org/licenses/by/4.0/).

MDPI
St. Alban-Anlage 66
4052 Basel
Switzerland
Tel. +41 61 683 77 34
Fax +41 61 302 89 18
www.mdpi.com

Cancers Editorial Office
E-mail: cancers@mdpi.com
www.mdpi.com/journal/cancers

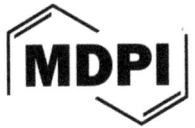

www.ingramcontent.com/pod-product-compliance
Lightning Source LLC
LaVergne TN
LVHW070655100526
838202LV00013B/969